Gastrointestinal Imaging

A CORE REVIEW

Second Edition

Editors

Wendy C. Hsu, MD

Teaching Coordinator, Gastrointestinal Imaging
Section Chief, Ultrasound
Department of Radiology
Virginia Mason Medical Center
Seattle, Washington

Felicia P. Cummings, MD

Teaching Coordinator, MRI
Section Chief, Fluoroscopy
Department of Radiology
Virginia Mason Medical Center
Seattle, Washington

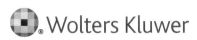 Wolters Kluwer

Philadelphia · Baltimore · New York · London
Buenos Aires · Hong Kong · Sydney · Tokyo

Acquisitions Editor: Nicole Dernoski
Development Editor: Eric McDermott
Editorial Coordinator: Vinoth Ezhumalai
Marketing Manager: Kirsten Watrud
Production Project Manager: David Saltzberg
Design Coordinator: Stephen Druding
Manufacturing Coordinator: Beth Welsh
Prepress Vendor: SPi Global

Second Edition

9 8 7 6 5 4 3 2

Printed in The United States of America

Cataloging-in-Publication Data available on request from the Publisher

ISBN: 978-1-9751-4777-8

shop.lww.com

To mom and dad, two of the bravest people I know.

—WENDY C. HSU

To my amazing men David, Nathan, and Cameron, with love and gratitude

—FELICIA P. CUMMINGS

CONTRIBUTORS

Michael A. Cecil, MS, RT (R) (MR)

Director of Advanced Imaging
Department of Radiology
Virginia Mason Medical Center
Seattle, Washington

Kevin J. Chang, MD, FACR, FSAR

Associate Professor of Radiology
Boston University School of Medicine
Adjunct Associate Professor of Diagnostic Imaging
The Warren Alpert Medical School of Brown University
Director of MRI
Boston Medical Center
Boston, Massachusetts

Anil Chauhan, MD, FSAR, FSRU

Associate Professor of Radiology
Division of Abdominal Imaging
Department of Radiology
University of Minnesota
Minneapolis, Minnesota

Ahmad F. Haidary, MD

Assistant Professor of Radiology
Case Western Reserve University
Staff Radiologist
Division of Emergency Radiology
Department of Radiology
University Hospitals Health System
Cleveland, Ohio

Michael F. McNeeley, MD

Radiologist
Department of Body Imaging
Center for Diagnostic Imaging
St. Louis Park, Minnesota

Shuchi K. Rodgers, MD

Clinical Associate Professor of Radiology
Sidney Kimmel Medical College at Thomas Jefferson
University
Associate Chair, Body Imaging
Department of Radiology
Einstein Medical Center
Philadelphia, Pennsylvania

Claire K. Sandstrom, MD

Associate Professor of Radiology
Emergency and Trauma Radiology
Harborview Medical Center
University of Washington School of Medicine
Seattle, Washington

The second edition of the *Gastrointestinal Imaging: A Core Review* builds on the success of the first edition by covering the vast field of gastrointestinal imaging in a manner that serves as a guide for residents to assess their knowledge and review the material in a format that is similar to the ABR core examination.

The print copy of the *Gastrointestinal Imaging: A Core Review*, second edition, still contains 300 questions. Some questions from the first edition have been kept and some have been removed due to no longer being relevant in current practice. Nearly 30% of new questions have been added to the second edition, with the e-book containing an additional 88 questions to the 300 questions in print.

The coeditors, Dr. Hsu and Dr. Cummings, have done an excellent job in producing a book that exemplifies the philosophy and goals of the *Core Review Series*. They have done a meticulous job in covering key topics and providing quality images. The questions have been divided logically into chapters so as to make it easy for learners to work on particular topics as needed. There questions are multiple-choice. Each question has a corresponding answer with an explanation of not only why a particular option is correct but also why the other options are incorrect. There are also references provided for each question for those who want to delve more deeply into a specific subject.

The intent of the *Core Review Series* is to provide the resident, fellow, or practicing physician a review of the important conceptual, factual, and practical aspects of a subject with multiple choice questions in a format similar to the ABR core examination. The *Core Review Series* is not intended to be exhaustive but to provide material likely to be tested on the ABR core examination and that would be required in clinical practice.

As series editor of the *Core Review Series*, it has been rewarding to not only be a coeditor of one of the books in this series but to work with so many talented individuals in the profession of radiology across the country. This series represents countless hours of work and involvement by many, and it would not have come together without their participation. It has been very gratifying to receive numerous positive comments from residents of the difference they feel the series has made in their board preparation.

I would like to thank all the coeditors for their dedication to the series and for doing an exceptional job on the second edition. I believe *Gastrointestinal Imaging: A Core Review*, second edition, will serve as a valuable resource for residents during their board preparation and a useful reference for fellows and practicing radiologists.

Biren A. Shah, MD, FACR
Clinical Professor of Radiology
Wayne State University School of Medicine
Associate Residency Program Director
Section Chief, Breast Imaging
Detroit Medical Center

Preparing for the ABR Core or Certifying examinations can be an intimidating prospect. The study guides offer a bare outline of potential topics and comprehensive textbooks an overwhelming amount of material. How then to confront this daunting task?

A questions-based approach is a good place to start. In this second edition of Gastrointestinal Imaging: A Core Review, we present a bank of 300 questions that are largely image-based, along with knowledge questions including imaging techniques and physics. We have focused on cases that every diagnostic radiologist should be familiar with and a selection of other cases, which though less commonly encountered, are perennial examination favorites.

Gastrointestinal radiology is a rapidly evolving subspecialty. For the practitioner, in addition to knowledge of anatomy and radiographic presentation of disease processes, challenges include working with an ever-changing bank of tools: new imaging sequences, techniques, contrast, and molecular imaging agents. Within our own discipline, we continually strive to improve the sensitivity and specificity of our examinations. With our clinical colleagues, we communicate more clearly by adopting the lexicon and terminology recommended by multidisciplinary consensus. We increase the relevance of our oncologic interpretations by recognizing the nexus points of tumor staging. We aid the general practitioner with follow-up imaging recommendations according to best practice guidelines.

All of these challenges require a commitment to lifelong learning. But the opportunities to make a positive contribution to patient care and to education are presented to us every day, with every case, quotidian or exotic. For your investment of time, you cannot ask for a better reward than that.

Wendy C. Hsu
Felicia P. Cummings

CONTENTS

1 Pharynx and Esophagus

1 A 50-year-old male presents with a 10-year history of intermittent substernal chest pain. An esophagram is performed.

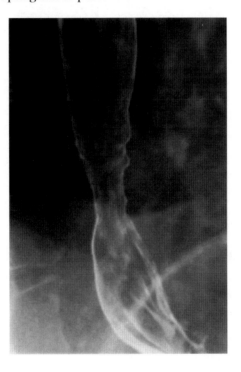

What is the most likely diagnosis?

A. Varices
B. Caustic ingestion
C. Gastroesophageal reflux disease (GERD)
D. Pill esophagitis

2   On these barium esophagram studies (A through E), which of the following
entities is **NOT** typically associated with gastroesophageal reflux disease (GERD)?

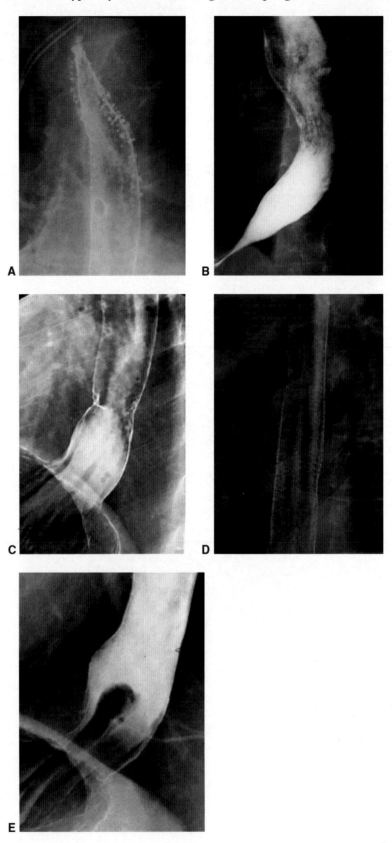

3 A 56-year-old male presents with history of chronic substernal chest pain and belching following weight gain over the past 5 years. The following image is obtained. What is the next best step?

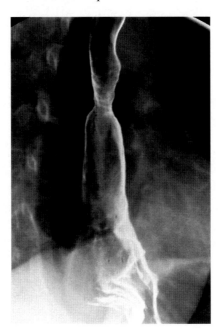

A. Follow the patient clinically as he is improving on medical therapy.
B. Recommend endoscopic evaluation with biopsy.
C. Refer to a surgeon for findings concerning for malignancy.
D. Obtain a 24-hour pH monitoring test to confirm suspicion of gastroesophageal reflux.

4 A 56-year-old female presents with history of gastroesophageal reflux disease. A double-contrast esophagram was performed. What is the correct diagnosis?

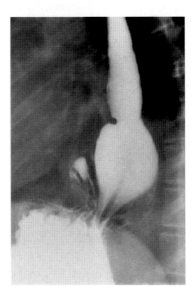

A. Type I hiatal hernia
B. Type II hiatal hernia
C. Type III hiatal hernia
D. Type IV hiatal hernia

5 A 63-year-old female presents with epigastric pain and nausea. A double-contrast upper GI study was performed. What is the correct diagnosis?

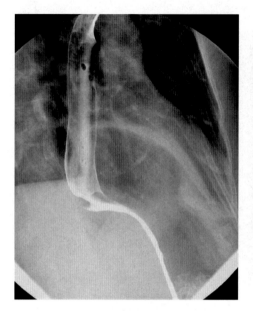
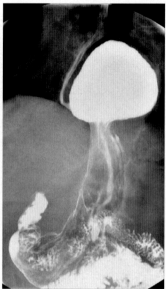

A. Type I hiatal hernia
B. Type II hiatal hernia
C. Type III hiatal hernia
D. Type IV hiatal hernia

6 A patient with a history of a Nissan fundoplication 5 years earlier returns with recurrent reflux symptoms. What finding is depicted?

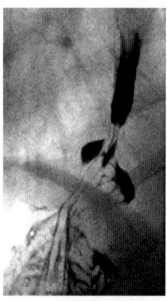
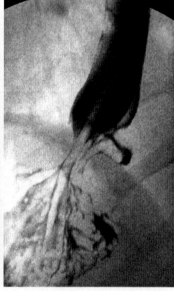
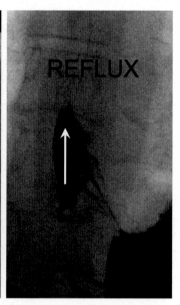

A. The fundoplication is intact and normal in position with no recurrent hernia.
B. The fundoplication is intact and normal in position with a recurrent hernia.
C. The fundoplication is intact with no recurrent hernia but is above the diaphragm.
D. The fundoplication is completely disrupted with a recurrent hernia.

7 A 56-year-old man presents with dysphagia to solid foods. What is the most likely diagnosis?

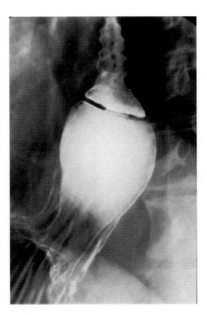

A. Caustic ingestion
B. Esophageal carcinoma
C. Schatzki ring
D. Esophageal web

8a Patient with a history of longstanding dysphagia to solids and liquids and regurgitation of undigested food undergoes an esophagram. At fluoroscopy, peristaltic stripping activity is markedly diminished.

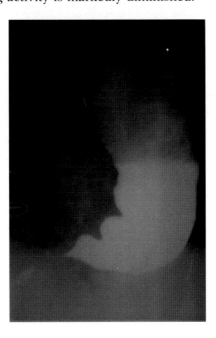

The most likely diagnosis is

A. Achalasia
B. Peptic stricture
C. Progressive systemic sclerosis
D. Esophageal carcinoma
E. Caustic ingestion

8b A 57-year-old male with a history of progressive dysphagia over 3 months is referred to a gastroenterologist. The patient has a presumptive diagnosis of achalasia based upon an initial esophagram. A review of the esophagram is requested. What features of the images suggest an alternate diagnosis?

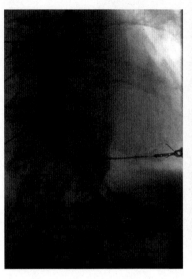 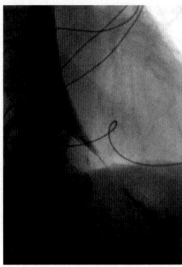

A. Presence of a polypoid mass at the gastroesophageal junction.

B. Absence of esophageal dilatation and length of the stricture.

C. Presence of a hiatal hernia suggesting a peptic stricture.

D. No features suggest an alternative diagnosis, as the appearance is classic for achalasia.

8c A patient from El Salvador presents with findings on esophagram of a markedly dilated, aperistaltic esophagus similar to achalasia. What infectious entity may be responsible?

A. *Schistosoma mansoni*

B. *Trichuris trichiura*

C. *Strongyloides stercoralis*

D. *Entamoeba histolytica*

E. *Trypanosoma cruzi*

9 In classic primary achalasia, what will be the most typical finding on esophageal manometry?

A. Hyperperistalsis in the lower two-thirds of the esophagus

B. Abnormally low resting pressure at the lower esophageal sphincter

C. Simultaneous contractions in multiple segments of the esophagus

D. Incomplete relaxation of the lower esophageal sphincter

10 A 76-year-old male with a history of longstanding dysphagia has an esophagram from 10 years earlier shown below. He presents currently with significantly worsening dysphagia over the past 2 months. What complication is demonstrated on the CT images?

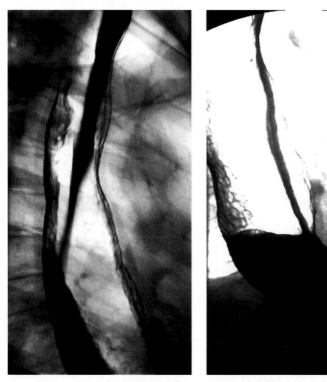

Esophagram from 10 years earlier

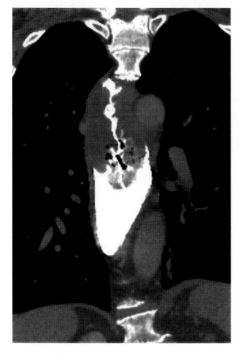
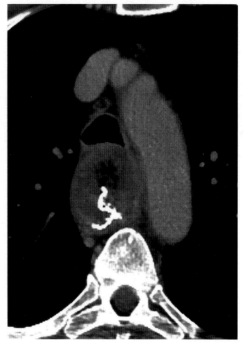

A. Food impaction
B. Candida infection
C. Esophageal neoplasm
D. Peptic stricture

11a A 45-year-old female presents with dysphagia. An esophagram is performed.

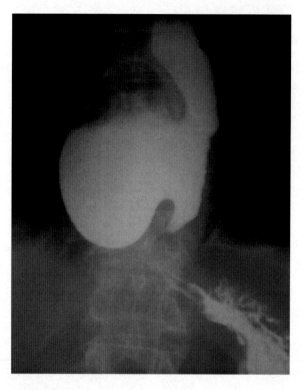

What finding is shown on this esophagram?

A. Type I hiatal hernia
B. Type II paraesophageal hernia
C. Type III paraesophageal hernia
D. Epiphrenic diverticulum

11b The most common association of this finding is with

A. Esophageal reflux disease
B. Primary motility disorder of the esophagus
C. Chronic granulomatous infection
D. Trauma

12 The most significant risk factors for development of esophageal adenocarcinoma include

A. GERD, obesity, cigarette smoking
B. Alcohol, cigarette smoking
C. High fat consumption and alcohol
D. *Helicobacter pylori* infection, alcohol, and cigarette smoking

13 A 44-year-old female presents with several month history of worsening substernal chest discomfort. A barium esophagram demonstrates loss of the peristaltic stripping wave from the level of the aortic arch inferiorly. The gastroesophageal junction is widely patulous, and free gastroesophageal reflux is noted. What diagnosis may be suggested?

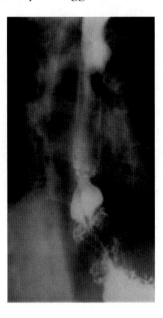

A. Progressive systemic sclerosis
B. Achalasia
C. Presbyesophagus
D. Myasthenia gravis

14 A 32-year-old male with poorly controlled diabetes and dysphagia has a barium esophagram. What is the most likely diagnosis?

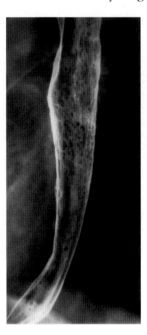

A. Cytomegalovirus esophagitis
B. Herpes simplex virus esophagitis
C. Glycogenic acanthosis
D. Candida esophagitis
E. Squamous papillomatosis

15 A 45-year-old man who has undergone allogenic bone marrow transplantation now presents with odynophagia. What is the most likely infectious etiology?

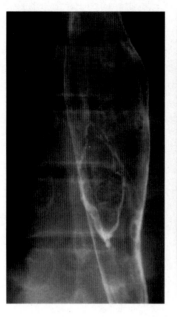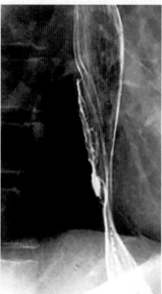

    A. Cytomegalovirus
    B. Herpes simplex virus
    C. Candidiasis
    D. Epstein-Barr virus
    E. Human papillomavirus

16 A 42-year-old male presents with chest pain after severe vomiting. He undergoes a fluoroscopic esophagram with water-soluble contrast followed by a CT. What portion of the esophagus is typically involved in this syndrome?

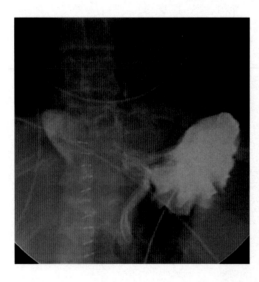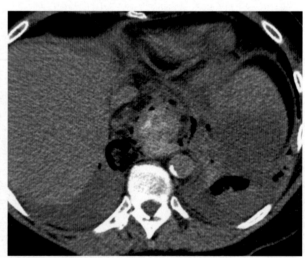

    A. Left posterolateral wall of the mid esophagus
    B. Left posterolateral wall of the distal esophagus
    C. Right posterolateral wall of the mid esophagus
    D. Right posterolateral wall of the distal esophagus

17a A 40-year-old man suffered blunt trauma to the neck from a cap propelled off a high-pressure gas can. For respiratory distress, endotracheal and right chest tubes were emergently placed. Selected axial images from contrast-enhanced CT are shown.

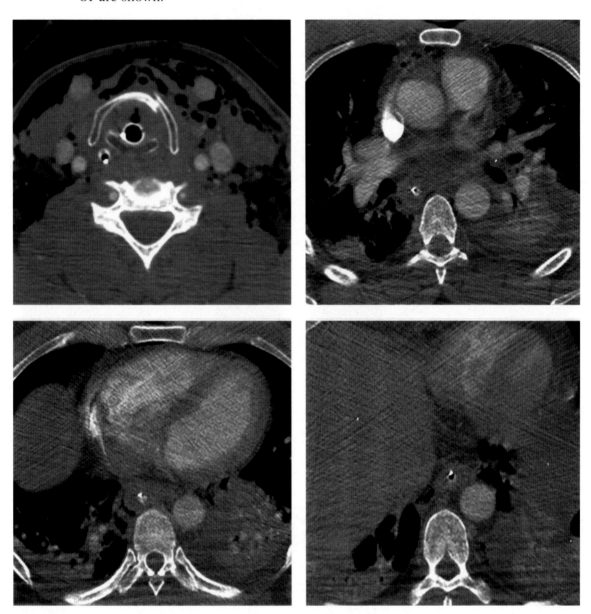

What is the most likely origin of pneumomediastinum in this patient?

A. Laryngeal fracture
B. Macklin phenomenon
C. Tracheal rupture
D. Esophageal perforation
E. Traumatic intubation

17b The patient subsequently underwent this examination with water-soluble contrast injected via enteric tube. What is the next step?

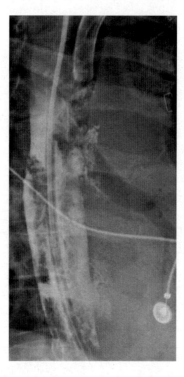

    A. Repeat injection with barium contrast
    B. Bronchoscopy
    C. Diagnostic endoscopy
    D. Endoscopic stent placement
    E. Thoracotomy

18a A 25-year-old patient presents with reflux symptoms. A barium esophagram is performed followed by a CT of the chest.

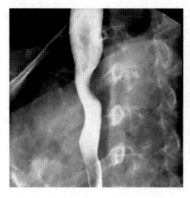 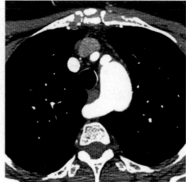 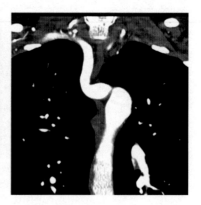

What is the diagnosis?

    A. Leiomyoma
    B. Double aortic arch
    C. Aberrant left subclavian artery
    D. Aberrant right subclavian artery

18b A 78-year-old patient presents with dysphagia to solid foods. A barium esophagram and CT are performed. What is the diagnosis?

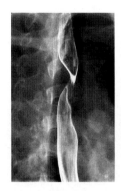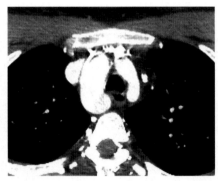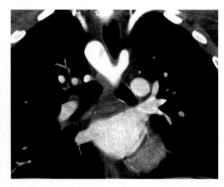

    A. Leiomyoma
    B. Double aortic arch
    C. Pulmonary sling
    D. Aberrant right subclavian artery

19a A 36-year-old male with a history of hematemesis and abdominal distention presents for evaluation with a double-contrast upper GI study and contrast-enhanced abdominal MRI. What is the salient finding that may be contributing to his symptoms?

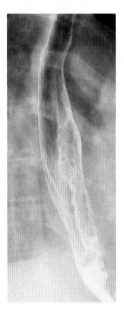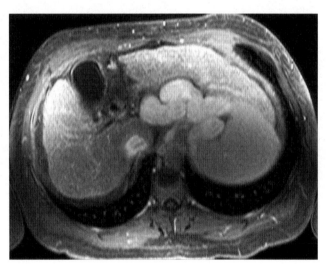

    A. Esophageal carcinoma
    B. Gastroesophageal varices
    C. Mediastinal lymphadenopathy
    D. Normal examination

19b When performing an esophagram, which technique will make the varices more apparent?

    A. Upright double-contrast view
    B. Semiprone (right anterior oblique) full column esophagus with full distention
    C. Semiprone (right anterior oblique) collapsed esophagus with mucosal relief
    D. Upright collapsed esophagus

20a A 67-year-old male with a recent diagnosis of cancer in the midesophagus (squamous cell) on endoscopy undergoes staging studies. What is the main role of CT in the staging of his cancer?

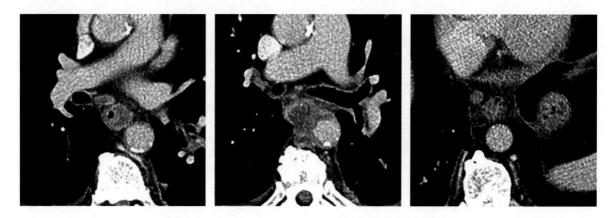

A. The CT helps distinguish between invasion of the submucosa and muscularis propria.

B. The CT assesses invasion of local mediastinal structures.

C. The CT identifies a malignant distal esophageal node.

D. The CT identifies a potential percutaneous approach to a nodal biopsy.

20b A PET CT scan was also performed. What is the main role of the PET CT in the staging of his cancer?

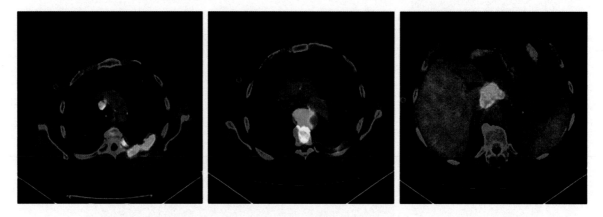

A. The PET CT identifies uptake in mediastinal nodes adjacent to the primary tumor.

B. The PET CT assesses depth of tumor invasion into the wall of the esophagus.

C. The PET CT identifies a potential distant metastatic focus in the pleural space.

D. The PET CT distinguishes between left gastric and celiac nodal disease.

21 A 57-year-old female patient with a history of breast cancer presents with recent onset solid food dysphagia. Endoscopy reveals a mid-esophageal stricture with normal overlying mucosa with biopsies revealing normal squamous epithelium. A barium esophagram followed by a chest CT is performed. What is the most likely diagnosis?

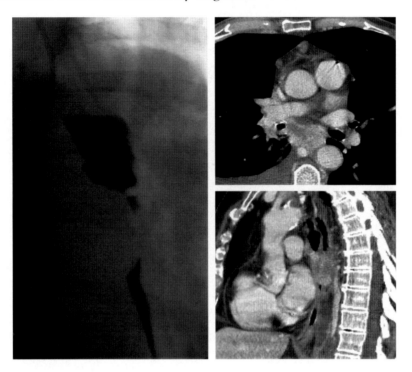

A. Peptic stricture
B. Esophageal varices
C. Leiomyoma
D. Metastasis
E. Esophageal carcinoma

22 A 29-year-old male with a history of dysphagia has a double-contrast barium esophagram. What is the most likely diagnosis?

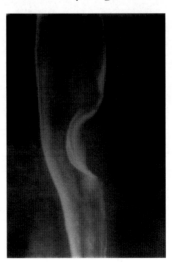

A. Granular cell tumor
B. Fibrovascular polyp
C. Gastrointestinal stromal tumor (GIST)
D. Leiomyoma

23 A 22-year-old-male presents with a long history of solid-food dysphagia and occasional food impaction. He undergoes a barium esophagram. What is the most likely diagnosis?

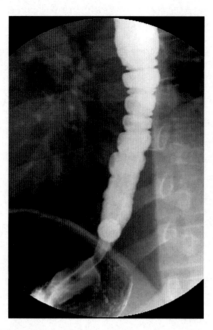

A. Peptic strictures from GERD
B. Caustic ingestion
C. Pill esophagitis
D. Eosinophilic esophagitis

24 A 34-year-old female has an esophagram. What is the most likely etiology for this finding?

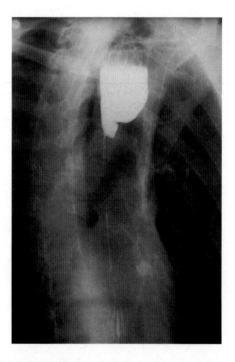

A. Chronic indwelling nasogastric tube
B. Gastroesophageal reflux and Zollinger-Ellison syndrome
C. Caustic ingestion
D. Eosinophilic esophagitis

25 A 75-year-old male with a history of esophageal cancer treated at an outside institution presents with a history of intermittent painless regurgitation. He undergoes a barium esophagram.

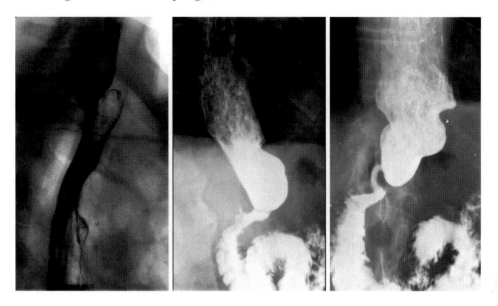

What do the images show?

A. Marked esophageal dilatation and distal narrowing, likely achalasia
B. Esophagectomy changes with colonic interposition
C. Esophagectomy changes with gastric pull-up
D. Partial gastrectomy with esophagojejunal anastomosis
E. Large hiatal hernia containing most of the stomach

26 A 82-year-old female has symptoms of severe dysphagia to liquids and solids. The patient undergoes a single-contrast esophagram. Which antecedent history may be associated with the findings seen?

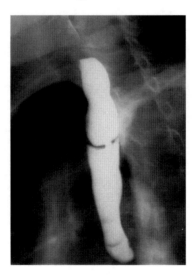

A. Prolonged ICU stay with indwelling nasogastric tube
B. History of bullous skin disorder
C. Chronic severe GERD
D. Radiation therapy for lymphoma
E. Zollinger-Ellison syndrome

27a A patient with a history of a stroke and chronic cough has a videofluoroscopic swallowing study performed. The patient swallows a sip of thin barium with images from the lateral pharyngogram below. What finding is illustrated in this case?

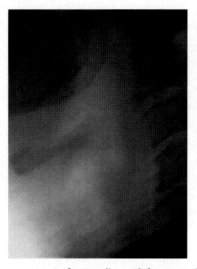 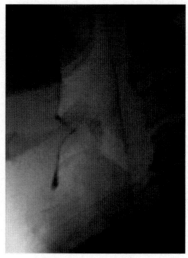

Left: Baseline. **Right**: Post single swallow thin barium.

A. Normal
B. Shallow laryngeal penetration
C. Deep laryngeal penetration
D. Aspiration

27b Which action listed below is not involved in the pharyngeal phase of a normal swallow?

A. Elevation of the soft palate
B. Depression of the hyoid bone with posterior and inferior movement of the larynx
C. Epiglottic inversion
D. Adduction of the vocal cords
E. Relaxation of the upper esophageal sphincter

28 A 85-year-old female presents with a history of dysphagia and regurgitation of undigested material. She undergoes a barium pharyngoesophagram. What is the most likely diagnosis?

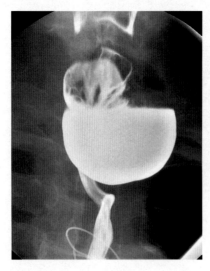 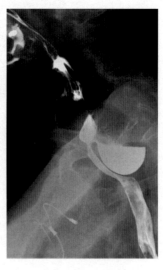

A. Killian-Jamieson diverticulum
B. Lateral pharyngeal pouch
C. Lateral pharyngeal diverticulum
D. Zenker diverticulum

29 A 31-year-old female complains of a sensation of dysphagia in the cervical region. She is otherwise healthy. A pharyngogram is performed, and manometric measurements demonstrate increased upper esophageal sphincter (UES) pressure at rest and failure of the UES to completely relax. What additional condition is likely to be present?

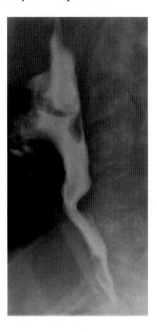

A. Zenker diverticulum
B. Gastroesophageal reflux disease
C. Cranial nerve dysfunction
D. Recurrent pneumonias from aspiration

ANSWERS AND EXPLANATIONS

1 **Answer C.** On this double-contrast esophagram, the findings are of distal esophageal stricture, shallow ulcerations, mucosal nodularity, and sacculations caused by adjacent scarring. These findings in the distal esophagus are typical for **gastroesophageal reflux disease (GERD) with a peptic stricture**. Caustic ingestion typically results in a long stricture, and an appropriate history is usually declared. Varices present as irregular serpentine filling defects, not as a stricture. Pill esophagitis typically occurs in the midesophagus due to delay in passage of a pill (e.g., tetracycline, quinidine, potassium chloride) at points of extrinsic compression on the esophagus from the aortic arch or left mainstem bronchus.

Gastroesophageal reflux disease (GERD) is the most common gastrointestinal disorder presenting in outpatient visits. Up to 20% of adults in the United States report having experienced chronic heartburn, the classic symptom of GERD. The actual prevalence of GERD is hard to document, because the correlation between symptoms and endoscopic findings of the disease are not perfect; a significant number of people who have endoscopic evidence of Barrett esophagus or esophagitis are asymptomatic.

References: Kahrilas PJ, Kim HC, Pandolfino JE. Approaches to the diagnosis and grading of hiatal hernia. *Best Pract Res Clin Gastroenterol* 2008;22(4):601–616.

Shaheen NJ, Hansen RA, Morgan DR, et al. The burden of gastrointestinal and liver diseases, 2006. *Am J Gastroenterol* 2006;101(9):2128–2138.

2 **Answer B.** In answer B, the dilated esophagus with a bird's beak configuration of the lower esophageal sphincter (LES) is the classic appearance of **achalasia**. This condition is associated with failure of the lower esophageal sphincter (LES) to relax; with gastroesophageal reflux, the LES is patulous.

Answer A demonstrates **esophageal intramural pseudodiverticulosis (EIP)**, an uncommon finding in which dilated mucous glands are found in association with reflux esophagitis. While *Candida* may be cultured in a significant number of patients with EIP, this is felt to be more likely a secondary infection.

Answer C shows a **sliding type I hiatal hernia** which is commonly found in patients who have significant GERD. Whether the hiatal hernia causes the gastroesophageal reflux is controversial; inflammation from the gastroesophageal reflux causes longitudinal shortening of the esophagus, which disrupts the anchoring ligaments at the LES and may actually cause the hernia. The intrinsic dysfunction of the LES is the primary determinant of gastroesophageal reflux.

Answer D demonstrates the uniform, fine transverse folds that are seen transiently during an esophagram known as "**feline esophagus**," which have a high association with gastroesophageal reflux.

Answer E demonstrates a gastric fold extending into the distal esophagus with a clubbed terminus, known as an **inflammatory esophagogastric polyp**, or polyp-fold complex. This is a benign regenerative mucosal response to esophagitis, most commonly in the setting of GERD. While it is itself benign, it is a marker of significant reflux esophagitis, for which endoscopic evaluation is warranted.

Findings of Reflux Esophagitis on Barium Studies

Findings	Description
Abnormal motility	Diminished peristalsis in up to 50% patients; nonpropulsive contractions common
Mucosal filling defects	Nodular, granular, or plaque-like appearance
Ulceration	Usually shallow, may be linear or stellate
Sacculations	Recesses caused by redundant wall adjacent to thick folds
Thick longitudinal folds	Regular fold thickening best seen on collapsed view
Transverse folds - transient	Shortening of longitudinal folds causes transient, uniform, thin transverse folds ("feline esophagus")
Transverse folds - fixed	Thick, irregular, eccentric folds
Intramural pseudodiverticula	Dilated intramural mucous glands appear to "float" outside the lumen due to non-visualized connecting neck
Inflammatory esophagogastric polyp	Polypoid extension of thickened gastric fold into the distal esophagus
Stricture	Typically in the distal esophagus and associated with an axial hiatal hernia; if mid-esophageal, increased association with Barrett esophagus

References: Gore RM, Levine MS. *Textbook of gastrointestinal radiology*, 4th ed. Philadelphia, PA: Elsevier/Saunders, 2015.

Levine MS, Rubesin SE. Diseases of the esophagus: diagnosis with esophagography. *Radiology* 2005;237(2):414–427.

3 **Answer B.** The findings are of a mid-esophageal stricture in the setting of a patulous gastroesophageal junction and a history suggesting GERD. The **high location of the strictures** is atypical for uncomplicated GERD and should raise concern for **Barrett esophagus**, a premalignant condition which requires further investigation. The next best step would involve **endoscopy with biopsy**. A 24-hr pH monitoring for confirmation of reflux is likely redundant at this stage. Surgical consultation may be needed eventually depending upon biopsy results for consideration of esophagectomy or anti-reflux procedure. A mucosal reticular appearance on double-contrast esophagography is a finding more specific for Barrett esophagus, especially in combination with a high stricture. These more specific findings are seen in a minority (5% to 30%) of patients with Barrett esophagus however, with other findings of a hiatal hernia, gastroesophageal reflux, distal esophageal peptic stricture, and ulcerations common in patients with Barrett's but overlapping with uncomplicated GERD.

Barrett esophagus represents metaplasia of the normal esophageal squamous epithelium to columnar epithelium. Studies have shown a minority (6% to 12%) of patients with prolonged GERD symptoms have Barrett esophagus, mostly in males >50 years of age. The true prevalence of Barrett esophagus in the general population may be higher, as a significant percentage of patients with Barrett esophagus are asymptomatic. Barrett esophagus may progress from metaplasia through varying degrees of dysplasia to frank adenocarcinoma. The annual risk of developing adenocarcinoma from nondysplastic Barrett esophagus is low (less than 0.4%), but the risk increases with up to 5% annual risk for cancer when high-grade dysplasia is present. For patients with nondysplastic Barrett's, endoscopic screening is recommended every 3 years. Despite screening, 80% to 90% of esophageal adenocarcinoma will occur in patients without Barrett esophagus.

References: Hvid-Jensen F, Pedersen L, Drewes AM, et al. Incidence of adenocarcinoma among patients with Barrett's esophagus. *N Engl J Med* 2011;365(15):1375–1383.

Rustgi AK, El-Serag HB. Esophageal carcinoma. *N Engl J Med* 2014;371(26):2499–2509.

4 **Answer A.** Fluoroscopic spot image from a double-contrast esophagram demonstrates upward herniation of the stomach into the chest with superior migration of the gastroesophageal junction. This is compatible with a **type I hiatal hernia**, also called a **sliding hiatal hernia**. Type I hiatal hernias account for over 90% of all hiatal hernias and are associated with diffuse weakening of the phrenicoesophageal membrane, which normally acts to fix the distal esophagus near the hiatus. This laxity allows the upward displacement of the gastroesophageal junction and stomach into the chest through the diaphragmatic hiatus. Patients with type I hiatal hernias also can have diminished lower esophageal sphincter tone and therefore **often present with symptoms of gastroesophageal reflux.**

The other types of hernias listed (Types II-IV) are paraesophageal hernias and will be discussed in a later question.

References: Abbara S, Kalan MM, Lewicki AM. Intrathoracic stomach revisited. *AJR Am J Roentgenol* 2003;181(2):403–414.

Kahrilas PJ, Kim HC, Pandolfino JE. Approaches to the diagnosis and grading of hiatal hernia. *Best Pract Res Clin Gastroenterol* 2008;22(4):601–616.

5 **Answer B.** Fluoroscopic spot image from double contrast upper GI study demonstrates a **normally positioned gastroesophageal junction** (image on left) with adjacent herniation of the gastric fundus above the diaphragm (image on right). This is compatible with a **type II paraesophageal hiatal hernia**. Paraesophageal hernias result from a focal defect in the phrenicoesophageal membrane that provides a small opening for upward gastric herniation, generally beginning with the gastric fundus.

Hiatal hernias are generally classified into two major groups:

- Type I (sliding or axial) hiatal hernia
- Types II-IV (paraesophageal hernias)
  - Type II (paraesophageal or rolling hernia)
    - Focal defect in the anterolateral phrenicoesophageal membrane.
    - Gastric cardia and esophagogastric junction remain subdiaphragmatic.
    - Fundus is usually the first portion herniated.
  - Type III (mixed or compound)
    - Most common type of paraesophageal hernia with features of type 1 and 2
    - Associated with gastric rotation
    - Usually large
  - Type IV
    - Marked widening of the diaphragmatic hiatus containing other organs (colon, omentum, pancreas, small bowel, liver)

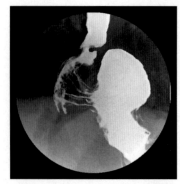

Type III hiatal hernia (mixed).

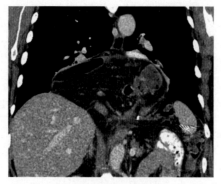

Type IV hernia coronal.

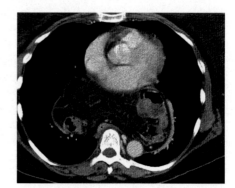

Type IV hernia axial.

References: Abbara S, Kalan MM, Lewicki AM. Intrathoracic stomach revisited. *AJR Am J Roentgenol* 2003;181(2):403–414.

Kahrilas PJ, Kim HC, Pandolfino JE. Approaches to the diagnosis and grading of hiatal hernia. *Best Pract Res Clin Gastroenterol* 2008;22(4):601–616.

6 **Answer B.** The fundoplication is intact and normal in position (infradiaphragmatic) but there is a recurrent type I hernia and gastroesophageal reflux is demonstrated. Antireflux surgery is a common and effective treatment for gastroesophageal reflux disease (GERD). Patients who fail medical therapy or have complications of GERD including stricture, Barrett metaplasia, or other changes of significant esophagitis may be considered for a surgical fundoplication.

The **Nissan fundoplication** is the most common anti-reflux procedure performed currently. It consists of reduction of any hiatal hernia and repair of a crural defect if present, return of the distal 3 to 4 cm of esophagus to the abdomen, recreation the esophagogastric angle (angle of His) that acts as an antireflux valve mechanism, and creation of a gastric fundal wrap that encompasses the distal esophagus (360 degrees wrap). For patients with poor esophageal motility, a partial wrap may be preferred, such as a **Toupet procedure** (270-degree wrap). The procedure has a high success rate, but a small percentage may have complications and need a redo fundoplication.

Causes of Failed Fundoplications

- Too tight fundoplication
- Too loose fundoplication
- Wrap disruption, partial or complete (Hinder type I)
- Supradiaphragmatic gastric slippage (Hinder type 2)
- Slipped Nissan with gastric pouch above wrap but below diaphragm (Hinder type 3)
- Supradiaphragmatic wrap migration (Hinder type 4)

References: Carbo AI, Kim RH, Gates T, et al. Imaging findings of successful and failed fundoplication. *Radiographics* 2014;34(7):1873–1884.

Hinder RA, Perdikis G, Klinger PJ, et al. The surgical option for gastroesophageal reflux disease. *Am J Med* 1997;103(5A):144S–148S.

7 **Answer C.** Images from a barium esophagram shows a large sliding hiatal hernia with focal, concentric narrowing at the esophagogastric junction, consistent with a **narrowed lower esophageal B ring**. Because the patient is symptomatic, this finding may appropriately be referred to as a **Schatzki ring**. For comparison, normal lower esophageal B ring is shown below. The abnormal thickening of the Schatzki ring results from **chronic inflammation from gastroesophageal reflux**; sliding hiatal hernias are a commonly associated finding. Symptoms are generally associated with luminal narrowing <13 mm and are rare with luminal diameter >20 mm. Large food boluses such as poorly chewed meat can lead to impaction and the "steakhouse syndrome."

Caustic strictures usually involve a long segment of the esophagus. Esophageal carcinoma usually shows a more asymmetric and irregular contour. Esophageal webs are typically located in the cervical esophagus.

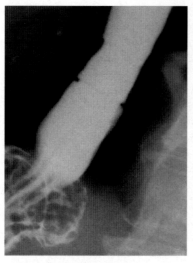
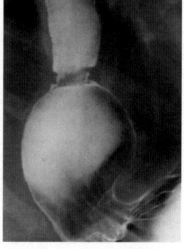

Normal B ring. Thickened and narrowed B ring.

References: Norton RA, King GD. "Steakhouse Syndrome": the symptomatic lower esophageal ring. *Lahey Clin Found Bull* 1963;13:55–59.

Smith MS. Diagnosis and management of esophageal rings and webs. *Gastroenterol Hepatol (N Y)* 2010;6(11):701–704.

8a **Answer A.** The barium esophagram demonstrates a **markedly dilated esophagus with short, smooth tapered narrowing at the gastroesophageal junction, a "bird's beak" appearance due to failure of the lower esophageal sphincter to relax.** The findings are consistent with **classic achalasia**.

A peptic stricture typically does not cause this degree of dilatation. While dilatation and diminished peristaltic activity may be seen with progressive systemic sclerosis (PSS), also known as scleroderma, the lower esophageal sphincter is widely patulous in PSS as opposed to narrowed (although a secondary peptic stricture may develop with longstanding reflux). The smooth stricture in this case would be atypical for a stricture associated with an esophageal malignancy. Caustic ingestion typically produces a very long stricture.

The etiology of primary achalasia is unknown, but the pathogenesis involves degeneration of myenteric ganglia in the esophageal wall. Circulating antibodies to enteric neurons suggest a possible autoimmune etiology. The upper esophageal sphincter also may not relax normally in achalasia, contributing to increased intraluminal pressure which causes dilatation. The onset of the disease is insidious, and patients often experience symptomatology for years before seeking care. The diagnosis is established by esophageal manometry, with findings of elevated LES resting pressure, failure of the LES to relax, and diminished peristalsis in the distal two-thirds of the esophagus.

There are **variants of achalasia** aside from the classic appearance, which is known as type I. Type III involves spastic, nonpropulsive contractions of the body of the esophagus in conjunction with a hypertensive LES (formerly called "vigorous achalasia"). Type II has features of both types I and III.

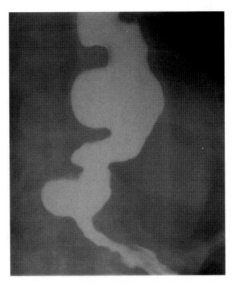

Type III achalasia.

8b **Answer B.** The images show a distal esophageal stricture with tapering smooth margins. No hiatal hernia or polypoid mass is demonstrated. **The appearance superficially resembles classic achalasia, except that the stricture is longer than expected, and there is no dilatation.** These features along with the relatively short onset of symptoms does not suggest a long-standing process. Mucosal irregularities if present would also suggest pseudoachalasia. In this case, biopsies of the stricture revealed adenocarcinoma. FDG PET study performed demonstrated elevated activity in the region of the tumor.

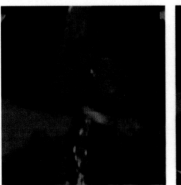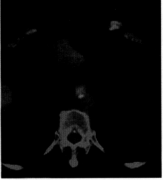

Secondary achalasia (or sometimes called **pseudoachalasia**) due to malignancy may be caused by macroscopic tumor infiltration into the wall restricting distensibility or dysfunction of the myenteric neuronal plexus due to microinvasion or paraneoplastic release of tumoral factors. Tumors that produce this appearance include carcinomas of the esophagus, stomach, lung, pancreas as well as lymphoma.

8c **Answer E.** While all of the listed parasites affect the intestinal tract, the appearance of a dilated esophagus is typical for **Chagas disease**. Chagas disease (common in South America, Central America, and Mexico) is caused by the flagellate protozoan ***Trypanosoma cruzi***, which is transmitted to humans via an insect vector (reduviid or kissing) bug. **Involvement of the enteric nervous system results in radiologic appearance of a megaesophagus similar to achalasia**, although lower esophageal sphincter pressure is decreased relative to normal in Chagas disease, in contrast to idiopathic achalasia.

References: Boeckxstaens GE, Zaninotto G, Richter JE. Achalasia. *Lancet* 2014;383(9911):83–93.

Goldenberg SP, Burrell M, Fette GG, et al. Classic and vigorous achalasia: a comparison of manometric, radiographic, and clinical findings. *Gastroenterology* 1991;101(3):743–748.

Matsuda NM, Miller SM, Evora PR. The chronic gastrointestinal manifestations of Chagas disease. *Clinics (Sao Paulo)* 2009;64(12):1219–1224.

Woodfield CA, Levine MS, Rubesin SE, et al. Diagnosis of primary versus secondary achalasia: reassessment of clinical and radiographic criteria. *AJR Am J Roentgenol* 2000;175(3):727–731.

9   **Answer D.** The typical manometric features of **primary achalasia** include **absence of primary peristalsis increased or normal resting pressure of the lower esophageal sphincter, and incomplete or absent relaxation in response to a swallow**. Variants with atypical manometric findings include vigorous achalasia or Type III achalasia (see discussion for question 8), in which simultaneous, high-amplitude, repetitive contractions are seen (Answer C) and early achalasia, in which primary peristalsis is decreased but LES relaxation is normal. Another motility disorder diffuse esophageal spasm (DES) involves simultaneous nonpropulsive contractions, which may be lumen obliterating, leading to the classic corkscrew appearance on barium studies. Classic DES was thought not to involve the LES, but recent studies have shown a frequent association with LES dysfunction. Some investigators now believe that achalasia and DES represent a spectrum of esophageal motility disorders that are related.

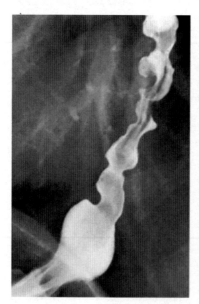 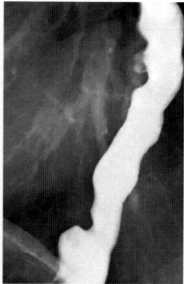

Diffuse esophageal spasm (DES).

References: Boeckxstaens GE, Zaninotto G, Richter JE. Achalasia. *Lancet* 2014;383(9911):83–93.

Prabhakar A, Levine MS, Rubesin S, et al. Relationship between diffuse esophageal spasm and lower esophageal sphincter dysfunction on barium studies and manometry in 14 patients. *AJR Am J Roentgenol* 2004;183(2):409–413.

10   **Answer C.** The esophagram from 10 years earlier show a dilated esophagus with a smooth, short tapering narrowing at the gastroesophageal junction consistent with classic achalasia. The current CT images demonstrate a dilated contrast-filled esophagus and a new mid-esophageal mass with abrupt shoulders and luminal narrowing. This mass is not seen above a stricture, which would be expected with impacted food. While candida esophagitis may be present in patients with achalasia, inflammation may cause wall thickening but not a bulky mass. The findings are consistent with an **esophageal neoplasm**.

There is an **increased risk for esophageal neoplasm in patients with long-standing achalasia, with both adenocarcinoma and squamous cell carcinoma found.** A mid-esophageal location is common. Chronic stasis with inflammation is thought to be responsible for the neoplastic transformation.

References: Gore RM, Levine MS, Laufer I. *Textbook of gastrointestinal radiology.* Philadelphia, PA: W.B. Saunders Co., 1994.

Nesteruk K, Spaander MCW, Leeuwenburgh I, et al. Achalasia and associated esophageal cancer risk: what lessons can we learn from the molecular analysis of Barrett's-associated adenocarcinoma? *Biochim Biophys Acta Rev Cancer* 2019;1872(2):188291.

11a **Answer D.** There is a large saccular outpouching at the level of the distal esophagus. This closely resembles a type II paraesophageal hernia, especially when the location of the gastroesophageal junction is ambiguous. **Evaluation for gastric folds in the sac and identifying the relationship to the gastroesophageal junction are important to determine whether this finding arises from the esophagus or represents a herniated portion of the stomach.** In this case, the gastroesophageal junction is below the outpouching, and its smooth contours are absent of gastric folds, establishing the diagnosis of an **epiphrenic diverticulum**.

11b **Answer B.** Epiphrenic diverticula are pulsion diverticula caused by increased intraluminal pressure. These have a **strong association with primary neuromuscular motility disorders of the esophagus such as achalasia**. These are pseudodiverticula as they consist only of mucosal and submucosal layers. As they do not have a muscularis layer, they tend to retain ingested material. Other than esophageal motility disorders, esophageal strictures may also be associated with pulsion diverticula.

Other diverticular-like outpouchings of the esophageal wall may be caused by adjacent mediastinal inflammation from granulomatous infection such as tuberculosis or histoplasmosis. These tend to occur in the mid esophagus (adjacent to carinal lymph nodes involved by infection) and not the distal esophagus. These post-inflammatory diverticula are caused by traction and tend to have a triangular configuration with a wide base at the esophageal origin narrowing to a pointed apex distant from the lumen.

Small pulsion diverticula are usually asymptomatic. Large diverticula may be associated with dysphagia, regurgitation of undigested food, and halitosis. These may perforate (especially with endoscopy or nasogastric tube placement). Rarely these may develop neoplasm, potentially related to stasis and chronic inflammation. Epiphrenic diverticula have a tendency to enlarge and are treated by diverticulotomy which may be performed by surgery or endoscopy.

References: Fasano NC, Levine MS, Rubesin SE, et al. Epiphrenic diverticulum: clinical and radiographic findings in 27 patients. *Dysphagia* 2003;18(1):9–15.

Tedesco P, Fisichella PM, Way LW, et al. Cause and treatment of epiphrenic diverticula. *Am J Surg* 2005;190(6):891–894.

12 **Answer A. The major risk factors for adenocarcinoma are GERD, obesity, and cigarette smoking**. The relationship of GERD and adenocarcinoma, especially in the setting of Barrett esophagus, is well established. Abdominal obesity may lead to increased intragastric pressure, which relaxes the lower esophageal sphincter and may promote gastroesophageal reflux. The risk for adenocarcinoma of the esophagus is twice as high in smokers compared to never smokers, although smoking is a stronger risk factor for squamous cell carcinoma. Alcohol intake does not appear to elevate the risk for adenocarcinoma. Interestingly, the presence of *Helicobacter pylori* infection is actually associated with a decreased risk for adenocarcinoma, potentially due to the ultimate reduction in acid production seen in patients with *H. pylori*–induced gastric atrophy from chronic gastritis.

Although **squamous cell cancer accounts for 90% of esophageal cancers worldwide**, the **incidence of adenocarcinoma has been increasing rapidly within the past generation and has now surpassed squamous cell cancer in several parts of North America and Europe**.

The major risk factors for developing **squamous cell carcinoma** are **smoking and alcohol**. Additional less common causes include: GERD, head and neck tumors, achalasia, caustic ingestion, radiation, celiac disease, Plummer Vinson syndrome, tylosis, and autoimmune mucocutaneous blistering disease (e.g., bullous pemphigus).

References: Levine MS, Rubesin SE. Diseases of the esophagus: diagnosis with esophagography. *Radiology* 2005;237(2):414–427.

Rustgi AK, El-Serag HB. Esophageal carcinoma. *N Engl J Med* 2014;371(26):2499–2509.

13 **Answer A. Progressive systemic sclerosis (scleroderma)** is an autoimmune disorder that affects skin, the gastrointestinal system, lungs, and multiple other organs. **In the gastrointestinal tract, the esophagus is the most common site of involvement.** The condition causes atrophy of smooth muscle, which is located in the distal two-thirds of the esophagus. The gastroesophageal junction is widely patent, and gastroesophageal reflux is common. In severe cases, fibrosis replaces the atrophied smooth muscle and causes **esophageal shortening, which may pull a hiatal hernia into the thorax**, as seen in this case. Eventually, the patulous gastroesophageal junction may be replaced by a peptic stricture from chronic reflux.

Achalasia may demonstrate absent peristalsis, but the lower esophageal sphincter is narrowed with a smooth tapered ("birds beak") configuration, rather than appearing patulous. Presbyesophagus may be associated with diminished peristalsis but is a motor dysfunction seen with aging. Myasthenia gravis involves the proximal esophagus and striated muscle.

Reference: Boland, GW. *Gastrointestinal imaging: the requisites.* Philadelphia, PA: Elsevier Saunders, 2014.

14 **Answer D.** The esophagram demonstrates **multiple filling defects in the esophagus with a background of relatively normal mucosa**. Appearance is typical for **early candida esophagitis**. Candida esophagitis is the most common type of infectious esophagitis and occurs in patients who are immunosuppressed. Early changes involve mucosal plaques; ulcerations develop with more advanced disease, with severe involvement leading to a "shaggy" appearance. Cytomegalovirus (CMV) most commonly presents as solitary large ulcers in AIDS patients. Herpes simplex virus (HSV) typically causes shallow ulcers, sometimes linear or stellate with a surrounding halo of edema. Glycogenic acanthosis is a benign degenerative condition in which the epithelial cells accumulate glycogen causing mucosal plaques that may resemble early candidiasis; this condition is found in older asymptomatic patients. Squamous papillomatosis, a premalignant condition, also causes small plaques but is very rare.

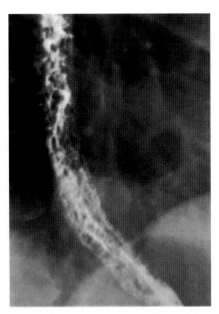

Shaggy esophagus of late *Candida* esophagitis.

Reference: Roberts L Jr, Gibbons R, Gibbons G, et al. Adult esophageal candidiasis: a radiographic spectrum. *Radiographics* 1987;7(2):289–307.

15 **Answer A.** Frontal and left-posterior oblique images from a double-contrast esophagram show a large, flat, diamond-shaped ulcer projecting from the posterior wall of the mid-esophagus. The remainder of the visualized mucosa is normal, and there is no associated mass lesion. This imaging appearance is typical for **cytomegalovirus (CMV) esophagitis**; identical findings may be seen with the human immunodeficiency virus (HIV). Because the treatment for CMV esophagitis (ganciclovir) is fairly toxic, confirmation with brushings, biopsy, or culture obtained by endoscopy will be needed.

Herpes simplex virus (HSV) usually results in multiple tiny and superficial ulcers surrounded by a radiolucent halo of edema. Candidal esophagitis manifests as multiple plaques (rather than true ulcers) oriented along the long axis of the esophagus. Epstein-Barr virus (EBV) infection results in deep linear ulcers, as opposed to the flat and ovoid ulcers associated with CMV and HIV esophagitis. Infection with human papillomavirus (HPV) may result in clusters of tiny polypoid lesions.

Reference: Levine MS, Rubesin SE. Diseases of the esophagus: diagnosis with esophagography. *Radiology* 2005;237(2):414–427.

16 **Answer B.** Single contrast upper GI shows extraluminal contrast leakage along the right posterolateral aspect of the esophagus. This is confirmed on noncontrast CT with pneumomediastinum surrounding the esophagus. This is a less common location for an esophageal tear in **Boerhaave syndrome (spontaneous esophageal perforation)**, which usually presents with the tear originating from the **left posterolateral wall of the distal esophagus**. Esophageal perforation is caused by forceful ejection of gastric contents from an unrelaxed esophagus against a closed glottis. The classic clinical presentation is with vomiting, chest pain, and subcutaneous emphysema (Mackler's triad). The transmural tears are typically vertically oriented and 1 to 4 cm in length. Timely detection of a perforation is critical, as **mortality is high, and survival rates may fall to 20% after 24 hours**.

CXR findings are nonspecific but may include pneumomediastinum, pneumothorax, and a pleural effusion. The fluoroscopic esophagram may show the location of the contrast leakage from the distal esophagus into the mediastinum. There is a 10% to 38% false-negative rate for leakage detection on conventional fluoroscopy, so CT is recommended in addition to or in lieu of the fluoroscopic study if the patient is clinically unstable. In addition to detecting subtle pneumomediastinum or a small pneumothorax, CT may show a contained leak missed on fluoroscopy if the tear is small and sealed-off from the lumen.

References: Gimenez A, Franquet T, Erasmus JJ, et al. Thoracic complications of esophageal disorders. *Radiographics* 2002;22(Spec No):S247–S258.

Tonolini M, Bianco R. Spontaneous esophageal perforation (Boerhaave syndrome): diagnosis with CT-esophagography. *J Emerg Trauma Shock* 2013;6(1):58–60.

17a **Answer D.** Esophageal perforation.

This patient does have a laryngeal fracture, shown as step-off of the left thyroid cartilage on the upper left image. However, the volume of pneumomediastinum is greater than expected for this finding alone and increases in volume moving inferiorly in the mediastinum. Therefore, other causes of pneumomediastinum must be considered.

Indirect findings of esophageal perforation on MDCT include periesophageal air, periesophageal fluid, and esophageal wall thickening, all three of which are present on this scan. A full-thickness laceration of the esophageal wall may be identified on CT (but not in this case), and if administered, oral contrast may leak from the esophagus.

The other answer choices are possible causes of pneumomediastinum, but there are no CT signs of tracheal injury; traumatic intubation should not result in the mediastinal findings noted above; and Macklin phenomenon (alveolar rupture leading to pulmonary interstitial emphysema and pneumomediastinum) is a diagnosis of exclusion.

References: de Lutio di Castelguidone E, Merola S, Pinto A, et al. Esophageal injuries: spectrum of multidetector row CT findings. *Eur J Radiol* 2006;59:344–348.

Young CA, Menias CO, Bhalla S, et al. CT features of esophageal emergencies. *Radiographics* 2008;28:1541–1553.

17b **Answer E.** The contrast esophagram shows two sites of thoracic esophageal perforation. Free perforation of the esophagus is usually considered a surgical emergency, requiring **thoracotomy** to repair the esophageal wall defect, debride necrotic tissue, and irrigate the mediastinum and, if necessary, the pleural space.

Confirmation of esophageal perforation should be performed with **water-soluble contrast only**. Barium should only be administered if the examination is negative for perforation after the initial water-soluble contrast portion. **Leaked barium in the mediastinum can cause chemical mediastinitis, and retained barium can cause artifact on CT**. In this case also bronchoscopy and diagnostic endoscopy are unnecessary for diagnosis of the perforation. Endoscopic stent placement would not allow wash-out of the mediastinal or pleural contamination and is therefore not advised in isolation.

Reference: Nirula R. Esophageal perforation. *Surg Clin North Am* 2014;94:35–41.

18a **Answer D.** Images from the esophagram demonstrate a smooth extrinsic impression on the posterior thoracic esophagus. An arterial structure extending from the left-sided arch posterior to the esophagus demonstrated on the CT, consistent with an aberrant right subclavian artery.

The left aortic arch with aberrant right subclavian artery is the most common anomaly of the aortic arch found in 0.5% to 2% of the population. The right subclavian artery usually arises from the brachiocephalic artery, continuing as the axillary artery after passing the right first rib. **The aberrant right subclavian artery arises from the aortic arch distal to the left subclavian artery origin and passes posterior to the esophagus** (in 80% of cases) prior to continuing its normal course. Less commonly, the aberrant artery will pass between the esophagus and the trachea (15%) or anterior to the trachea (5%). This anomaly is thought to be caused by abnormal involution of the fourth right aortic arch in embryogenesis. The anomaly is usually sporadic, but it may be associated with Trisomy 21. Most patients are asymptomatic, since the ductus arteriosus is left-sided and a full vascular ring is not formed.

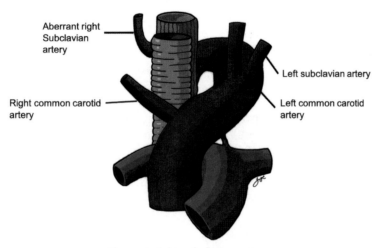

Aberrant right subclavian artery.

18b **Answer B.** Images demonstrate both left and right aortic arches which encircle the trachea and esophagus forming a true vascular ring. **The double aortic arch (DAA) is the most common *symptomatic* vascular ring**. The dysphagia associated with a vascular ring is known as "dysphagia lusoria" (derived from "lusus naturae" or "freak or jest of nature"). Onset of dysphagia may be in late adulthood with loss of peristalsis with aging and progressive vascular aneurysmal dilatation exacerbating the extrinsic compression of the esophagus.

This anomaly is due to persistence of both right and left fourth aortic arches and dorsal aortae during embryonic development. Tracheal and esophageal compression are common in patients with DAA. The double aortic arch may demonstrate posterior and bilateral impressions on the esophagus and the trachea.

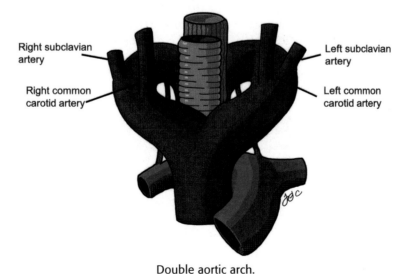

Double aortic arch.

References: Dandelooy J, Coveliers JP, Van Schil PE, et al. Dysphagia lusoria. *CMAJ* 2009;181(8):498.

Etesami M, Ashwath R, Kanne J, et al. Computed tomography in the evaluation of vascular rings and slings. *Insights Imaging* 2014;5(4):507–521.

Li YL, Yam MK, Yu JM. A rare cause of dysphagia. *BMJ Case Rep* 2017;2017:bcr2017220773.

19a **Answer B.** Fluoroscopic spot image from double-contrast upper GI demonstrates serpentine filling defects coursing longitudinally in the distal esophagus. Axial postcontrast T1-weighted MRI image demonstrates numerous enhancing **varices** in the upper abdomen, including around the gastroesophageal junction. Gastroesophageal varices that occur as a result of portal hypertension are sometimes referred to as **uphill varices** because of the direction of blood flow away from the abdomen cephalad into the chest. Venous return from the portal vein extends through the left gastric (coronary) vein into the periesophageal venous plexus and then into the azygous vein and superior vena cava (SVC).

Downhill varices are much less common and are associated with obstruction of the SVC. These varices involve the venous plexus surrounding the upper and middle third of the esophagus with blood flow in a caudal direction. Blood flows through the azygous system into the SVC downstream of the obstruction. If the azygous or inferior SVC below the level of the azygous entrance is also obstructed the flow must extend into the distal esophageal plexus and enter the portal vein, where it flows into the inferior vena cava. These varices would involve the entire thoracic esophagus.

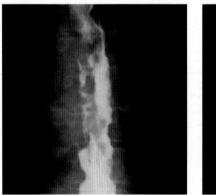 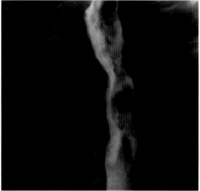

Downhill varices, AP and lateral barium esophagram.

19b **Answer C.** Esophageal varices may be difficult to visualize during a barium examination if the right technique is not utilized. In fact, their variable appearance on different positioning may help confirm the diagnosis. Detection is aided by a semiprone (rather than upright) position to increase venous return from the extremities and a **collapsed** esophageal lumen (rather than full distention).

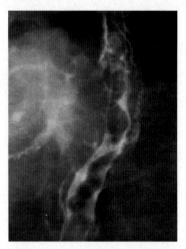

Esophageal varices on RAO prone esophagram with nondistended lumen.

Note that some esophageal carcinomas may have a serpentine tubular morphology resembling varices. These will not change with the maneuvers described above.

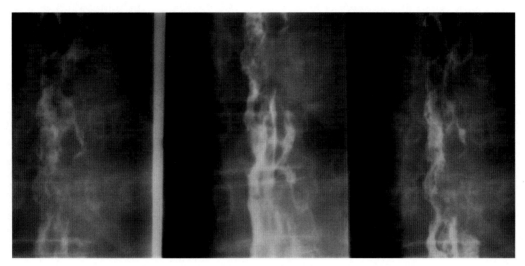

Varicoid carcinoma.

References: Levine MS. Radiology of esophagitis: a pattern approach. *Radiology* 1991;179(1):1–7.

Levine MS, Rubesin SE. Diseases of the esophagus: diagnosis with esophagography. *Radiology* 2005;237(2):414–427.

20a **Answer B.** CT images demonstrate circumferential thickening of the mid-esophageal wall with an adjacent enlarged subcarinal lymph node (left image). The tumor contacts the aorta involving 180 degrees with loss of intervening fat plane (center image). There is a rounded subcentimeter distal periesophageal lymph node (right image).

Surgical resection of esophageal cancer and adjacent malignant lymph nodes offers the only possibility for cure. Accurate staging is essential for determining appropriate treatment. Staging modalities include endoscopic ultrasound, CT, and PET CT. Clinical staging of esophageal cancer is assessed with the TNM system as developed by the AJCC.

Endoscopic ultrasound is the primary means for assessing the T stage. It can ascertain depth of tumor invasion into the wall layers and distinguish T1, T2, and T3 disease, which CT or PET CT cannot. **In assessment of the primary tumor, CT is most useful for detection of T4 disease (Answer B), with loss of fat planes between the tumor and adjacent mediastinal structures.** As demonstrated in this case, aortic involvement is suggested when the tumor contacts 90 degrees or more of the aortic wall (arrowheads) or there is involvement of the fat space between the aorta, esophagus, and the spine (arrow).

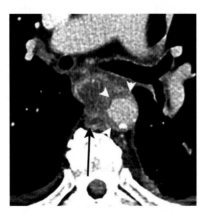

CT has limited sensitivity and specificity for detecting nodal metastases, given the primary criterion for an abnormal node is size of 1 cm or greater. As with other neoplasms, metastases in small nodes and benign changes in enlarged nodes limit the accuracy of CT for nodal staging. Endoscopic ultrasound is superior to CT for detection of nodal metastases, and fine-needle aspiration is most readily accomplished with endoscopic ultrasound (not percutaneously, as suggested in Answer D).

20b **Answer C.** The PET CT images demonstrate intense uptake in the primary mid-esophageal tumor (left image), a right paratracheal lymph node and the left pleural space (center image), and in a gastrohepatic/celiac nodal mass (right image).

As with standard CT, PET CT does not accurately assess depth of tumor invasion into the wall, unless there is involvement of local structures. Locoregional lymph node involvement may be difficult to detect with PET CT as the intense uptake at the primary tumor may obscure adjacent regional metastases. PET has a high sensitivity for detection of distant nodal and nonnodal metastases. Although in this case, the patient was deemed unresectable by virtue of the aortic involvement, the PET CT demonstrated an area of metastatic involvement (left pleural metastases) that might need future local symptomatic treatment.

Distinction between left gastric and celiac axis lymphadenopathy has been traditionally important clinically as the latter was considered to be unresectable. This may be changing as new outcomes data emerge. Due to the close proximity of these nodal stations however, this distinction may be difficult on any imaging study.

References: Esophagus and esophagogastric junction. In: Edge, SB, Byrd DR, Compton CC, et.al., eds. *AJCC cancer staging manual*, 7th ed. New York, NY: Springer, 2010:103–111.

Kim TJ, Kim HY, Lee KW, et al. Multimodality assessment of esophageal cancer: preoperative staging and monitoring of response to therapy. *Radiographics* 2009;29(2):403–421.

21 **Answer D.** Esophagram image demonstrates a midesophageal nearly obstructing stricture with relatively smooth mucosal appearances, as was noted on endoscopy. Mucosal changes would be expected findings in a peptic stricture, as well as a malignant stricture due to primary esophageal carcinoma. The annular localized stricture and obstruction would be atypical for a leiomyoma. Varices would not obstruct and are not likely to be confined to a short segment as in this case. In this patient with a history of another primary tumor (breast cancer), the most likely etiology is a **metastasis from breast cancer**.

Metastases to the esophagus from a distant primary are rare. Lung cancer is the most common primary origin for esophageal metastases, but metastases from breast, ovarian, thyroid, pharyngeal, stomach, and other sites have been reported. Most patients have metastatic involvement to other sites. Breast cancer is the most common neoplasm in women and while typically metastasizing to lung, bones, brain, and liver may also involve the gastrointestinal tract (most commonly the stomach).

References: Nazareno J, Taves D, Preiksaitis HG. Metastatic breast cancer to the gastrointestinal tract: a case series and review of the literature. *World J Gastroenterol* 2006;12(38):6219–6224.

Simchuk EJ, Low DE. Direct esophageal metastasis from a distant primary tumor is a submucosal process: a review of six cases. *Dis Esophagus* 2001;14(3–4):247–250.

22 **Answer D.** The double-contrast barium esophagram demonstrates a lesion in the midesophagus with a **smooth surface and a right angle interface with the wall, findings typical for a submucosal lesion**.

Leiomyomas are the most common benign esophageal neoplasm, accounting for 50% of all such tumors. Tumors usually occur in the middle and distal esophagus (corresponding to the segments with smooth muscle). These range in size from 2 to 8 cm in diameter, usually 3 cm or smaller; they rarely ulcerate. Leiomyomas follow muscle signal on MRI (see arrow on MRI below on a different patient), unlike carcinomas which tend to be higher signal on T2 compared to the esophageal wall (see example below on a different patient). They are isoechoic with muscle on endoscopic ultrasound.

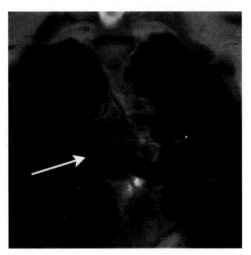

T2-weighted image MRI mid-esophageal leiomyoma.

Diffuse esophageal leiomyomatosis is an unusual form of esophageal leiomyomas, which is histologically identical to the typical localized mass. These may be seen in association with Alport syndrome (glomerulonephritis, hearing loss, various eye diseases, and esophageal and female genital tract leiomyomatosis).

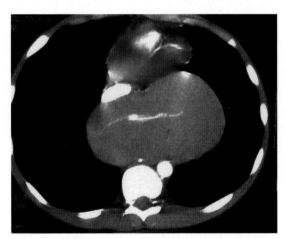

Diffuse esophageal leiomyomatosis.

Granular cell tumors resemble leiomyomas morphologically but tend to be smaller and are much less common. Originally, they were thought to arise from muscle and were formerly called granular cell myoblastomas, but the correct origin is the Schwann cell.

A fibrovascular polyp originates from the cervical esophagus or lower hypopharynx. They are composed of adipose and fibrovascular tissue covered by normal squamous epithelium. They are soft tumors which elongate into an intraluminal mass.

Gastrointestinal stromal tumors (GST) are another common mesenchymal tumor of the gastrointestinal tract. The esophagus is the only segment of the gastrointestinal tract where leiomyomas are more common than GISTs.

References: Jang KM, Lee KS, Lee SJ, et al. The spectrum of benign esophageal lesions: imaging findings. *Korean J Radiol* 2002;3(3):199–210.

Lewis RB, Mehrotra AK, Rodriguez P, et al. From the radiologic pathology archives: esophageal neoplasms: radiologic-pathologic correlation. *Radiographics* 2013;33(4): 1083–1108.

23 **Answer D.** The findings on the barium enema demonstrate multiple short concentric rings of the esophagus, typical for **eosinophilic esophagitis**. Eosinophilic esophagitis can present with segmental strictures in the upper, mid, or less commonly distal esophagus, or as a diffusely gracile narrow-caliber esophagus, findings which overlap with those seen in some of the other entities listed. Eosinophilic esophagitis may also present with a unique ringed or corrugated appearance as in this example, not found with the other entities.

Eosinophilic esophagitis is an idiopathic chronic inflammatory condition which has been increasingly diagnosed in the past two decades likely both to an increasing prevalence and greater awareness of the entity. It is characterized clinically by symptoms of esophageal dysfunction and histologic findings of eosinophilic-predominant esophageal inflammation. It is seen in the pediatric and adult population and has a high (though not universal) association with food allergies. Patients may have a **general atopic history** as well, including asthma and seasonal allergies. A seasonal variation in food-induced eosinophilic esophagitis has been described in some patients. Although eosinophilic esophagitis is seen as a distinct entity, eosinophilic infiltrate may also be present in GERD, and understanding of the relationship between eosinophilic esophagitis and GERD is still under evolution.

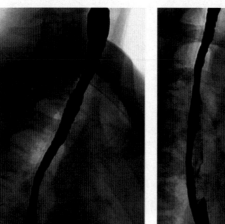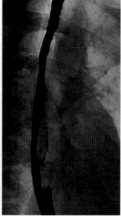

Eosinophilic esophagitis with gracile esophagus.

References: Moawad FJ, Veerappan GR, Wong RK. Eosinophilic esophagitis. *Dig Dis Sci* 2009;54(9):1818–1828.

Zimmerman SL, Levine MS, Rubesin SE, et al. Idiopathic eosinophilic esophagitis in adults: the ringed esophagus. *Radiology* 2005;236(1):159–165.

24 **Answer C.** The barium esophagram demonstrates diffusely severe narrowing of the esophagus and dilatation of the more proximal esophagus. With a **severe stricture of this length, the primary consideration is caustic or corrosive ingestion**, which is the diagnosis in this case. Pertinent history is usually available prior to the examination. Severe gastroesophageal reflux, most commonly caused by an indwelling nasogastric tube, or rarely by high acid content associated with Zollinger-Ellison syndrome and gastroesophageal reflux may result in severe long strictures. Eosinophilic esophagitis may produce a diffusely gracile esophagus. None of the other conditions is likely to result in as severe a stricture as in this case.

Ingestion of a strong alkali agent such as lye (concentrated sodium hydroxide) will cause liquefactive necrosis and a severe ulcerative esophagitis acutely, with a full-thickness injury produced by a 30% sodium hydroxide solution in 1 second. Fibrosis and severe scarring may develop 1 to 3 months later. Injury from acid ingestion tends to be less severe. Aside from causing mechanical obstruction, the injury **increases the risk for developing a malignancy by 1,000-fold** for 10 to 25 years after the acute event.

References: Luedtke P, Levine MS, Rubesin SE, et al. Radiologic diagnosis of benign esophageal strictures: a pattern approach. *Radiographics* 2003;23(4):897–909.

Lupa M, Magne J, Guarisco JL, et al. Update on the diagnosis and treatment of caustic ingestion. *Ochsner J* 2009;9(2):54–59.

25 **Answer C.** The barium esophagram demonstrates absence of most of the normal thoracic esophagus and replacement with a conduit with anastomosis in the upper mediastinum. The conduit can be recognized as a vertically oriented stomach given the presence of rugal folds, continuity with the pylorus and duodenal bulb, and absence of the stomach in the expected infradiaphragmatic location. This procedure is performed for pathology involving the mid and distal esophagus, most commonly esophageal cancer. The stomach is the most common choice for a conduit given the relative ease of preservation of the vascular supply. Less commonly, the colon or jejunum is used as the conduit.

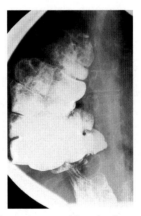

Esophagectomy with colonic conduit.

The most common operation using a gastric conduit (also known as a gastric pull-up) is the Ivor Lewis procedure. This involves a laparotomy for mobilization of the esophagus and stomach, possible tubulation of the stomach, an abdominal lymphadenectomy, and a possible pyloroplasty or pylorotomy. Through a right thoracotomy, the esophagus is removed en bloc with adjacent tissue, a mediastinal lymphadenectomy is performed, and the stomach is pulled up into the chest and anastomosed with the proximal remaining esophagus.

Pulmonary complications (pneumonia, aspiration, acute respiratory distress syndrome, ventilator dependence) and anastomotic leaks are the most common postoperative complications. Delayed gastric emptying due to vagotomy may occur. Gastroesophageal reflux is very common following this procedure.

References: Flanagan JC, Batz R, Saboo SS, et al. Esophagectomy and gastric pull-through procedures: surgical techniques, imaging features, and potential complications. *Radiographics* 2016;36(1):107–121.

Huang L, Onaitis M. Minimally invasive and robotic Ivor Lewis esophagectomy. *J Thorac Dis* 2014;6(Suppl 3):S314–S321.

26   **Answer B. Autoimmune mucocutaneous blistering diseases are a group of conditions which involve bullae and blisters of the skin and mucous membranes.** These can also involve the pharynx and the upper esophagus. Rupture and healing of the bullae can lead to strictures and web formation. **Bullous pemphigoid** is the most common example, typically seen in elderly females, with epidermolysis bullosa a rare related condition. Other conditions including graft versus host disease, toxic epidermal necrolysis, and Stevens-Johnson syndrome that cause desquamation can have similar esophageal involvement with strictures and webs forming in the healing phase.

The other answer choices listed are less likely to result in the findings seen. Strictures associated with indwelling nasogastric tubes are long and involve the distal esophagus Zollinger-Ellison syndrome may also produce long strictures of the distal esophagus due to the increased acidity of refluxed material. GERD is unlikely to involve a segment as high as seen in this example. Appropriate ports for radiation of cervical lymphadenopathy should be able to avoid the hypopharynx and esophagus.

Other causes of high esophageal web formation include heterotopic gastric mucosa, which may be seen in the cervical esophagus on endoscopy in up to 10% of patients. This is typically asymptomatic but can be associated with scarring and web formation due to acid production.

Plummer-Vinson syndrome involves cervical esophageal webs, iron deficiency anemia, and glossitis. Patients have dysphagia related to the webs and are at increased risk for hypopharyngeal and esophageal cancer.

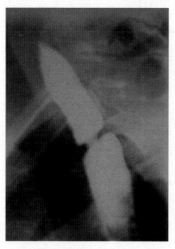 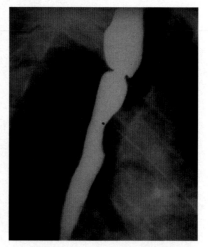

Heterotopic gastric mucosa.   Plummer-Vinson syndrome.

References: Akbayir N, Alkim C, Erdem L, et al. Heterotopic gastric mucosa in the cervical esophagus (inlet patch): endoscopic prevalence, histological and clinical characteristics. *J Gastroenterol Hepatol* 2004;19(8):891–896.

Ergun GA, Lin AN, Dannenberg AJ, et al. Gastrointestinal manifestations of epidermolysis bullosa. A study of 101 patients. *Medicine (Baltimore)* 1992;71(3):121–127.

27a **Answer C.** Penetration of ingested material into the upper laryngeal vestibule may be shallow and clear with progression of the swallow ("flash" penetration) and can be a normal finding. In this case however, the image demonstrates abnormal **deep laryngeal penetration** of barium into the lower laryngeal vestibule just above the vocal cords. No subglottic extension of barium is seen in this case, but if the penetrated material is not ejected, this material may be aspirated.

Swallowing (deglutition) is a complex process. Aside from structural or anatomic causes, a large number of neuromuscular disorders of the oral cavity and pharynx may affect swallowing. These include oral stasis, delayed swallow initiation, premature spillage into the pharynx, nasopharyngeal reflux, pharyngeal stasis, laryngeal penetration, and aspiration. These disorders may be caused by an abnormality of the central nervous system or peripheral disorders. Central nervous system causes include stroke, Parkinson disease, Alzheimer's and other dementias, cerebral palsy, intracranial trauma, amyotrophic lateral sclerosis, or demyelinating disease. Peripheral causes include myasthenia gravis, striated muscular disorders including muscular dystrophy, polymyositis, and metabolic or hormonal conditions affecting muscle such as thyroid disorders.

27b **Answer B.** The process of normal deglutition (swallowing) involves complex volitional and reflexive neuromuscular activity. Many conditions, including cognitive impairment, neuromuscular abnormalities (such as stroke or intrinsic muscle weakness), or structural abnormalities (e.g., strictures, diverticula, masses) can interfere with the normal swallowing mechanism. Swallowing is divided into oral, pharyngeal, and esophageal phases. A bolus is created in the oral phase and propelled by the tongue toward the pharynx. The pharyngeal phase involves elevation of the soft palate to seal the nasopharynx, **elevation and anterior movement of the hyoid and larynx**, adduction and apposition of the vocal cords and laryngeal closure, epiglottic inversion, and upper esophageal sphincter relaxation (hence all actions except that described in answer B are true). The bolus then enters into the esophagus where it is propelled toward the stomach by peristaltic waves.

References: Carucci LR, Turner MA. Dysphagia revisited: common and unusual causes. *Radiographics* 2015;35(1):105–122.

Gates J, Hartnell GG, Gramigna GD. Videofluoroscopy and swallowing studies for neurologic disease: a primer. *Radiographics* 2006;26(1):e22.

Harris JA, Bartelt D, Campion M, et al. The use of low-osmolar water-soluble contrast in videofluoroscopic swallowing exams. *Dysphagia* 2013;28(4):520–527.

28 **Answer D.** On a barium pharyngoesophagram, there is a diverticulum originating from the posterior hypopharyngeal wall above a prominent cricopharyngeal muscle, representing a **Zenker diverticulum**. A Zenker diverticulum is a pulsion pseudodiverticulum that involves herniation of mucosa and submucosa through **Killian's dehiscence**, a posterior defect between the horizontal and oblique fibers of the inferior constrictor muscle in the region of the cricopharyngeus muscle. The diverticulum extends inferiorly below the level of the cricopharyngeus posterior to the cervical esophagus. When small, the diverticulum may remain midline; as it enlarges, it may extend laterally. The pathogenesis of the diverticulum formation is uncertain, but associated cricopharyngeal spasm or incoordination of upper esophageal sphincter opening with swallowing have been implicated. Gastroesophageal reflux (GERD) disease and esophageal dysmotility are commonly associated with a Zenker diverticulum; GERD is also associated with cricopharyngeal spasm. The patient may present with halitosis and regurgitation of undigested food. Secondary aspiration of diverticulum contents may occur. When large, a palpable neck mass may be found.

A Killian-Jamieson diverticulum extends laterally from the cervical esophagus below the cricopharyngeus (through the Killian-Jamieson space, distinct from Killian's dehiscence). Although the example below is large, this diverticulum is usually small and asymptomatic, may be bilateral, and is less common than a Zenker diverticulum.

Lateral pharyngeal pouches are focal bulges in the lateral pharyngeal wall in the region of the thyrohyoid membrane; these are usually bilateral. When pharyngeal mucosa herniates through the thyrohyoid membrane, a fixed lateral pharyngeal diverticulum with a narrow neck (usually unilateral) may develop; these may be symptomatic with dysphagia and aspiration. Lateral pharyngeal diverticula are commonly associated with increased intraluminal pressure (e.g., horn players and glass blowers).

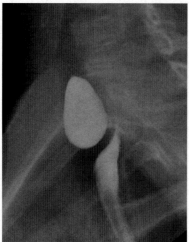 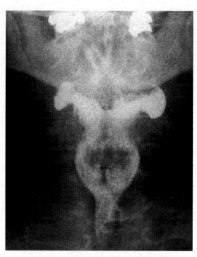

Killian-Jamieson diverticulum.   Lateral pharyngeal pouches.

References: Gore RM, Levine MS. *Textbook of gastrointestinal radiology*, 4th ed. Philadelphia, PA: Elsevier/Saunders, 2015.

Rubesin SE, Levine MS. Killian-Jamieson diverticula: radiographic findings in 16 patients. *AJR Am J Roentgenol* 2001;177(1):85–89.

29 **Answer B.** The lateral pharyngogram demonstrates a prominent posterior impression at the junction of the hypopharynx and esophagus at the C5-C6 level consistent with a **prominent cricopharyngeus muscle (also called a cricopharyngeal bar)**. The cricopharyngeus muscle is usually contracted at rest and relaxes with initiation of a swallow. While it may be seen in asymptomatic people, it is commonly related to gastroesophageal reflux disease (GERD). The cricopharyngeus serves as a barrier to prevent retrograde flow of ingested material and stomach acid into the airway and to prevent air entry into the esophagus. Note that cricopharyngeal bars may also be asymptomatic and incidental findings.

Increased tone of the muscle at rest may lead to a **Zenker diverticulum** but is not demonstrated on this examination. A brainstem infarct with lower cranial nerve dysfunction may lead to pharyngeal paresis with an associated cricopharyngeal bar but is not necessarily associated with increased pressure on manometry and would be unlikely in the patient's age group. While cricopharyngeal muscle dysfunction may be associated with aspiration pneumonias, this patient's clinical presentation is not consistent.

References: Cook I. Cricopharyngeal bar and Zenker diverticulum. *Gastroenterol Hepatol (N Y)* 2011;7(8):540.

Tao TY, Menias CO, Herman TE, et al. Easier to swallow: pictorial review of structural findings of the pharynx at barium pharyngography. *Radiographics* 2013;33(7):e189–e208.

QUESTIONS

1 A 78-year-old female with epigastric discomfort undergoes an upper GI study.

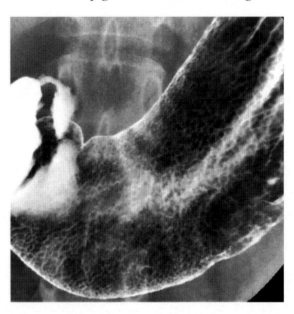

What does the mucosal pattern represent?

A. Areae gastricae
B. Hypertrophic sessile polyps
C. Atrophic gastritis
D. Ménétrier gastropathy

2   A 69-year-old female with a history of breast cancer presents for evaluation of nausea, vomiting, and poor oral intake. An upper GI study and contrast-enhanced CT scan were performed. What is the correct diagnosis?

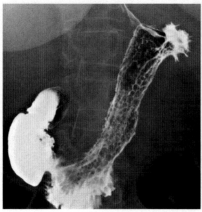 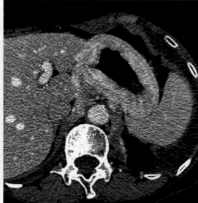 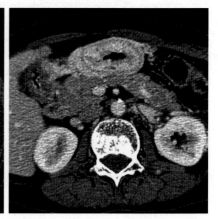

A. Chemotherapy toxicity
B. Gastric ulcer
C. Linitis plastica
D. Gastric varices

3   A 67-year-old patient presents with hematemesis. Endoscopic evaluation demonstrates marked fold thickening with ulcerations, and biopsy is consistent with lymphoma. The CT and PET scan obtained for staging is shown below. Regarding primary gastric lymphoma, which of the following statements is TRUE?

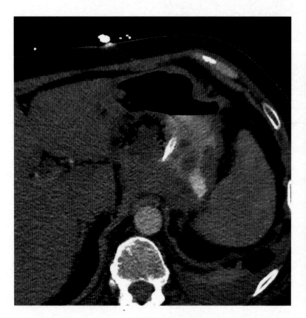 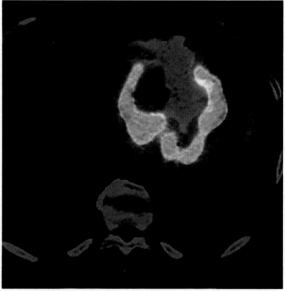

A. Most primary gastric lymphomas are Hodgkin lymphoma.
B. Lymphoma is the most common type of gastric malignancy.
C. Transpyloric spread of a gastric mass favors the diagnosis of lymphoma over adenocarcinoma.
D. Eradication of *H. pylori* infection may cause regression of low-grade MALT lymphoma.

4 An upper GI is performed on a 72-year-old male with epigastric pain. What is the appropriate next step in management?

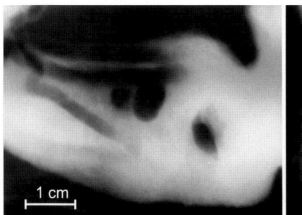 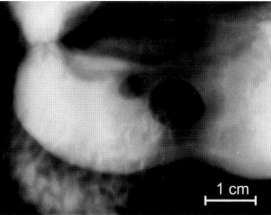

A. Examination should be repeated with double-contrast technique to better characterize the polyps.

B. Polyps have definitive benign features and need no further workup.

C. Endoscopy is required for diagnosis and potential treatment.

D. Polyps have malignant features and as endoscopic biopsy may be prone to sampling error and false-negative results, surgical consultation is needed.

5a A 45-year-old male presents with left upper quadrant pain, melena, and a hematocrit of 30. An endoscopy reveals an ulcerated gastric mass. Immunohistochemistry of the biopsy is strongly positive for CD117. A CT scan is performed for staging purposes. What type of tumor is this most likely?

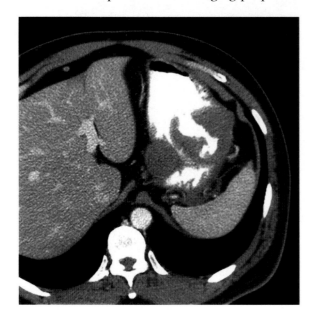 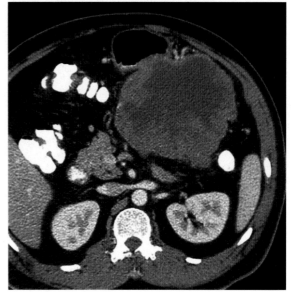

A. Leiomyosarcoma

B. Adenocarcinoma

C. Lymphoma

D. Gastrointestinal stromal tumor (GST)

5b A factor which determines for malignant potential of gastric GSTs is

A. Size
B. Ulceration
C. Degree of enhancement
D. Adjacent mesenteric fat stranding

5c Where is this tumor most likely to metastasize?

A. Liver
B. Lungs
C. Lymph nodes
D. Brain

6 A 45-year-old female presents with epigastric pain. She undergoes a single-contrast barium UGI examination. Based upon the finding, which of the following statements is most accurate?

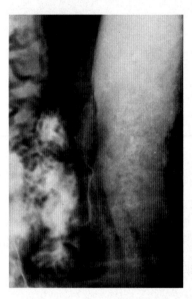
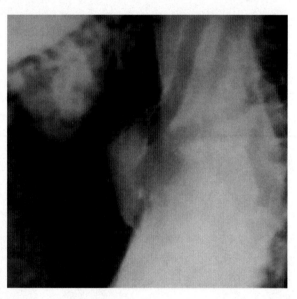

A. The ulcer appears benign because it extends beyond the expected lumen of the stomach.
B. The ulcer appears malignant because it is associated with a mass.
C. The ulcer appears malignant because it is located in the body of the stomach.
D. The ulcer is indeterminate and has no features suggestive of a benign or malignant nature.

7 A radiologist is performing an UGI study and sees a possible small ulceration in the stomach. The finding is subtle and she chooses a smaller field of view (FOV) to better visualize the finding. As a consequence of this magnification, which of the following statements is TRUE?

A. The spatial resolution is decreased.
B. The dose to the patient is increased.
C. The magnification gain is higher.
D. There is a decrease in the kVp.

8 A 22-year-old male with vague upper abdominal pain undergoes an upper GI examination. No additional lesions were seen. What is the most likely diagnosis?

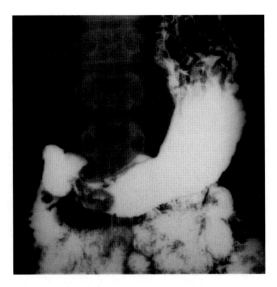 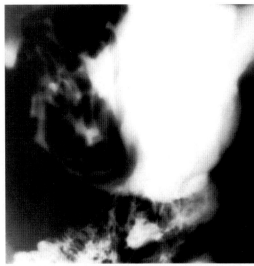

A. Metastatic melanoma
B. Gastrointestinal stromal tumor (GIST)
C. Lymphoma
D. Ectopic pancreatic rest

9 A 56-year-old male with a history of abdominal discomfort has a CT. A urea breath test is reported as abnormal. What is the most likely diagnosis?

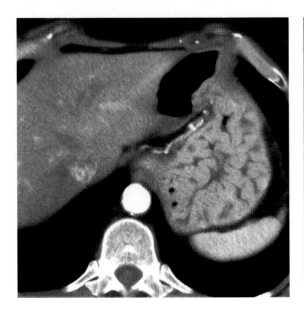 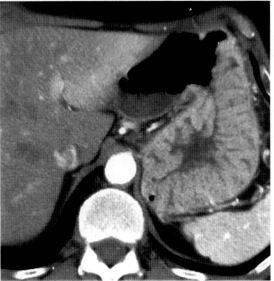

A. *Helicobacter pylori* gastritis
B. Ménétrier disease
C. Gastric lymphoma
D. Zollinger-Ellison syndrome

10a A 41-year-old female presents with a history of chronic abdominal pain. A contrast-enhanced CT scan was obtained, followed by an In-111 Octreotide SPECT study. What is the best diagnosis?

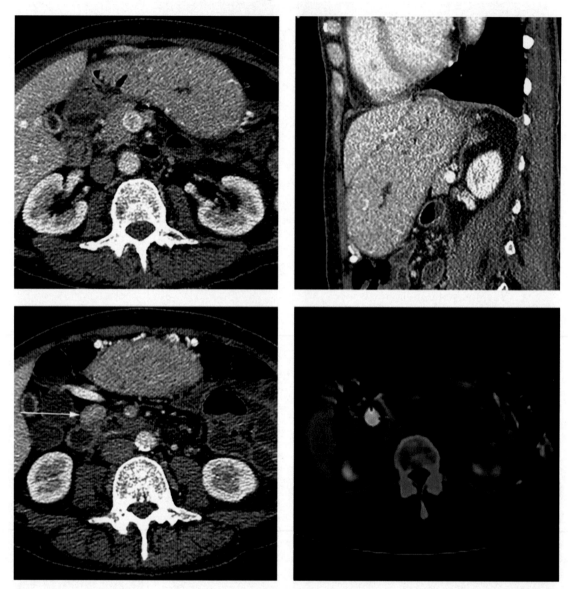

A. *H. pylori* gastritis
B. Ménétrier disease
C. Gastric lymphoma
D. Zollinger-Ellison syndrome

10b The mass identified in this patient is located in the gastrinoma triangle, which is bounded medially by the junction of the pancreatic neck–body and inferiorly by the junction of the second-third portions of the duodenum. What comprises the superior margin of the gastrinoma triangle?

A. Falciform ligament
B. Junction of common hepatic artery and gastroduodenal artery
C. Junction of cystic duct and common bile duct
D. Right portal vein

11a A 53-year-old male presented with epigastric discomfort. An endoscopy reveals a gastric mass. An MRI of the abdomen is performed with the following T1-weighted sequences post contrast.

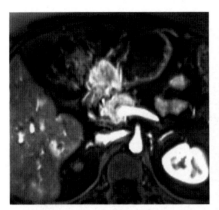 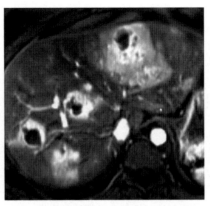 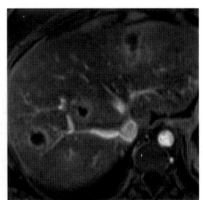

Arterial phase.   Arterial phase.   Venous phase.

What is the most likely etiology for the findings?

A. Lymphoma
B. Gastrointestinal stromal tumor
C. Gastric adenocarcinoma
D. Gastric carcinoid

11b Following a partial gastrectomy, later staging studies included a gallium-68 DOTATATE PET-CT. What receptor is bound by this radiotracer?

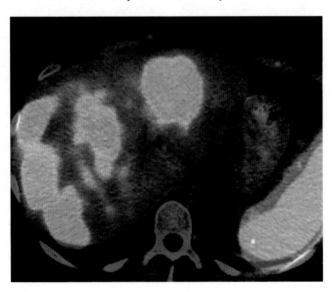

A. Somatostatin
B. Gastrin
C. Vasoactive intestinal peptide (VIP)
D. Glucagon-like peptide 1 (GLP-1)

12 In these cases of gastric outlet obstruction, match the following images with the best diagnosis. Each answer may be used once only.

Patient 1: A 39-year-old male with a history of vomiting after an ERCP.

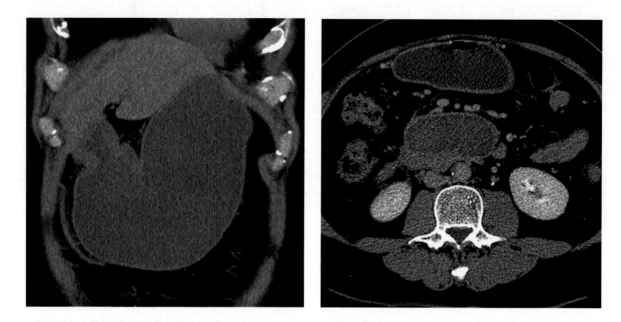

Patient 2: A 31-year-old male recently begun on a proton pump inhibitor with postprandial bloating.

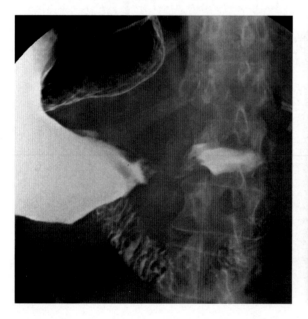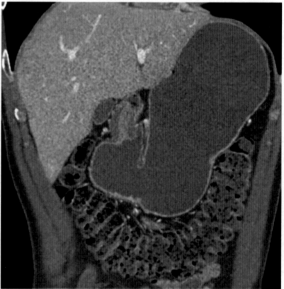

Patient 3: A 78-year-old female with early satiety.

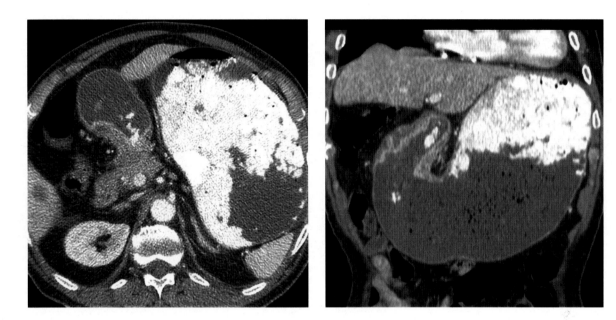

Patient 4: A 40-year-old male with severe acute abdominal pain.

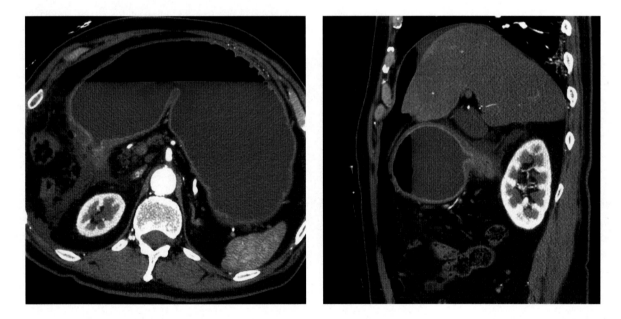

A. Gastric carcinoma involving the antrum and duodenal bulb
B. Adult hypertrophic pyloric stenosis
C. Perforated duodenal ulcer
D. Duodenal hematoma

13 Identify the following bariatric surgical procedures:

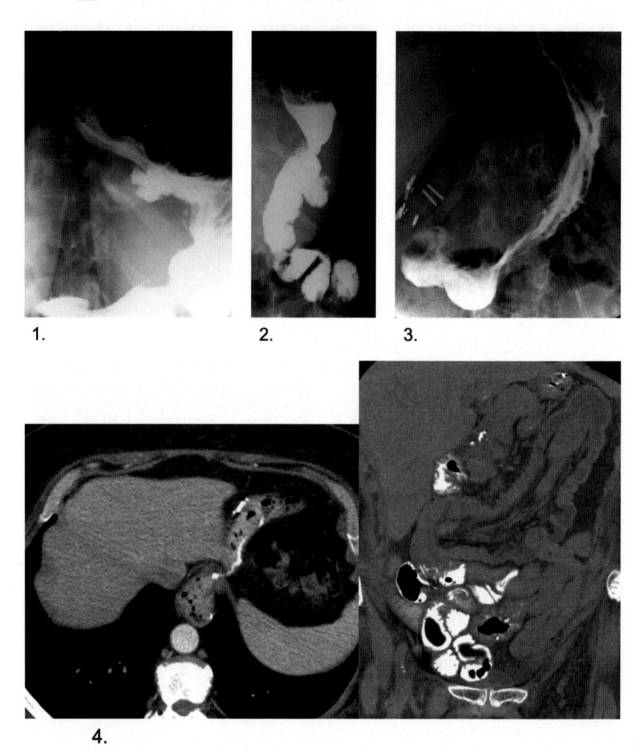

1.

2.

3.

4.

A. Roux-en-Y gastric bypass
B. Sleeve gastrectomy
C. Adjustable gastric band (lap band)
D. Biliopancreatic diversion with duodenal switch

14 A 53-year-old female with a history of laparoscopic gastric band placement for morbid obesity presents with increased vomiting and poor oral intake. An upper GI study was performed. What is the most likely diagnosis?

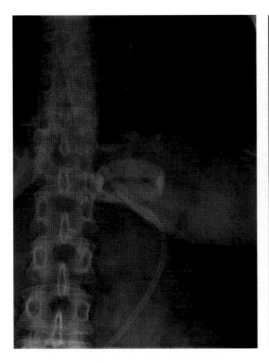 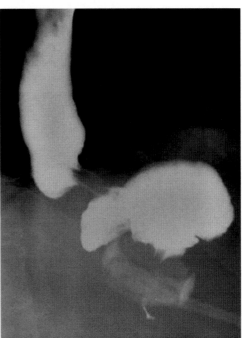

   A. Gastric band slippage
   B. Gastric perforation
   C. Intraluminal band erosion
   D. Normal appearance

15 A 60-year-old female who had a sleeve gastrectomy performed 5 days ago undergoes a routine postoperative upper GI study. What is the diagnosis?

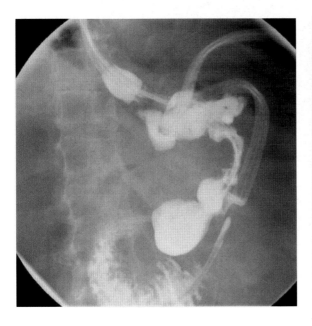 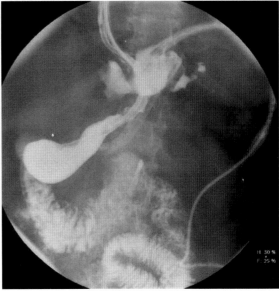

   A. Normal postoperative appearance
   B. Staple line leak
   C. Gastrocolic fistula
   D. Gastric obstruction

16 A 50-year-old female with a history of laparoscopic Roux-en-Y gastric bypass presents with a history of persistent abdominal pain and poor weight loss. An upper GI study was performed. What finding is demonstrated?

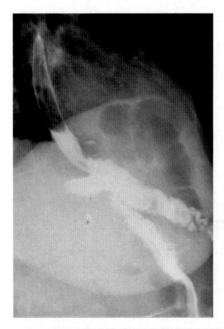 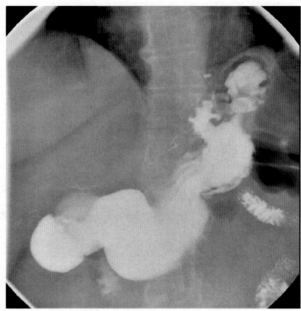

    A. Esophageal reflux

    B. Gastrocolic fistula

    C. Gastrogastric fistula

    D. Efferent limb obstruction

17 What type of artifact is illustrated in the CT scan below?

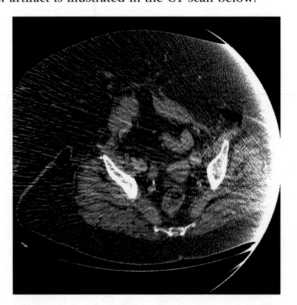

    A. Quantum mottle

    B. Wrap-around artifact

    C. Truncation artifact

    D. Beam hardening

18 A 26-year-old female presents with cramping epigastric pain. An upper GI and small bowel follow-through examination is performed. What is the most likely diagnosis?

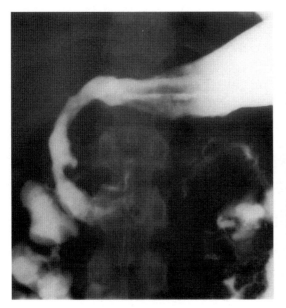 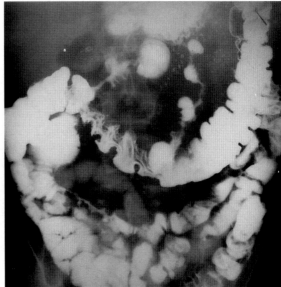

A. *H. pylori* gastroduodenitis
B. Crohn disease
C. Eosinophilic gastroenteritis
D. Pancreatitis

19 An 86-year-old female with symptoms of mild early satiety has an upper GI barium examination. What is the name for the gastric abnormality seen?

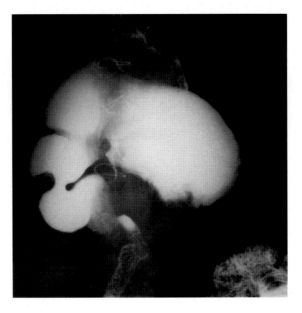

A. Organoaxial rotation
B. Mesenteroaxial rotation
C. Borchardt hernia
D. Bochdalek hernia

20 A 74-year-old female with a history of hiatal hernia presents to the emergency department with acute onset of nausea and vomiting. An upper GI study was performed. Based on these results, the most appropriate treatment strategy is

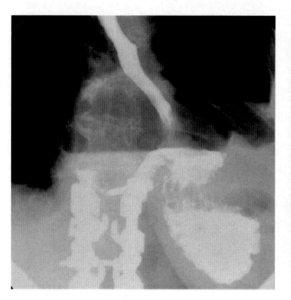 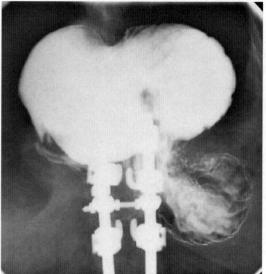

A. Discharge to home with prescription for proton pump inhibitor.
B. Obtain a CT scan of the chest and abdomen.
C. Admit to internal medicine service for observation.
D. Obtain surgical consultation for urgent operation.

21 A 77-year-old male underwent ERCP for suspected choledocholithiasis. Cannulation of the bile duct was technically challenging. He was afebrile and clinically stable at the time of the follow-up CT. What is the most likely cause of the finding below?

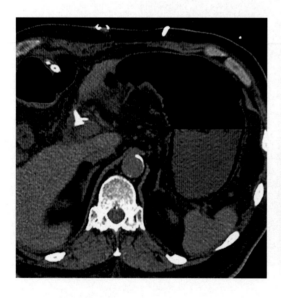 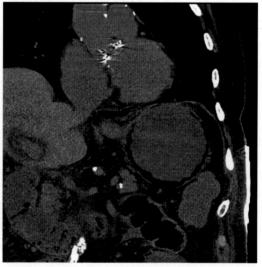

A. Clostridium infection
B. Ischemia
C. Iatrogenic from the ERCP
D. Benign pneumatosis related to underlying COPD

22 An image from an abdominal CT is shown. What features produce this artifact?

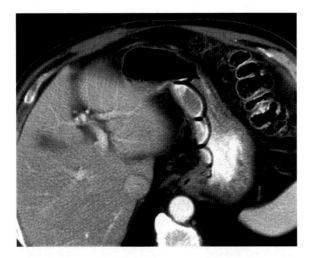

    A. The artifact is a result of both image acquisition and reconstruction processes.

    B. The artifact may be eliminated by slower scanning.

    C. The artifact is caused by the presence of stationary gas bubbles.

    D. The artifact is increased with solid food ingestion.

23 An 81-year-old male presents to the emergency department with a history of acute abdominal pain after several hours of severe intermittently productive retching. He becomes hypotensive and a CT without contrast is obtained, due to renal impairment. What is the diagnosis?

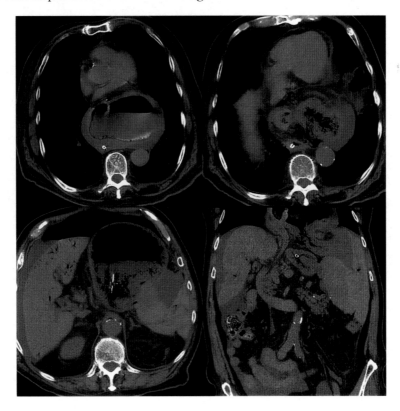

    A. Large sliding hiatal hernia with pneumobilia

    B. Nasogastric tube perforation of the esophagus with mediastinal abscess

    C. Large paraesophageal hernia with gastric ischemia and perforation

    D. Achalasia with perforation

24   A 38-year-old female with epigastric pain undergoes an upper GI study. What is the most likely diagnosis?

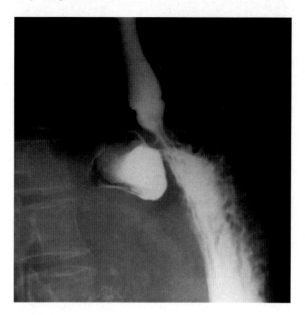

A. Epiphrenic diverticulum
B. Gastric diverticulum
C. Slipped fundoplication
D. Gastric fundal ulcer

25   A 20-year-old female presents with a 2-week history of abdominal pain and nausea. On examination, she has a palpable periumbilical mass. She has a CT scan performed. She is not diabetic and is on no medications that would affect gastric motility. What should be recommended as the next step in evaluation?

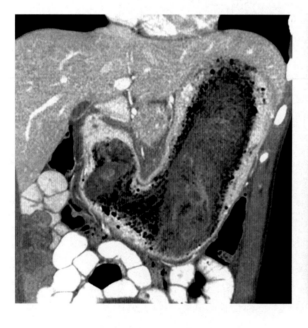
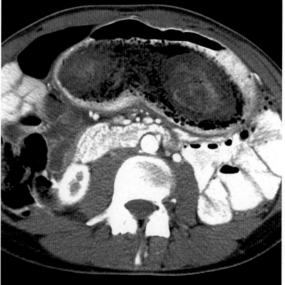

A. Endoscopic evaluation
B. Surgical consultation
C. PET scan
D. Gastric emptying study

26 Regarding gastric erosions, which of the following statements is TRUE?

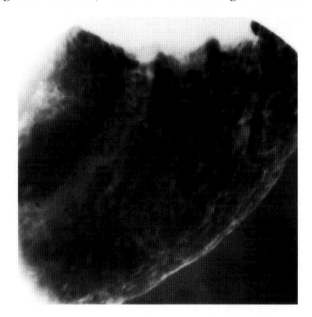

A. Gastric erosions are best visualized on single-contrast UGI.
B. Gastric erosions are the most common radiographic manifestation of gastritis due to *H. pylori* infection.
C. Gastric erosions are most commonly located in the stomach fundus.
D. Gastric erosions are nonspecific and may be seen with a number of different etiologies.

ANSWERS AND EXPLANATIONS

1 **Answer A.** The upper GI study demonstrates a confluent reticular appearance of the gastric mucosa with the intersecting furrows outlining regular ovoid or polygonal structures 1 to 5 mm in size, known as areae gastricae. The other conditions listed result in a different mucosal appearance: hypertrophic polyps are seen on a background of flatter mucosa; atrophic gastritis has smooth featureless mucosa; and Ménétrier gastropathy results in a thickened wall and rugal folds.

When **involvement is limited, areae gastricae are considered a normal finding** and an indication of good mucosal coating using double-contrast technique. They are more commonly demonstrated in older patients, and when enlarged or more extensive (as in this case), they are thought to indicate thinning of the mucus coating of the stomach lining and are associated with gastric hypersecretion. Areae gastricae on radiographic studies correspond to a mosaic mucosal pattern on endoscopy which is associated with *H. pylori* infection.

References: Charagundla SR, Levine MS, Langlotz CP, et al. Visualization of areae gastricae on double-contrast upper gastrointestinal radiography: relationship to age of patients. *AJR Am J Roentgenol* 2001;177(1):61–63.

Watanabe H, Magota S, Shiiba S, et al. Coarse areae gastricae in the proximal body and fundus: a sign of gastric hypersecretion. Radiological and endoscopic correlation. *Radiology* 1983;146(2):303–306.

2 **Answer C.** Fluoroscopic spot image from a double-contrast upper GI demonstrates nodular pattern of the wall and diffuse narrowing of the stomach lumen. Axial contrast-enhanced CT image demonstrates diffuse wall thickening and enhancement. No ulceration is demonstrated, and gastritis from chemotherapy or other causes would involve fold thickening but not the nodularity demonstrated in this case. Varices are usually found in the proximal stomach and would not cause the diffuse luminal restriction. The imaging features are most compatible with **linitis plastica**, in this case from metastatic breast carcinoma.

Linitis plastica is characterized by loss of normal gastric distensibility as a result of infiltrative tumor, leading to a "leather bottle" appearance of the stomach. The degree of gastric distensibility is variable, ranging from a quite subtle limitation to severe rigidity. This may occur in the setting of advanced scirrhous gastric carcinoma as in this case below from a different patient. Note the invariant gastric contours on the AP (left) and RAO (right) images.

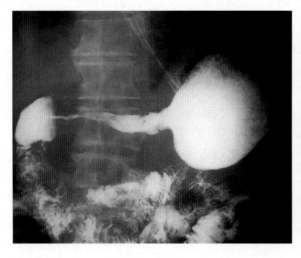 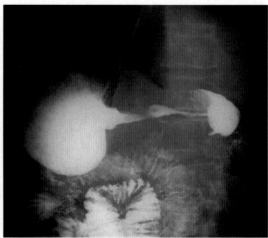

A linitis plastica appearance can also be seen with lymphoma or metastatic disease (most commonly of breast and lung origin). Imaging plays an important role in diagnosis, as up to 30% of cases may have a false-negative endoscopic biopsy due to the tumor's deep and infiltrative behavior.

References: Levine MS. Stomach. In: Levine MS, Ramchandani P, Rubesin SE, eds. *Practical fluoroscopy of the GI and GU tracts.* New York, NY: Cambridge University Press; 2012:73–104.

Taal BG, Peterse H, Boot H. Clinical presentation, endoscopic features, and treatment of gastric metastases from breast carcinoma. *Cancer* 2000;89(11):2214–2221.

3 **Answer D.** Primary gastric lymphoma is the most common type of extranodal lymphoma, accounting for 50% to 70% of all primary gastrointestinal lymphomas. Gastrointestinal lymphoma is nearly always of the non-Hodgkin type. **Lymphoma is much less common than adenocarcinoma in the stomach**, accounting for only 1% to 5% of all gastric malignancies. Adenocarcinoma and lymphoma may present with similar radiographic features, including fold thickening, polypoid masses, and ulceration. Severe infiltration with lymphoma may even produce a linitis plastica appearance, although in distinction from adenocarcinoma, gastric distention is usually relatively preserved. Note that while transpyloric spread is more common in lymphoma than adenocarcinoma, a tumor showing such transpyloric spread is still more likely to be adenocarcinoma, given its much higher prevalence.

Of the primary gastric lymphomas, a large proportion (50% to 72%) are mucosa-associated lymphoid tissue (MALT)–type lymphomas. **MALT-type lymphomas are associated with chronic *H. pylori* infection** and are classified into low-grade and high-grade histologic categories. **Eradication of *H. pylori* infection with antibiotics and proton pump inhibitors is the first line of therapy for low-grade tumors and may cause complete tumor regression.**

Radiographically most low-grade MALT lymphomas may show superficial spreading lesions with mucosal nodularity, shallow ulcerations, and mild fold thickening on barium studies, whereas high-grade tumors are associated with formation of masses or marked wall thickening.

References: Choi D, Lim HK, Lee SJ, et al. Gastric mucosa-associated lymphoid tissue lymphoma: helical CT findings and pathologic correlation. *AJR Am J Roentgenol* 2002;178(5):1117–1122.

Ghai S, Pattison J, Ghai S, et al. Primary gastrointestinal lymphoma: spectrum of imaging findings with pathologic correlation. *Radiographics* 2007;27(5):1371–1388.

4 **Answer C.** There are multiple polyps in the gastric antrum, incompletely characterized with regard to morphology on this single-contrast study. Gastric polyps are common findings on endoscopy and upper gastrointestinal fluoroscopic studies. 90% are asymptomatic and do not have malignant potential, but some do require intervention. **Detection of polyps on radiographic studies should prompt endoscopic evaluation.** Certain morphologic features are associated with different rates of malignancy. Pedunculated or larger polyps are more commonly adenomatous, which are considered premalignant, and small sessile polyps are more likely hyperplastic and benign. Morphologic features are not sufficient however to determine management; therefore characterization on imaging studies with optimized technique (e.g., double-contrast) will not preclude the need for endoscopy. **Hyperplastic polyps are a response to chronic inflammation, and there is an increased risk for a synchronous gastric cancer when atrophic**

gastritis is present. For this reason, even though small sessile polyps are themselves likely benign, endoscopy is still warranted to evaluate for separate cancers. Polypectomy is indicated for larger (≥1 cm) polyps; smaller solitary polyps may be resected or biopsied. In addition, the surrounding mucosa is sampled to rule out dysplasia, underlying atrophic gastritis, and to assess for *Helicobacter pylori*.

Polyps may be classified by their tissue type of origin: epithelial, hamartomatous, or mesenchymal. **Epithelial** polyps include hyperplastic polyps, fundic gland polyps, and adenomatous polyps. Hyperplastic polyps are seen in the setting of chronic inflammation (such as atrophic gastritis), *H. pylori* infection, pernicious anemia, and adjacent to ulcers. They are generally benign but have some risk for malignant potential (between 1 and 20%, with increased risk for polyps >1 cm).

Fundic gland polyps are the most common type in Western countries where *H. pylori* infection rates are lower. These are sporadic or may be associated with polyposis syndromes. Long-term proton pump inhibitor (PPI) use is associated with an increased risk of fundic gland polyps. Fundic gland polyps that are sporadic or associated with PPI use have no significant malignant potential. In patients with familial adenomatous polyposis (FAP), there is a greater incidence of dysplasia present in the fundic gland polyps (usually low grade with progression to malignancy rare).

Adenomas are seen typically in a background of chronic atrophic gastritis with intestinal metaplasia. Eight to fifty-nine percent of adenomas are associated with a synchronous gastric carcinoma. Increased risk of invasive carcinoma in an adenoma is correlated with larger size, villous morphology, and the degree of dysplasia.

Hamartomatous polyps are seen in Peutz-Jeghers syndrome, juvenile polyposis, and Cowden disease.

Mesenchymal tissues may give rise to a number of polyp types. Inflammatory fibroid polyps are rare mesenchymal tumors that arise in the submucosa and mucosa and are considered nonneoplastic. Other mesenchymal origin polyps include gastrointestinal or gut stroma tumors (GST), leiomyomas, and granular cell tumors.

References: Carmack SW, Genta RM, Schuler CM, et al. The current spectrum of gastric polyps: a 1-year national study of over 120,000 patients. *Am J Gastroenterol* 2009;104(6):1524–1532.

Feczko PJ, Halpert RD, Ackerman LV. Gastric polyps: radiological evaluation and clinical significance. *Radiology* 1985;155(3):581–584.

5a **Answer D.** The CT scan demonstrates a mass centered in the gastric body wall with an endoluminal component that has a large ulceration, likely the cause of the bleeding. The mass also has a large exophytic component extending inferiorly. These morphologic features favor a gastrointestinal stromal tumor over the other choices. **Gastrointestinal stromal tumors (GSTs) also called gut stroma tumors are the most common mesenchymal tumor of the gastrointestinal tract.** They are defined by the positive immunoreactivity to CD117 (KIT), a tyrosine kinase growth factor receptor. Other mesenchymal tumors are negative or only weakly positive for CD117.

Ulcerations are common, seen in 50% of GSTs. The exophytic growth pattern is also common. The tumors have a tendency to hemorrhage. Enhancement tends to be heterogeneous, but more pronounced peripherally. Aside from the immunohistochemistry marker, no lymphadenopathy is seen that might be associated with lymphoma or adenocarcinoma.

5b **Answer A.** The malignant potential for GSTs is based upon **size and mitotic rate**. Tumors <5 cm in diameter with five or fewer mitoses per 50 consecutive high power fields (HPFs) have a very low risk for malignant behavior. Tumors >10 cm with more than five mitoses per HPF are considered to be at high risk. Tumors that fall in between these categories are of uncertain or intermediate risk. The risk of malignant potential is also related to location. In the small intestine, a GST may have a more aggressive behavior compared to a tumor of the same size in the stomach.

5c **Answer A.** GSTs most commonly metastasize to **liver** and intraabdominally within the **peritoneal cavity**. **Lymph node metastases are rare**, and lymph node metastases are not performed routinely at resection. Lung and brain metastases are unusual as well. With tyrosine kinase inhibitor therapy, liver metastases may become almost completely cystic.

References: Kim HC, Lee JM, Kim KW, et al. Gastrointestinal stromal tumors of the stomach: CT findings and prediction of malignancy. *AJR Am J Roentgenol* 2004;183(4):893–898.

Sandrasegaran K, Rajesh A, Rydberg J, et al. Gastrointestinal stromal tumors: clinical, radiologic, and pathologic features. *AJR Am J Roentgenol* 2005;184(3):803–811.

6 **Answer A.** The UGI study demonstrates an ulcer crater along the lesser curvature of the stomach. This ulcer extends beyond the expected lumen of the stomach, has no associated mass, and is consistent with a **0** ulcer. Additional features favoring a benign nature include its regular ovoid shape, folds radiating to the edge of the crater, and smooth ulcer collar. Benign ulcers are more common in the antrum and lesser curvature, but location in the stomach is not a reliable indicator of benignity versus malignancy. Duodenal ulcers are almost invariably benign.

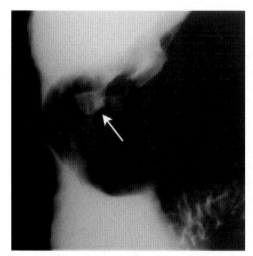 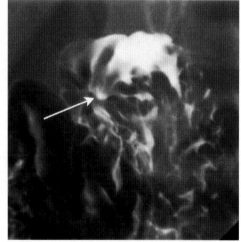

Malignant ulcer in a gastric mass.   Benign duodenal ulcer.

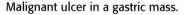

Ulcer Features	
Features of Benign Gastric Ulcer	**Features of Malignant Gastric Ulcer**
No mass present	Mass present
Extension beyond the expected lumen of the stomach	Location within the expected lumen of the stomach
Folds radiate smoothly to edge of crater	Folds end in clubbed or nodular contours and do not reach edge of crater
Round or ovoid regular shape	Irregular shape
Hampton's line (intact mucosa with undermined submucosa) or thicker but smooth ulcer collar	Irregular thick rim

Helicobacter pylori infection is a major etiologic cause of duodenal and gastric ulcers. One current approach to evaluating patients with initial presentation of dyspepsia is to screen for *H. pylori* infection with noninvasive tests (stool antigen and urea breath test) or to try empiric proton pump inhibitor (PPI) therapy. For patients who are older than age 55 or have alarm features (such as unintended weight loss, GI bleeding, family history of GI malignancy), endoscopy is usually recommended. Barium studies have been supplanted by endoscopy in the past 30 years, partly due to early reports of relative lack of sensitivity and specificity for detection of gastric malignancy. These data were based on comparison of endoscopy with single-contrast barium technique, and although double-contrast technique has been since shown to have comparable sensitivity and specificity to endoscopy for detection and characterization of most ulcers, the bias toward endoscopy remains. Nevertheless, as some patients may not tolerate endoscopy, the ability to characterize ulcers by barium radiography remains important.

References: Gore RM, Levine MS. *Textbook of gastrointestinal radiology.* 4th ed. Philadelphia, PA: Elsevier/Saunders, 2015.

Talley NJ, American Gastroenterological Association. American Gastroenterological Association medical position statement: evaluation of dyspepsia. *Gastroenterology* 2005;129(5):1753–1755.

7 | **Answer B.** When a smaller field of view is chosen by the fluoroscopist, the image intensifier electronically alters the size of the input radiation field of view while keeping the output field fixed. This will increase the spatial resolution performance. The minification gain is defined as the input phosphor area/output phosphor area, thus decreasing the input area will decrease the minification gain.

As the input field of view is decreased, a smaller area of the input phosphor is being irradiated. This decreases the brightness gain, so in compensation the automatic brightness control feedback circuit increases the exposure rate to maintain the brightness at the output phosphor. The **dose to the patient is increased**, and as a rule of thumb, the dose generally increases as the square of the ratios of the image intensifier diameters. Use of magnification modes in fluoroscopy is usually accompanied by an increase in kVp in order to reduce the entrance skin air kerma. In addition, the kVp increases in order to keep the tube current low and not overheat the x-ray tube.

References: Bushberg JT. *The essential physics of medical imaging*, 3rd ed. Philadelphia, PA: Wolters Kluwer Health/Lippincott Williams & Wilkins, 2012.

Mahesh M. Fluoroscopy: patient radiation exposure issues. *Radiographics* 2001;21(4):1033–1045.

8 | **Answer D.** The finding on the upper GI examination is an approximately 2 cm smooth submucosal mass in the gastric antrum containing a central collection of barium. This lesion with a target appearance is most likely an **ectopic pancreatic rest**. As a solitary lesion in a young patient, lymphoma and metastases would be unlikely. While a solitary GIST is a more common submucosal mass, lesions of this size do not typically ulcerate.

Pancreatic rests are uncommon, reported as present in up to 0.21% at autopsy. They are most commonly located in the gastric antrum within 6 cm of the pylorus, with the duodenum the next most common site. A rudimentary duct forms a central umbilication in 50% of lesions. Pancreatic rests are usually asymptomatic, but they can develop pancreatitis and consequent gastric outlet obstruction, and there are rare reports of carcinoma arising from the rest.

References: Jeong HY, Yang HW, Seo SW, et al. Adenocarcinoma arising from an ectopic pancreas in the stomach. *Endoscopy* 2002;34(12):1014–1017.

Kilman WJ, Berk RN. The spectrum of radiographic features of aberrant pancreatic rests involving the stomach. *Radiology* 1977;123(2):291–296.

Yuan Z, Chen J, Zheng Q, et al. Heterotopic pancreas in the gastrointestinal tract. *World J Gastroenterol* 2009;15(29):3701–3703.

9 **Answer A.** Contrast-enhanced CT images through the stomach demonstrate marked gastric fold thickening, which predominantly involves the gastric fundus and body. The gastric antrum appears relatively spared. Gastric fold thickening is nonspecific and differential includes *H. pylori* gastritis, Ménétrier disease, gastric lymphoma, and Zollinger-Ellison syndrome. The **urea breath test is a simple and highly accurate method for clinical assessment of *H. pylori* infection**. Ingested urea that is labeled with carbon isotopes is rapidly converted to carbon dioxide due to the presence of urease in *H. pylori* species, which is subsequently exhaled by the patient in their breath and easily detected. Reported sensitivity and specificity values for the urea breath test both exceed 95%.

H. pylori is a common gram-negative bacillus in westernized populations, estimated to occur in >50% of patients over the age of 50 years. It is the **most common cause of chronic gastritis, and its presence can be documented in most cases of gastric and duodenal ulcers**. *H. pylori* gastritis is the number one cause of gastric fold thickening which can be either diffuse or localized. The degree of gastric fold thickening is often mild to moderate. However, marked fold thickening can be seen, and overlaps with other entities that result in giant gastric folds such as Ménétrier disease and Zollinger-Ellison syndrome. While *H. pylori* gastritis can result in localized symptoms of epigastric pain and dyspepsia, it is also an **important causative factor in the development of gastric carcinoma and gastric lymphoma**.

References: Levine MS. Stomach. In: Levine MS, Ramchandani P, Rubesin SE, eds. *Practical fluoroscopy of the GI and GU tracts*. New York, NY: Cambridge University Press; 2012:73–104.

Rubesin SE, Levine MS, Laufer I. Double-contrast upper gastrointestinal radiography: a pattern approach for diseases of the stomach. *Radiology* 2008;246(1):33–48.

10a **Answer D.** Axial and sagittal contrast-enhanced CT images (top left and right) demonstrate marked gastric fold thickening in the gastric fundus and body. There is an enlarged node near the pancreatic head (arrow, bottom left). Axial SPECT image from the In-111 Octreotide scan demonstrates a focus of avid tracer uptake in the right abdomen, corresponding to the enlarged node. The imaging features are compatible with **Zollinger-Ellison syndrome (ZES). ZES is a rare condition associated with an autonomous gastrin-producing neuroendocrine tumor, typically found in the pancreas or duodenum.** They are frequently multiple and often extrapancreatic in location. Laboratory tests often reveal elevated serum gastrin levels. This results in gastric hyperchlorhydria and can lead to ulcer disease in affected patients. Gastrinomas are malignant in over 50% of cases. Approximately 25% of patients will have multiple endocrine neoplasia type I. From an imaging standpoint, traditional cross-sectional techniques such as CT and MRI are less effective than somatostatin receptor scintigraphy for identification of the primary tumor and metastatic foci.

References: Ellison EC, Johnson JA. The Zollinger-Ellison syndrome: a comprehensive review of historical, scientific, and clinical considerations. *Curr Probl Surg* 2009;46(1):13–106.

Metz DC, Jensen RT. Gastrointestinal neuroendocrine tumors: pancreatic endocrine tumors. *Gastroenterology* 2008;135(5):1469–1492.

10b **Answer C.** The **gastrinoma triangle** is an important surgical space for patients with suspected gastrinomas, as most surgically apparent and visually occult gastrin-producing neoplasms occur in this space. The triangle is bounded medially by the pancreatic neck and body junction. The inferior margin is bounded by the junction of the second and third portions of the duodenal sweep. The superior margin is bounded by the junction of the cystic duct and common bile duct.

References: Howard TJ, Zinner MJ, Stabile BE, et al. Gastrinoma excision for cure. A prospective analysis. *Ann Surg* 1990;211(1):9–14.

Stabile BE, Morrow DJ, Passaro E Jr. The gastrinoma triangle: operative implications. *Am J Surg* 1984;147(1):25–31.

11a **Answer D.** There is a mass arising from the posterior gastric body wall, which demonstrates avid arterial enhancement. Multiple liver lesions consistent with metastases also demonstrate **intense arterial enhancement, which diminishes on venous phase imaging, features typical for a carcinoid tumor.** The other entities are not characterized by the same degree of arterial enhancement.

Carcinoids are well-differentiated neuroendocrine tumors that arise from amine precursor uptake and decarboxylation (APUD) cells. Gastrointestinal carcinoids account for the majority of all carcinoids (66.9%), followed by the tracheobronchial system (24.5%). Gastrointestinal carcinoids are a diverse group of tumors that may arise from a variety of endocrine cells throughout the gastrointestinal tract. Their biologic behavior and malignant potential depend upon the anatomic site of origin and cell type. The stomach is a relatively uncommon location, accounting for 8.7% of all gastrointestinal carcinoids.

Gastric carcinoids are divided into three subtypes: Type I associated with autoimmune chronic atrophic gastritis; Type II, associated with Zollinger-Ellison syndrome in patients with multiple endocrine neoplasia type 1 (MEN-1); and Type III, a sporadic type without the association with atrophic gastritis or hypergastrinemia. Type I and II carcinoids are multifocal, smaller (1 to 2 cm) with a tendency toward benign behavior, whereas Type III is solitary, large (>2 cm), with more aggressive behavior including a tendency to metastasize (as in this case).

11b **Answer A. Somatostatin** is an endogenous peptide secreted by neuroendocrine cells. Imaging of neuroendocrine tumors (NET) takes advantage of the **high expression of somatostatin receptors (SSTRs) on cell membranes of NETs.** Previously, the most common imaging study used forms of an indium-111–labeled octreotide, a synthetic somatostatin analog, combined with single photo emission computed tomography (SPECT). This has largely been replaced by imaging using Gallium-68 DOTATATE, a radiotracer with much higher affinity for the somatostatin receptor subtype 2 (SSTR2), in conjunction with the higher spatial resolution positron emission computed tomography (PET-CT).

References: Binstock AJ, Johnson CD, Stephens DH, et al. Carcinoid tumors of the stomach: a clinical and radiographic study. *AJR Am J Roentgenol.* 2001;176(4):947–951.

Hofman MS, Lau WF, Hicks RJ. Somatostatin receptor imaging with 68Ga DOTATATE PET/CT: clinical utility, normal patterns, pearls, and pitfalls in interpretation. *Radiographics* 2015;35(2):500–516.

Levy AD, Sobin LH. From the archives of the AFIP: gastrointestinal carcinoids: imaging features with clinicopathologic comparison. *Radiographics* 2007;27(1):237–257.

12 **Answers:**

Patient 1: D

Patient 2: B

Patient 3: A

Patient 4: C

In the adult, gastric outlet obstruction may be caused by a variety of neoplastic, inflammatory, posttraumatic conditions. Congenital abnormalities, not included here such as duodenal atresia and annular pancreas, are additional causes that may present earlier in life.

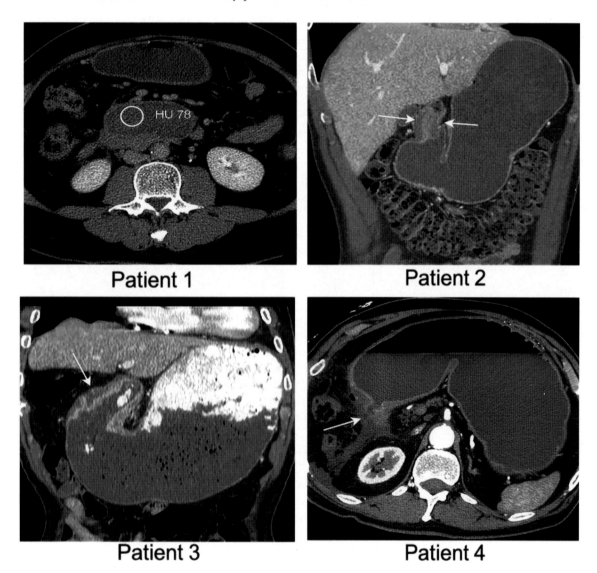

Patient 1: The CT demonstrates gastric distention and an ovoid circumscribed structure adjacent to the horizontal portion of the duodenum with mildly hyperdense contents consistent with a **hematoma**. These may be due to lap-belt injuries or other iatrogenic causes, as in this case with an ERCP.

Patient 2: The upper GI and CT demonstrate gastric distention and long smooth narrowing of the pylorus with smooth muscular hypertrophy seen as a hypodense parallel structures on the CT, suggesting **adult hypertrophic**

pyloric stenosis. This condition is rare, and the etiology is controversial with possible causes that include postinflammatory changes related to prior peptic ulcer disease, Crohn's, or other inflammatory conditions, and a persistence of the juvenile form into adult life.

Patient 3: The CT demonstrates gastric distention and a large amount of retained food not mixing with oral contrast. The antrum, pylorus, and bulb demonstrate irregular enhancing wall thickening and soft tissue infiltration around adjacent vessels highly suspicious for **neoplasm**. The wall thickening is more abrupt and the enhancement pattern more nodular than is seen in benign senile antral muscular hypertrophy. The most common malignant cause of gastric outlet obstruction is peripancreatic malignancy.

Patient 4: The CT demonstrates gastric distention, intraperitoneal free air, and retroperitoneal fluid consistent with an inflammatory process in the setting of a **perforated ulcer**. The duodenal ulcer crater is identified (arrow) in this case, although it may seal off and not be detectable in many cases. Peptic ulcer disease is the most common cause of gastric outlet obstruction in the adult.

References: Gibson JB, Behrman SW, Fabian TC, et al. Gastric outlet obstruction resulting from peptic ulcer disease requiring surgical intervention is infrequently associated with Helicobacter pylori infection. *J Am Coll Surg* 2000;191(1):32–37.

Horton KM, Fishman EK. Current role of CT in imaging of the stomach. *Radiographics* 2003;23(1):75–87.

Zarineh A, Leon ME, Saad RS, et al. Idiopathic hypertrophic pyloric stenosis in an adult, a potential mimic of gastric carcinoma. *Patholog Res Int* 2010;2010:614280.

13 **Answer: 1-C; 2-A; 3-B; 4-D**

Bariatric surgery is currently the most effective treatment for morbid obesity. The most commonly performed procedures are the Roux-en-Y gastric bypass (RYGB), sleeve gastrectomy, adjustable gastric banding, and biliopancreatic diversion with duodenal switch.

Example 1 demonstrates the adjustable gastric band performed laparoscopically (more commonly called the **lap band**), which involves placement of an inflatable band around the proximal stomach creating a small gastric pouch above the band. Advantages include easy reversibility with no resection of the stomach or intestine and lowest rate of early complications compared to all procedures. Later complications may be related to band slippage or erosion and less effective weight loss compared to other procedures.

Example 2 is the **Roux-en-Y gastric bypass** (RYGB) also called gastric bypass. This procedure involves division of the proximal stomach with creation of a small gastric pouch (~30 cc). The proximal jejunum is divided, and a roux limb is attached to the gastric pouch. The roux (alimentary) limb is anastomosed to the jejunal limb draining the excluded stomach and duodenum (pancreaticobiliary limb) with both limbs draining into a common channel. This commonly performed procedure is effective for both weight loss and metabolic changes (amelioration of type II diabetes) and has been until recently considered the standard for bariatric surgical procedures. It is technically more difficult than some of the other procedures and disrupts the normal access to the biliopancreatic ducts for endoscopic evaluation.

Example 3 shows a **sleeve gastrectomy** which involves a partial gastrectomy (~80% removed) with creation of a tubular stomach. This increasingly popular procedure is technically easier than some of the other procedures. It maintains the normal outlet anatomy, with preservation of access to the biliopancreatic ducts. Disadvantages are that it is nonreversible and has a longer staple line for potential disruption. It may be associated with increased gastroesophageal reflux.

Example 4 shows staples associated with a sleeve gastrectomy and oral contrast in the duodenum and distal small bowel, but not in the intervening small bowel which is bypassed. This is a **biliopancreatic diversion** (now most commonly performed with duodenal switch), which involves a sleeve gastrectomy and anastomosis of a short (250 cm) roux limb to the proximal duodenum, bypassing a long segment of the small intestine. The pancreaticobiliary limb is anastomosed approximately 50 cm proximal to the ileocecal valve. This procedure involves both restrictive and significant malabsorptive effects. It promotes the greatest weight loss but has a higher complication rate than the other procedures and is also associated with greater potential for nutritional deficiencies.

References: American Society for Metabolic and Bariatric Surgery. Bariatric Surgery Procedures. Available at: https://asmbs.org/patients/bariatric-surgery-procedures. Accessed June 4, 2020.

Levine MS, Carucci LR. Imaging of bariatric surgery: normal anatomy and postoperative complications. *Radiology* 2014;270(2):327–341.

14 **Answer A.** Scout image from upper GI study (figure on left) demonstrates a gastric band projecting over the epigastrium with a shallow, horizontal position. The band has a slightly circular/O-shape on this frontal view ("**O sign**"), rather than a rectangular appearance. Fluoroscopic spot image from upper GI study demonstrates gastric prolapse with pouch dilation above the gastric band and near-complete outlet obstruction at the level of the band itself. There are no signs of perforation (extraluminal contrast or gas) and the band appears to be extrinsic to the gastric lumen.

The laparoscopic gastric band procedure involves placement of an inflatable band approximately 2 cm below the gastroesophageal junction to create a small restrictive gastric pouch. The band may be adjusted through saline injection or withdrawal from the band via a subcutaneous port. Typically, the band is seen in near profile when viewed on a frontal radiograph of the abdomen. Slippage of the band will result in an oblique projection of the band, resulting in the O shape. A **φ angle** can be calculated by assessing the angle between the long axis of the band and the vertical axis of the spine (orientation of the spinous processes). Normal values should range between 4 and 58 degrees. The calculated φ angle for this patient is 88 degrees (see figure at presentation below). A change in band orientation on comparison studies is an additional valuable clue for assessing band slippage.

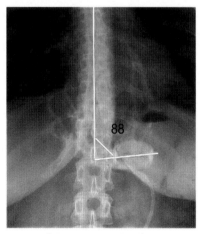

At presentation

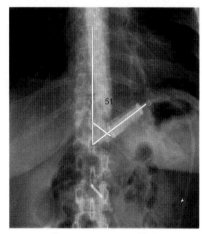

3 years earlier

Comparison scout image from upper GI study performed 3 years earlier, demonstrated normal rectangular appearance of the gastric band with a normal φ angle (51 degrees).

Band slippage can result in stomal narrowing and/or obstruction with upstream pouch dilation. As a rule, an ingested bolus of 15 to 20 mL should distend the proximal pouch no more than 4 cm in widest diameter, and the stomal diameter at the level of the pouch should be no more than 4 mm.

References: Levine MS, Carucci LR. Imaging of bariatric surgery: normal anatomy and postoperative complications. *Radiology* 2014;270(2):327–341.

Sonavane SK, Menias CO, Kantawala KP, et al. Laparoscopic adjustable gastric banding: what radiologists need to know. *Radiographics* 2012;32(4):1161–1178.

15 **Answer B.** Fluoroscopic spot images from single-contrast upper GI study demonstrate abnormal contrast accumulating around the proximal margin of the gastric sleeve, compatible with a **staple line leak** (arrows). Opacification of a surgical drain is seen in the figure on the right. No opacification of the colon is seen, and there is no gastric obstruction with filling of the small bowel shown.

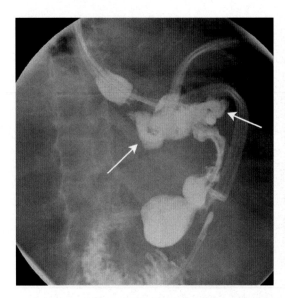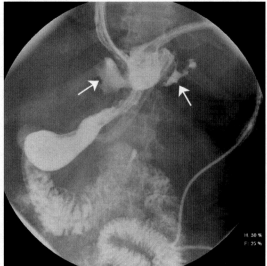

Sleeve gastrectomy originated as part of a staged duodenal switch procedure for bariatric surgery and became a stand-alone procedure due to advancements in laparoscopic technique and promising results after single-stage surgery. In this procedure, a small banana-shaped stomach is fashioned by resecting portions of the greater curvature. The resulting gastric sleeve is approximately 25% of the size of the original stomach and restricts intake. The complication rate for sleeve gastrectomy is low with reported leak rate of 1.3%. Leaks often occur near the proximal end of the staple line, toward the gastroesophageal junction. Patients may present with symptoms of abdominal infection or sepsis, including fever, leukocytosis, and abdominal pain.

Sleeve gastrectomies may also develop strictures along the staple line as in this case below. These may be treated endoscopically or surgically depending upon the severity.

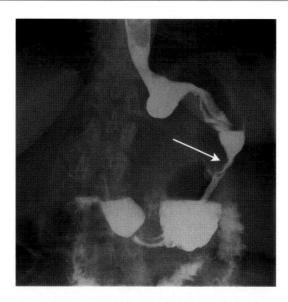

References: Deitel M, Gagner M, Erickson AL, et al. Third International Summit: current status of sleeve gastrectomy. *Surg Obes Relat Dis* 2011;7(6):749–759.

Levine MS, Carucci LR. Imaging of bariatric surgery: normal anatomy and postoperative complications. *Radiology* 2014;270(2):327–341.

16 **Answer C.** Fluoroscopic spot images from single-contrast upper GI study demonstrate postoperative changes compatible with Roux-en-Y gastric bypass surgery. There is prompt opacification of the gastric pouch in the figure on the left, along with opacification of the efferent limb of the gastrojejunostomy and simultaneous opacification of the excluded stomach, which progressively fills in the figure on the right. In Roux-en-Y gastric bypass surgery, a small gastric pouch is divided from the remainder of the stomach and drained via a gastrojejunostomy limb to create a restrictive bariatric effect (in addition to hormonal changes promoting loss of appetite). The gastric remnant remains in situ and drains through the normal anatomic route, including duodenal C-loop and proximal jejunum. After surgery, contrast should normally pass from the esophagus through the gastric pouch and into the efferent limb of the gastrojejunostomy. The gastric remnant should not opacify during ingestion of contrast material, although a small amount may appear on a delayed basis due to retrograde flow from the pancreaticobiliary limb at the jejunojejunostomy. A **gastro-gastric fistula** may occur as a result of gastric pouch staple line dehiscence (such as from pouch overdistention, infection, or ischemia) with organization and communication of the leak to the excluded stomach. Patients may present with poor postoperative weight loss.

References: Chandler RC, Srinivas G, Chintapalli KN, et al. Imaging in bariatric surgery: a guide to postsurgical anatomy and common complications. *AJR Am J Roentgenol* 2008;190(1):122–135.

Scheirey CD, Scholz FJ, Shah PC, et al. Radiology of the laparoscopic Roux-en-Y gastric bypass procedure: conceptualization and precise interpretation of results. *Radiographics* 2006;26(5):1355–1371.

17 **Answer C.** **Image truncation artifact** is illustrated on the left side of the images. When a patient's girth exceeds the field of view, the scan reconstruction assumes that the beam attenuation is caused by tissue within the field of view. The resulting reconstructed image will have high attenuation around the periphery of the image. The artifact may be eliminated by increasing the field of view to include all the tissues, but at a cost of decreasing the resolution and thus affecting the image quality negatively.

References: Fursevich DM, LiMarzi GM, O'Dell MC, et al. Bariatric CT imaging: challenges and solutions. *Radiographics* 2016;36(4):1076–1086.

Huda W, Scalzetti EM, Levin G. Technique factors and image quality as functions of patient weight at abdominal CT. *Radiology* 2000;217(2):430–435.

18 **Answer B.** The upper GI with small bowel follow-through demonstrates narrowing and deformity of the duodenal C-loop with thickened or effaced folds. The gastric antrum appears slightly coned as well. The small bowel follow-through demonstrates additional segments of small bowel abnormality, including marked narrowing at the terminal ileum with a "string sign" (arrow) and redundancy of portions of the small bowel wall with pseudosacculations (arrowheads).

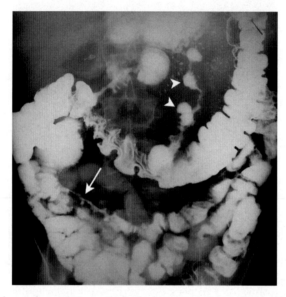

While a number of conditions included among the answer choices may cause gastroduodenal fold thickening, the only entity which would be associated with the more distal small bowel abnormalities is **Crohn disease**.

Clinically significant Crohn disease involving the stomach and duodenum is seen in up to 4% of patients, usually with other sites of involvement. Gastric wall and duodenal fold thickening is present, and the gastric antrum can have a rigid appearance (**ram's horn sign**).

Eosinophilic gastroenteritis is an uncommon condition associated with an eosinophilic infiltrate, peripheral eosinophilia; food allergies or other atopic history is common. Presentation can mimic peptic ulcer disease.

Pancreatitis commonly causes wall edema of the stomach and duodenum, and if severe can lead to outlet obstruction.

References: Farman J, Faegenburg D, Dallemand S, Chen CK. Crohn's disease of the stomach: the "ram's horn" sign. *Am J Roentgenol Radium Ther Nucl Med* 1975;123(2):242–251.

Kefalas CH. Gastroduodenal Crohn's disease. *Proc (Bayl Univ Med Cent)* 2003;16(2):147–151.

19 **Answer A.** On this patient's upper GI study, the stomach is located entirely within the chest. There is **organoaxial rotation** of the stomach and moderately gastric distention suggesting a partial obstruction. There is progression of barium through the pylorus however.

Abnormal rotation of the stomach may occur in two major forms: **organoaxial** and **mesenteroaxial**. With organoaxial rotation, the more common variant, the stomach rotates along its long axis with the greater curvature located cephalad to the lesser curvature as in this case. With a mesenteroaxial rotation, the stomach rotates along its short axis, with the antrum displaced above the gastroesophageal junction. Organoaxial rotation is often associated with a paraesophageal hernia or traumatic diaphragmatic defect. If the stomach rotates more than 180 degrees, a closed loop obstruction results and is called a volvulus. The term "volvulus" is commonly used to describe the abnormal rotation, but probably should be reserved for those cases which result in an obstruction.

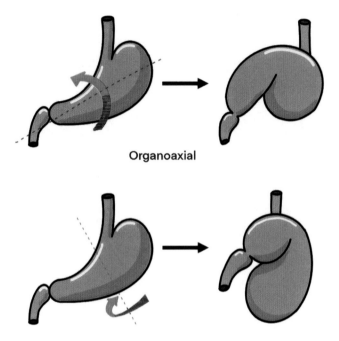

Organoaxial

Mesenteroaxial

The clinical triad of a complete volvulus with sudden epigastric pain, intractable nonproductive retching, and inability to pass a nasogastric tube is known as the Borchardt triad. **Complete gastric volvulus is a surgical emergency**, with the stomach at risk for ischemia and perforation if the volvulus is not repaired. **The mesenteroaxial variant has a higher risk** than organoaxial for a complete volvulus.

References: Abbara S, Kalan MM, Lewicki AM. Intrathoracic stomach revisited. *AJR Am J Roentgenol* 2003;181(2):403–414.

Peterson CM, Anderson JS, Hara AK, et al. Volvulus of the gastrointestinal tract: appearances at multimodality imaging. *Radiographics* 2009;29(5):1281–1293.

20 **Answer D.** Fluoroscopic spot images demonstrate a complex hernia. The ingested contrast enters from the esophagus into the proximal gastric body, which is located below the diaphragm (image on left), subsequently filling a large paraesophageal hernia that contains the distal gastric body and much of the antrum (image on right). The herniated stomach has rotated along the gastric short axis, with the pylorus now situated near the gastric fundus and the antrum above the level of the gastroesophageal (GE) junction. There is little passage of contrast through the pylorus into the duodenum. The clinical and imaging features in this patient with acute onset of vomiting are diagnostic of **gastric volvulus with acute obstruction**. Paraesophageal hernias are at risk for development of volvulus, which can result in gastric ischemia, necrosis, and perforation if left untreated. Although some patients with paraesophageal hernias may by asymptomatic or have intermittent mild symptoms, **patients with progressive symptoms or acute obstruction**

require emergent surgery. Below is an example of a mesenteroaxial rotation (note the cephalad antral position relative to the GE junction) without complete obstruction.

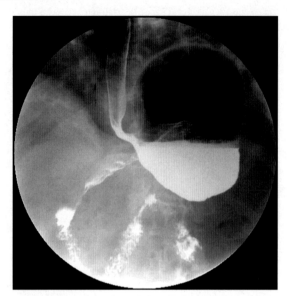

Mesenteroaxial volvulus.

References: Abbara S, Kalan MM, Lewicki AM. Intrathoracic stomach revisited. *AJR Am J Roentgenol* 2003;181(2):403–414.

Levine MS. Stomach. In: Levine MS, Ramchandani P, Rubesin SE, eds. *Practical fluoroscopy of the GI and GU tracts*. New York, NY: Cambridge University Press; 2012:73–104.

21   **Answer C.** Images from the CT demonstrate gas in the wall of the stomach, known as **gastric emphysema** (or **pneumatosis**). Gastric emphysema is an uncommon finding and has a number of causes which range from serious and life-threatening to benign and self-limited. When infection with a gas-forming organism is present, the condition has very high mortality rate (60% to 80%) and is called **emphysematous gastritis**. Of the possible visceral sites of involvement, the stomach is the least commonly affected. Caustic ingestion and alcohol abuse are the most common causes of mucosal injury–associated emphysematous gastritis. Causative bacteria include *Escherichia coli*, *Clostridium perfringens*, and *Staphylococcus aureus*.

This patient's improved clinical status does not fit the expected clinical course for either emphysematous gastritis or ischemia. Given his history, the findings more likely represent benign gastric emphysema, introduced during his unsuccessful endoscopic procedure. Intramural dissection during these procedures and high intraluminal pressure created by air insufflation lead to the ingress of intramural air. Traumatic nasogastric tube placements have been described as another procedural cause.

Benign gastric emphysema may also be seen in the setting of COPD, especially with persistent vigorous coughing, but this would likely cause more diffuse small bowel involvement than seen in this case. Gastric outlet obstruction from any cause can lead to increased intraluminal pressure. Mucosal disruption from an ulcer or tumor may be the entrance site for the gas.

References: Grayson DE, Abbott RM, Levy AD, et al. Emphysematous infections of the abdomen and pelvis: a pictorial review. *Radiographics* 2002;22(3):543–561.

Johnson PT, Horton KM, Edil BH, et al. Gastric pneumatosis: the role of CT in diagnosis and patient management. *Emerg Radiol* 2011;18(1):65–73.

22 **Answer A.** The CT shows a series of gas-attenuation semicircles along the lesser curvature of the contrast-filled stomach. This represents a **gas bubble motion artifact**.

A gas bubble motion artifact is described as an air-attenuation curvilinear structure that is created by a **moving gas bubble through a liquid**. The artifact is caused by both the image acquisition and reconstruction processes. The artifact is produced as the rotating gantry continuously measures the gas bubble during its trajectory. The reconstruction technique utilized assumes the attenuation measurement is from a stationary object. As the assumption is incorrect, the back projection maps the finding to an incorrect location. The shape and size of the artifact is affected by the bubble size and velocity, the scanner rotation speed, and the relative position of the X-ray tube. Theoretically scanning faster (not slower) should eliminate an artifact based upon motion although current scan acquisition times are still slightly too slow to accomplish this.

Reference: Liu F, Cuevas C, Moss AA, et al. Gas bubble motion artifact in MDCT. *AJR Am J Roentgenol* 2008;190(2):294–299.

23 **Answer C.** The CT study demonstrates distention of the stomach within a large paraesophageal hernia (note the nasogastric tube in the intact nondilated esophagus posterior to the hernia). There is pneumatosis in the gastric wall. In the abdomen, there is intraperitoneal free air and branching, peripheral gas within the liver consistent with portal venous gas. Absent another cause for **gastric ischemia,** the likely etiology in this patient is antecedent incarceration of the paraesophageal hernia.

Prior reports cited high lethal complication rates for incarcerated paraesophageal hernias as well as high operative mortality rates for emergent repair (56% in one series). Because of these reports, the prevailing recommendation has traditionally been for elective repair of most paraesophageal hernias, even if patients are asymptomatic. More recent series have suggested that both the rates of complications of unrepaired hernias and the surgical mortality have been overestimated, and that repair may be more selectively offered to patients who are symptomatic.

References: Schieman C, Grondin SC. Paraesophageal hernia: clinical presentation, evaluation, and management controversies. *Thorac Surg Clin* 2009;19(4):473–484.

Stylopoulos N, Gazelle GS, Rattner DW. Paraesophageal hernias: operation or observation? *Ann Surg* 2002;236(4):492–500; discussion 500–491.

24 **Answer B.** There is a large barium and gas containing structure extending posteriorly from the gastric fundus below the diaphragm. This is the typical location for a **gastric diverticulum**. This originates from the stomach, not the esophagus as would be expected for an epiphrenic diverticulum. This diverticulum is smoothly marginated and lined with normal-appearing mucosa, distinguishing it from a giant ulcer. The neck of the diverticulum is oriented in the vertical plane, orthogonal to the expected plane of a fundoplication impression.

Fundal diverticula are **congenital true diverticula containing all wall layers**. These are rare, present in 0.12% of patients on a large series of abdominal CTs. These are most commonly asymptomatic, although they may trap gastric contents, ulcerate, or rarely torse. The other described location of gastric diverticula is in the antrum; these are acquired pulsion-type outpouchings and are pseudodiverticula not containing all layers of the gastric wall.

References: Rashid F, Aber A, Iftikhar SY. A review on gastric diverticulum. *World J Emerg Surg* 2012;7(1):1.

Schramm D, Bach AG, Zipprich A, et al. Imaging findings of gastric diverticula. *ScientificWorldJournal* 2014;2014:923098.

25 **Answer A.** The CT demonstrates a stomach distended with a cast of mottled density material surrounded by a rim of oral contrast which does not mix with the central material suggesting a **bezoar**. Upon questioning, the patient admitted to a 7-year history of chewing her hair. Hair is not digestible in the gastrointestinal tract and will accumulate in the stomach. Endoscopy should be the next step in evaluation to confirm that the material is not ordinary ingested food and to attempt removal of the material. Ultimately however, most patients require a surgical removal of the bezoar.

Rapunzel syndrome refers to the condition of ingesting hair (trichophagia), often associated with a hair-pulling impulse control disorder (trichotillomania). The resulting trichobezoar consists of the large gastric portion and a long tail extending into the small bowel and possibly the right colon.

The other most common type of bezoar is known as a phytobezoar, composed of vegetable and fruit material (commonly persimmons). These may pass into the small bowel and cause obstruction.

CT is the ideal method of imaging bezoars, assessing for degree of obstruction, and identifying possible multiple bezoars.

References: Gaillard M, Tranchart H. Images in clinical medicine. Trichobezoar. *N Engl J Med* 2015;372(6):e8.

Ripolles T, Garcia-Aguayo J, Martinez MJ, et al. Gastrointestinal bezoars: sonographic and CT characteristics. *AJR Am J Roentgenol* 2001;177(1):65–69.

26 **Answer D.** The upper GI demonstrates multiple small collections of barium that are surrounded by a lucent halo of edema. These are **best seen with double-contrast technique**, although they may be seen on single-contrast examinations with the use of compression. Gastric erosions are most commonly seen in the antrum and have a tendency to line up along folds.

Gastric erosions are a nonspecific finding and may be seen in **gastritis** from a number of different etiologies. NSAIDs are the most common cause. Other causes include alcohol, stress, trauma, burns, viral or fungal infections, and Crohn disease. *H. pylori* infection causes gastritis with a number of radiographic features, of which thickened or polypoid folds are found to be the most commonly demonstrated feature.

References: Chen MY, Ott DJ, Clark HP, et al. Gastritis: classification, pathology, and radiology. *South Med J* 2001;94(2):184–189.

Ott DJ, Gelfand DW, Wu WC, et al. Sensitivity of single- vs. double-contrast radiology in erosive gastritis. *AJR Am J Roentgenol* 1982;138(2):263–266.

Sohn J, Levine MS, Furth EE, et al. *Helicobacter pylori* gastritis: radiographic findings. *Radiology* 1995;195(3):763–767.

QUESTIONS

1 Match the following images of patients with small bowel Crohn disease with the findings on MR enterography or CT enterography (each choice may be used only once):

Patient 1

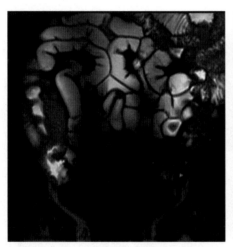

T1 post contrast.

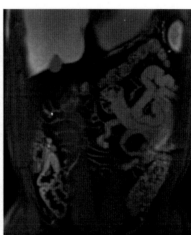

T2 fast spin echo.

Patient 2   Patient 3

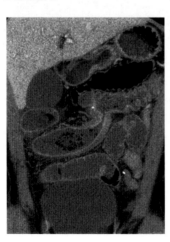   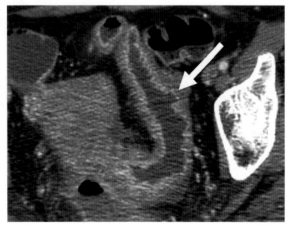

Patient 4

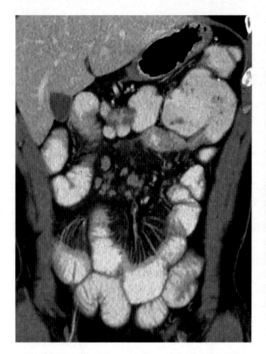

Patient 5

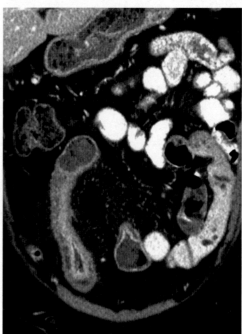

Patient 6

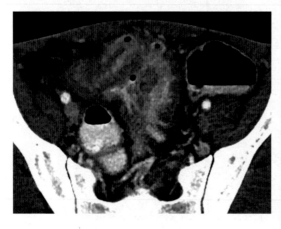

Patient 7

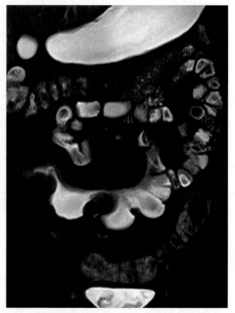

A. Pseudosacculations
B. Engorgement of vasa recta
C. Penetrating disease with fistulae and abscess
D. Intramural ulceration
E. Stricture
F. Mural enhancement
G. Fat halo and creeping fat

2a A 23-year-old female has a 5-year history of cramping abdominal pain and occasional diarrhea. Stool tests demonstrate increased fat. She undergoes a small bowel follow-through. What diagnosis is suggested by the findings?

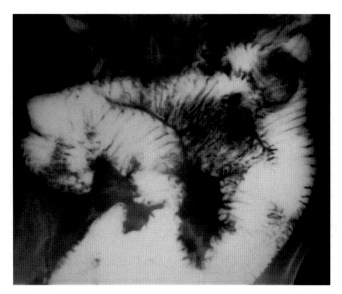

A. Celiac disease
B. Crohn disease
C. Zollinger-Ellison syndrome
D. Giardiasis

2b The most common malignancy associated with untreated celiac disease is

A. Squamous cell carcinoma of the esophagus
B. T-cell lymphoma of the small bowel
C. Adenocarcinoma of the small bowel
D. Ovarian carcinoma

3 A 33-year-old male presents with malaise, right lower quadrant pain, and high fever of 2 day's duration. He has a significant leukocytosis. He has been previously very healthy. An abdominal CT is performed. The most likely diagnosis is:

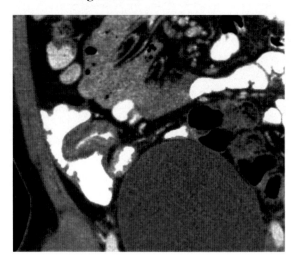 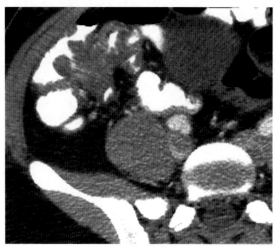

A. Ulcerative colitis with backwash ileitis
B. Infectious enterocolitis
C. Crohn disease
D. Lymphoma

4 A 33-year-old male with a history of asthma and multiple food allergies (but not to gluten) presents for evaluation of chronic intermittent abdominal pain. A small bowel follow-through and a CT scan are performed. What diagnosis may best fit this clinical presentation?

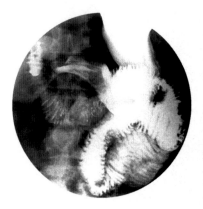
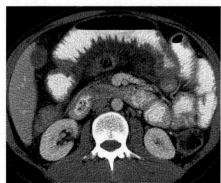
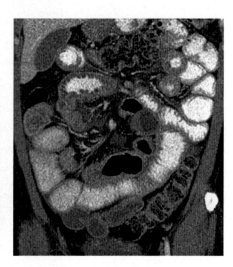

A. Zollinger-Ellison syndrome
B. Celiac sprue
C. Giardiasis
D. Eosinophilic enteritis

5 A 68-year-old female with a history of total abdominal hysterectomy and bilateral salpingo-oophorectomy for cervical cancer with positive nodes presents 3 years later with cramping abdominal pain. A CT is obtained. What is the most likely diagnosis?

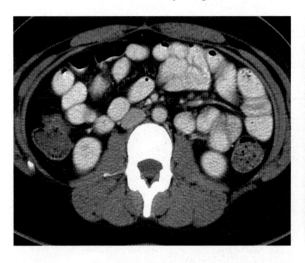
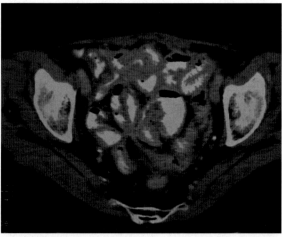

A. Graft versus host disease
B. Late-stage chemotherapy enteritis
C. Recurrent tumor
D. Chronic radiation enteritis

6 A 39-year-old female with a history of bloating and postprandial abdominal pain has a CT scan. A capsule endoscopy was originally planned, but based upon the CT findings, a small bowel follow-through was performed. What is a likely etiology for the findings?

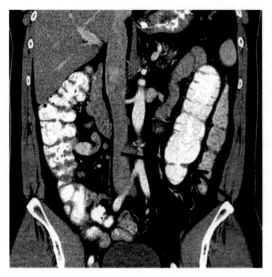
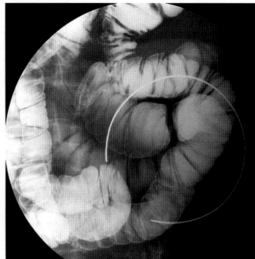

A. Adenocarcinoma
B. Congenital atresia
C. Crohn disease
D. Nonsteroidal anti-inflammatory drug (NSAID)

7 A 56-year-old male presented to the emergency department with a history of 2-day acute onset of severe abdominal pain and nausea. He is afebrile, in normal sinus rhythm, but has a mild leukocytosis. An abdominopelvic CT is performed. Images revealed no vascular occlusions. His medication list is reviewed. Which medication is most likely related to the findings on CT?

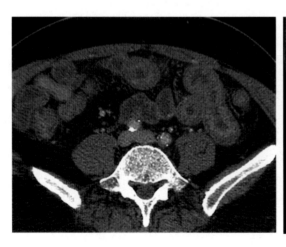
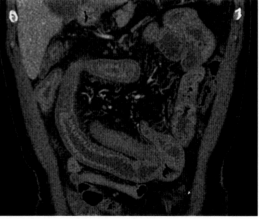

A. Aspirin
B. Propranolol (beta-blocker)
C. Lisinopril (angiotensin-converting enzyme inhibitor)
D. Omeprazole (proton pump inhibitor)

8 A 16-year-old male presents with chronic cramping abdominal pain. What is the diagnosis?

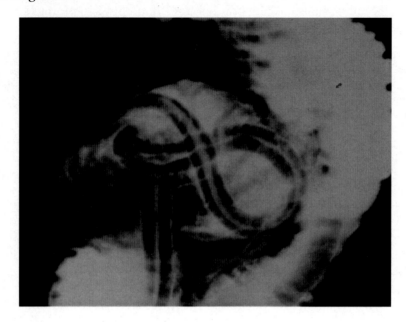

A. Anisakis
B. *Ascaris*
C. Hookworm
D. Trichuris

9 A 27-year-old female with a suspected Crohn disease underwent a video capsule endoscopy. An abdominal film was obtained 1 week later (Day 7) at which time the patient's symptoms were mild and stable. After another 2 weeks (Day 21), she is seen by her gastroenterologist with increasing cramping abdominal pain, new nausea and vomiting, and another abdominal film is obtained. What is the next best step in management?

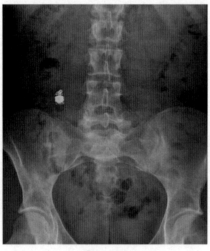
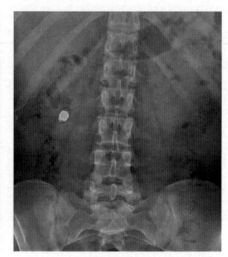

Day 7   **Day 21**

A. Repeat abdominal film in one more week
B. Standard CT abdomen and pelvis
C. MR enterography
D. Barium small bowel follow-through

10a A 50-year-old patient with a history of intermittent diarrhea and hot flushes undergoes a CT of the abdomen. No other abnormalities of the GI tract were present on other images. The patient denies any significant travel history. What is the most likely diagnosis?

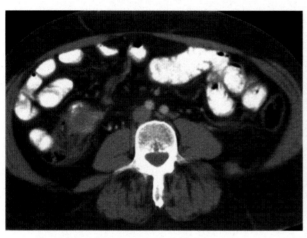 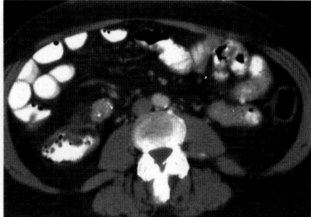

    A. Tuberculosis of distal ileum and associated nodal enlargement
    B. Small bowel lymphoma
    C. Ileal carcinoid and calcified nodal metastasis
    D. Crohn disease

10b What do the patient's presenting symptoms likely indicate?

    A. The tumor is metastatic to the liver.
    B. The tumor is metastatic to the lungs.
    C. The tumor is unresectable.
    D. The tumor is likely multifocal.

11 A 49-year-old male with abdominal pain, diarrhea, and weight loss has a CT showing a large mass involving the jejunum. What is the most likely diagnosis?

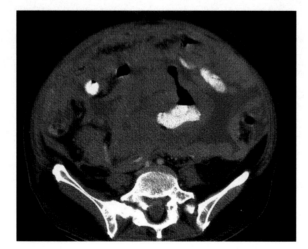

    A. Adenocarcinoma
    B. Gastrointestinal stromal tumor
    C. Non-Hodgkin lymphoma
    D. Carcinoid

12 A 53-year-old male with weight loss and worsening nausea and vomiting underwent a CT scan.

The most likely diagnosis is

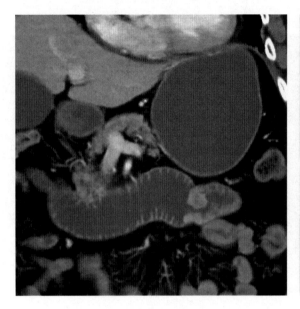 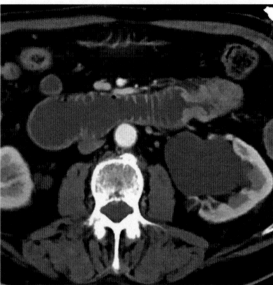

A. Duodenal atresia
B. Duodenal adenocarcinoma
C. Duodenal lymphoma
D. Stenosis associated with nonsteroidal anti-inflammatory agents

13 A 58-year-old male with a history of intermittent gastrointestinal bleeding has a CT enterography study. What is the finding?

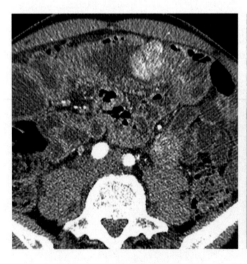 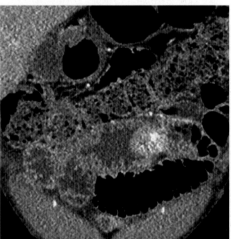

A. Annular mass
B. Polypoid mass
C. Small bowel obstruction without mass
D. Normal appearance

14 Match these duodenal filling defects with their diagnosis. Each choice may be used only once:

1.

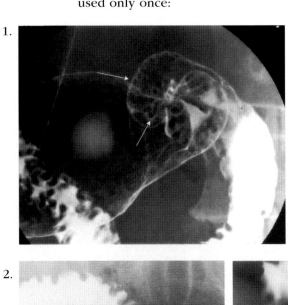

2.

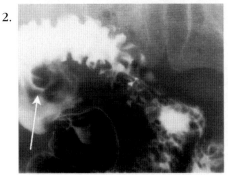 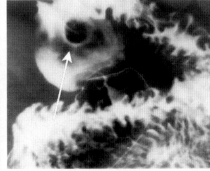 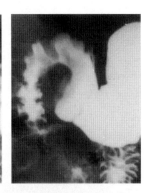

3.

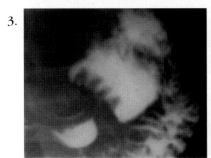 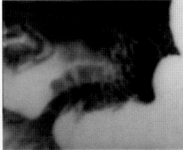 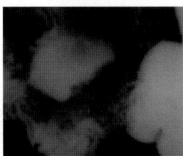

4.

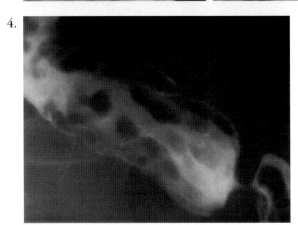

    A. Brunner gland hamartomas
    B. Heterotopic gastric mucosa
    C. Flexural pseudotumor
    D. Prolapsing gastric mucosa

15 A 41-year-old male presents with abdominal pain and fever. What is the likely diagnosis?

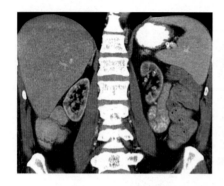 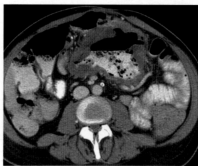 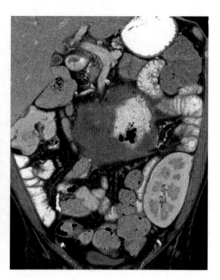

   A. Gastrointestinal stromal tumor
   B. Carcinoid
   C. Lymphoma
   D. Adenocarcinoma

16a The most common type of malignancy involving the small bowel is

   A. Gastrointestinal stromal tumor
   B. Lymphoma
   C. Carcinoid
   D. Metastases

16b A 48-year-old male presents with abdominal pain of 3 month's duration and has a CT scan. Which of the following cancers would be most likely to result in the finding?

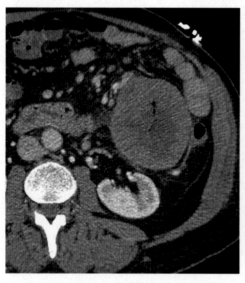 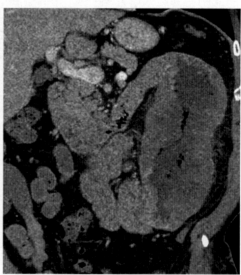

   A. Small bowel adenocarcinoma
   B. Metastatic melanoma
   C. Metastatic appendiceal cancer
   D. Metastatic gastric cancer

17a A 78-year-old male develops nausea, vomiting, and increased abdominal pain 2 days after a cystectomy. Supine and upright abdominal films are performed. The most appropriate test to order next would be

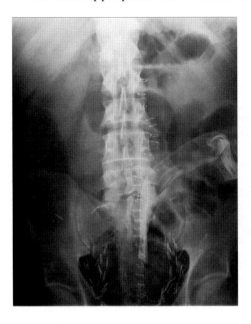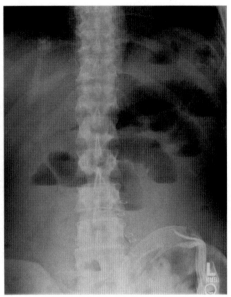

A. No further test needed, the examination is diagnostic
B. CT
C. Small bowel follow-through
D. MRI

17b The most common cause for small bowel obstruction in the United States is

A. Adhesions
B. Hernias
C. Neoplasm
D. Crohn disease

18a A 78-year-old female has a history of intermittent episodes of abdominal pain. An esophagogastroduodenoscopy (EGD) is negative. She undergoes a small bowel follow-through (SBFT). What description best fits the findings?

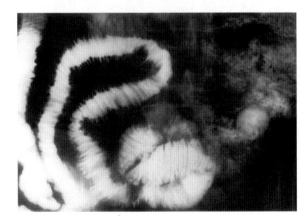

A. Small bowel folds are nodular and irregularly thickened.
B. Small bowel folds are thickened and closely spaced.
C. Small bowel folds are thin and widely spaced.
D. Small bowel folds are normal in thickness.

18b Which of the following is the most likely cause?

    A. Intramural hemorrhage

    B. Crohn disease

    C. Eosinophilic enteritis

    D. Progressive systemic sclerosis

19 Which of the following cases represents small bowel ischemia?

    A. A 52-year-old male with severe abdominal pain after prolonged hypotension.

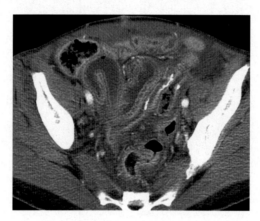

    B. A 75-year-old male with abdominal pain.

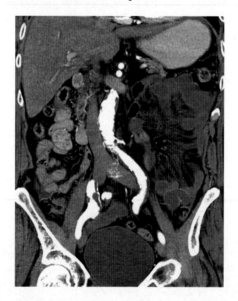

C. A 66-year-old female with breast cancer and abdominal pain.

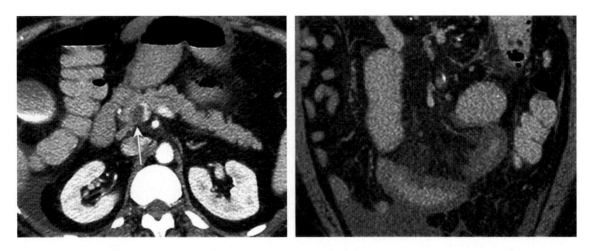

D. A 82-year-old male with sudden-onset abdominal and flank pain following cardiac catheterization.

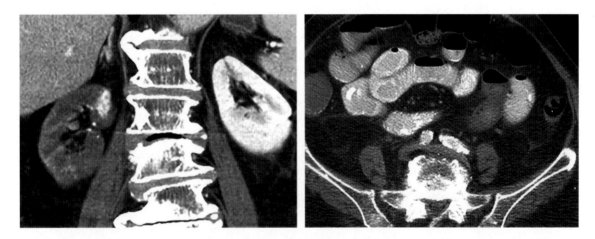

E. A 52-year-old female with hypotesion.

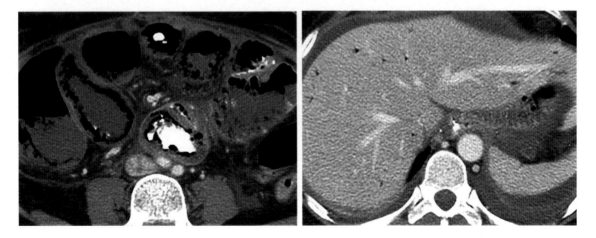

F.   All of the above.

20a A 65-year-old female presents with intermittent right upper quadrant colicky pain, nausea, vomiting, and abdominal distension. A CT scan is performed. What is the most likely diagnosis?

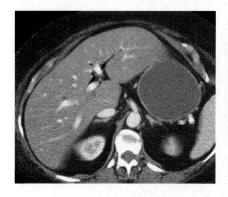 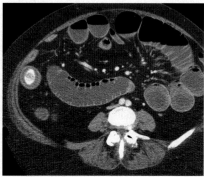 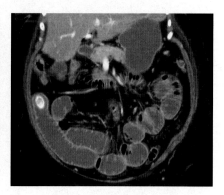

     A. Adynamic ileus
     B. Bezoar-induced small bowel obstruction
     C. Small bowel intussusception
     D. Gallstone ileus

20b Which of the following findings is not illustrated in the images shown but is still likely to be present?

     A. A distal ileal stricture
     B. A biliary enteric fistula
     C. A mesenteric arterial thrombus
     D. A distal ileal mass

21a A 48-year-old male underwent a CT scan after a motor vehicle collision. The incidental abnormality indicated by the arrows occurs via

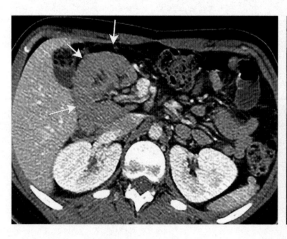 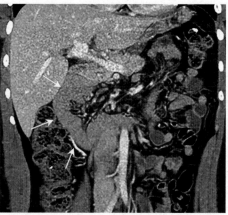

     A. The fossa of Landzert
     B. The fossa of Waldeyer
     C. The foramen of Winslow
     D. The mesocolic window

21b Right paraduodenal hernias account for what percentage of all paraduodenal hernias?

    A. 25

    B. 50

    C. 75

    D. 90

22 A 64-year-old male presents with bloody stools and a hematocrit of 22. He has no prior surgical history. He undergoes a CT of the abdomen and pelvis. What possible bleeding source is suggested by the findings?

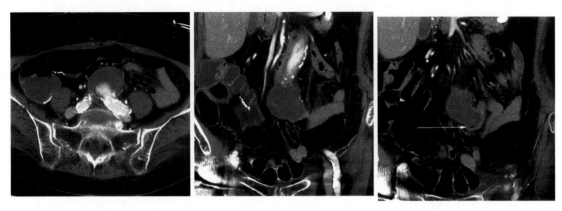

    A. Aortoenteric fistula

    B. Gastrointestinal stromal tumor

    C. Jejunal vascular malformation

    D. Small bowel lymphoma

23 A 90-year-old female developed nausea and vomiting 2 days after lifting a heavy box. On examination, she has a tender palpable mass in her right inguinal region. A CT scan is obtained. What is the diagnosis? (FV = femoral vein; IEV = inferior epigastric vessels; H = loop extending into hernia)

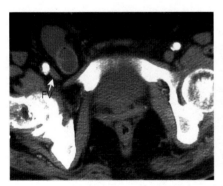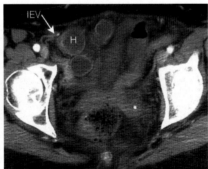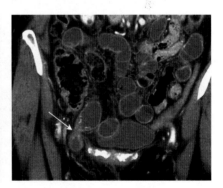

    A. Indirect inguinal hernia

    B. Direct inguinal hernia

    C. Spigelian hernia

    D. Femoral hernia

24 A 53-year-old female with a history of a Whipple procedure for pancreatic cancer presents at routine follow-up visit 2 years later with nausea, mild upper abdominal pain, and an elevated bilirubin and alkaline phosphatase. Her Ca 19-9 is normal. What is the likely diagnosis?

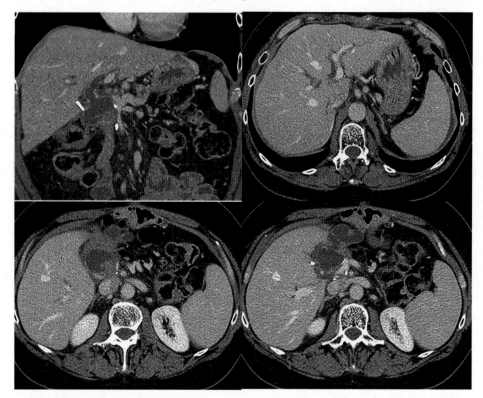

A. Hepaticojejunostomy stricture
B. Contained bile leak
C. Afferent limb syndrome
D. Pancreatitis with pseudocyst

25 During a basketball game, a 17-year-old male receives a direct blow to the abdomen from another player's knee. He presents with abdominal pain and undergoes a series of imaging studies.

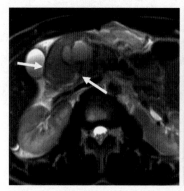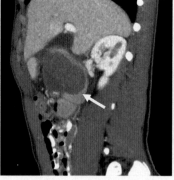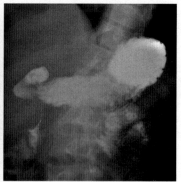

Left: MRI (axial T2 HASTE) perfomed day of presentation. **Center:** Sagittal CT with positive oral contrast performed Day 9 post trauma. **Right:** Upper GI performed day 15 post trauma.

Regarding the most likely diagnosis, which of the following statements is true?

A. It indicates need for immediate surgical exploration.
B. It is more likely in elderly patients following blunt trauma.
C. It is due to congenitally abnormal rotation of the pancreas.
D. The duodenum is the most common location for this entity in the GI tract.

26 A 39-year-old female with a history of Roux-en-Y gastric bypass surgery presents with increasing abdominal pain. A CT scan was performed, and coronal reformatted images were generated. What finding is demonstrated?

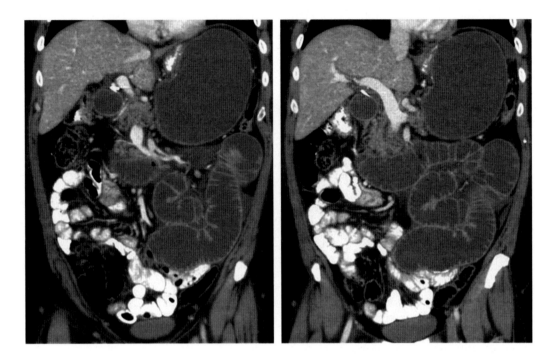

A. Small bowel obstruction with dilated alimentary/Roux limb
B. Small bowel obstruction with dilated biliopancreatic limb
C. Small bowel obstruction with dilated common enteric channel
D. Adynamic ileus

27 A 45-year-old female with a history of diarrhea undergoes a barium small bowel examination with the findings below. Which of the following statements is correct?

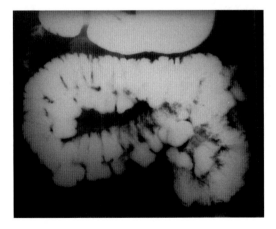

A. The findings are congenital and more commonly present in the pediatric population.
B. Treatment involves surgical resection of the involved segments.
C. CT would have been a better initial examination if this entity were suspected clinically.
D. This finding can be associated with malabsorption, bowel perforation, obstruction, or GI bleeding.

28 A 66-year-old female presents with nausea and epigastric pain of 1 day's duration. She was found to have a mild leukocytosis. A CT scan is obtained. Available for comparison is an upper GI study performed 1 year earlier.

What is the most likely diagnosis?

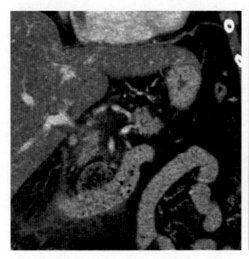 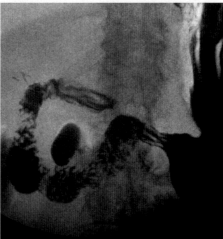

    A. Perforated duodenal ulcer

    B. Infected peripancreatic walled-off necrosis

    C. Bezoar in duodenal diverticulum with perforation

    D. Infected gut duplication cyst

29a What is the entrance exposure limit for standard operation of a fluoroscope?

    A. 1 R/min

    B. 5 R/min

    C. 10 R/min

    D. 20 R/min

29b Which of the following maneuvers will decrease the patient dose during fluoroscopy?

    A. Increasing the distance of the image intensifier from the patient

    B. Removing the grid

    C. Increasing the pulse rate using pulsed fluoroscopy

    D. Selecting a lower kilovolt peak

29c Reduction of the frame rate using pulse fluoroscopy from 30 frames per second to 15 frames per second

    A. Results in no dosage change

    B. Reduces the dosage by about 25%

    C. Reduces the dosage by about 50%

    D. Increases the dosage by about 50%

30 A 17-year-old female with a history of cramping abdominal pain undergoes a small bowel follow-through. A spot film of the ileocecal region is taken. What is the most likely diagnosis?

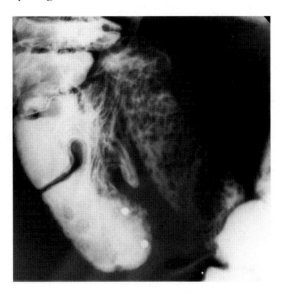

A. Crohn disease
B. Lymphoid nodular hyperplasia
C. Non-Hodgkin lymphoma
D. Carcinoid

31 A 45-year-old female presents for evaluation of chronic abdominal pain, which she states has been waxing and waning for 10 to 15 years and is exacerbated by meals. A small bowel follow-through was obtained. What finding is demonstrated?

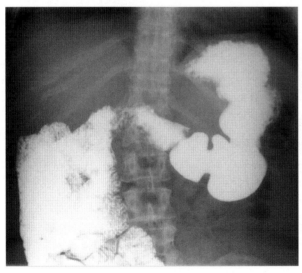

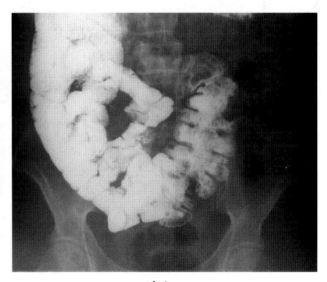

Early.

Later.

A. Small bowel obstruction
B. Intestinal malrotation
C. Increased number of small bowel folds
D. Multiple tiny colonic polyps

32a A 78-year-old female presents with abdominal pain and has a CT scan. What is the most likely etiology for the structure denoted by the arrow?

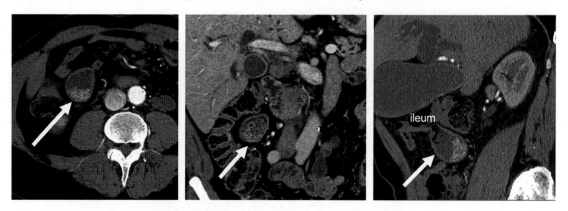

A. Gallbladder duplication
B. Teratoma
C. Meckel diverticulum
D. Appendicoliths in a dilated appendix

32b A 57-year-old male presented with GI bleeding. Upper endoscopy was negative, and colonoscopy demonstrated a pool of blood in the ileum without a clear source. A Technetium-99m red blood cell (^{99m}Tc RBC) scan followed by a CT enteroclysis are performed. What is the most likely diagnosis?

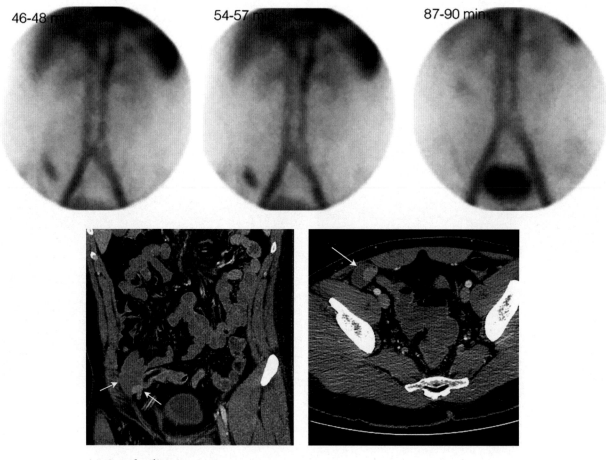

A. Gut duplication cyst
B. Meckel diverticulum with active bleeding
C. Meckel diverticulum without active bleeding
D. Appendiceal mucocele

32c What other anomaly may arise from the same embryologic origin as a Meckel diverticulum?

    A. Vitelline duct cyst
    B. Single umbilical artery
    C. Urachal cyst
    D. Unicornuate uterus

33 A 45-year-old female presents with cough, constipation, and substernal chest pain. A barium small bowel follow-through is performed. What is the best diagnosis?

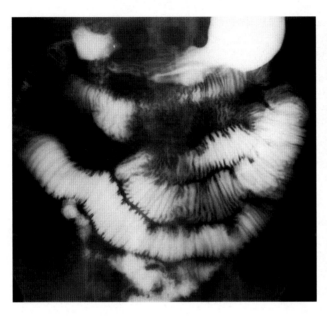 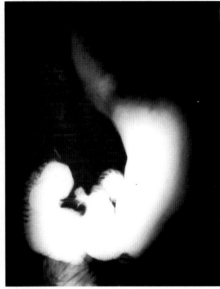

    A. Gastroesophageal reflux
    B. Gastric and small bowel ileus
    C. Small bowel obstruction
    D. Scleroderma

34a Early transient erythema is encountered at what approximate threshold dose?

    A. 0.2 Gy
    B. 2 Gy
    C. 20 Gy
    D. 200 Gy

34b For a patient of average build, at what approximate duration of fluoroscopy time does erythematous skin change become a risk?

    A. 5 minutes
    B. 20 minutes
    C. 1 hour
    D. 2 hours

35 A 29-year-old female presents with a progressive history of radiating back pain, nausea, and vomiting. Currently, the patient is only able to eat yogurt and juice consistencies. An upper GI procedure was performed. What is the best diagnosis?

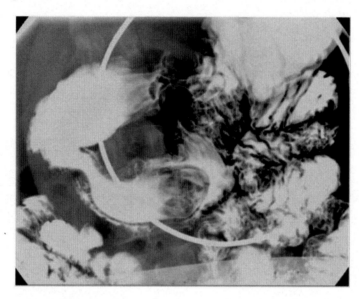

A. Duodenal carcinoma
B. Duodenal polyp
C. Duodenal ulcer
D. Duodenal intraluminal diverticulum

36 A 19-year-old female has a history of intermittent abdominal pain. On physical examination, she is noted to have pigmented lesions on her lips and oral mucosa. An MR enterography is performed.

The most likely diagnosis is

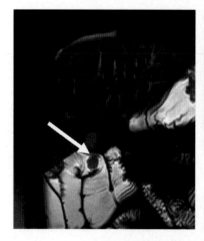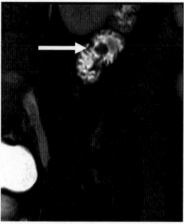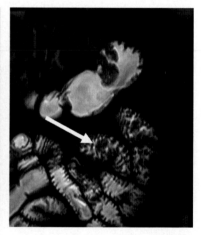

A. Neurofibromatosis type 1
B. Gardner syndrome
C. Metastatic melanoma
D. Peutz-Jeghers

37 A 24-year-old female with a history of anorexia nervosa presents with abdominal pain and vomiting. A CT scan is obtained. What anatomic factors may be responsible for these findings?

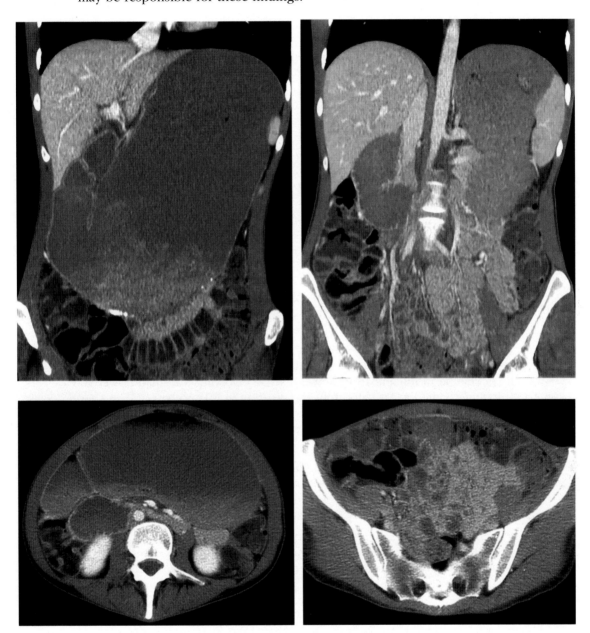

A. Presence of a median arcuate ligament
B. Narrowed angle between the superior mesenteric artery and aorta
C. Abnormal position of the ligament of Treitz
D. Retroaortic location of the left renal vein

ANSWERS AND EXPLANATIONS

1 **Answers:**

Patient 1: F. Mural enhancement. MR enterography demonstrates wall thickening of the terminal ileum on T2-weighted images. Postcontrast T1-weighted images demonstrate segmental mural wall hyperenhancement, which indicates active disease. The enhancement in this case is symmetric, but when asymmetric along the mesenteric border is even more specific for Crohn disease.

Patient 2: E. Stricture. Dilated small bowel loops with segmental stricture is seen. Small bowel stool sign indicates chronic obstruction. The term "luminal narrowing" is used when the luminal diameter is reduced at least 50% compared to normal adjacent bowel. The term "stricture" should be reserved for when luminal narrowing is accompanied by upstream luminal dilation (≥3 cm).

Patient 3: D. Intramural ulceration. In addition to the stratified mural wall thickening, there is a focal ulceration in the wall noted at the arrow.

Patient 4: B. Engorgement of vasa recta. Prominent mesenteric vessels supplying and draining a segment of inflamed bowel is also known as the "comb" sign.

Patient 5: G. Fat halo and creeping fat. Intramural fat deposition may be seen in chronic inflammatory conditions involving the gastrointestinal tract. It is common in inflammatory bowel disease involving the small bowel and colon, also called a "fat halo" appearance, though it is not specific and can be seen in other conditions (postinfectious or ischemic disease for example). Prominent fibrofatty proliferation of the mesentery adjacent to inflamed bowel loops is known as "creeping fat."

Patient 6: C. Penetrating disease with fistula and abscess. Extraluminal soft tissue tracts extending into the mesentery with a localized collection of oral contrast and gas is demonstrated. Penetrating disease associated with Crohn's includes fistulae, sinus tracts, inflammatory masses, and abscesses.

Patient 7: A. Pseudosacculations. Smooth wall thickening along the mesenteric border is seen with redundant wall on the antimesenteric border, resulting in a ruffled appearance, known as pseudosacculations. The redundant wall is the normal wall.

References: Bruining DH, Zimmermann EM, Loftus EV Jr, et al. Consensus recommendations for evaluation, interpretation, and utilization of computed tomography and magnetic resonance enterography in patients with small bowel Crohn's Disease. *Radiology* 2018;286(3):776–799.

Guglielmo FF, Anupindi SA, Fletcher JG, et al. Small bowel Crohn disease at CT and MR enterography: imaging atlas and glossary of terms. *Radiographics* 2020;40(2):354–375.

2a **Answer A.** The findings on this small bowel follow-through (SBFT) demonstrate dilated loops of jejunum with thin but relatively widely spaced folds (normal fold density is 4 to 6 per inch). A coiled-spring filling defect in a loop of jejunum is also present consistent with an intussusception. The findings are consistent with findings of celiac sprue. The other conditions listed, Crohn disease, Zollinger-Ellison syndrome, and giardiasis, are all associated with thickened folds.

Celiac sprue is an autoimmune disease resulting from a genetically based reaction to a protein component of gluten found in wheat, barley, and rye. Patients may present in early childhood or as young adults. Diagnosis is made with jejunal biopsy and serologic testing. Despite the relatively high prevalence of celiac disease in the US population (1 in 200), presentation is nonspecific, and diagnosis is often delayed.

Inflammation caused by the reaction to the protein leads to villous atrophy and malabsorption, especially to fats. **The classic findings on barium studies include dilution, dilatation, reversal of the normal fold pattern with decreased jejunal and increased ileal fold density (jejunization of the ileum), and transient jejunal intussusception.** As current practice has evolved, most patients presenting with abdominal pain will undergo a CT rather than a SBFT. Findings of small bowel dilatation, jejunization of the ileum, and intussusceptions may be recognized on CT. Other findings associated with celiac disease include prominent mesenteric lymph nodes and intramural fat deposition observed in the duodenum, jejunum, and colon, as seen with other chronic inflammatory conditions.

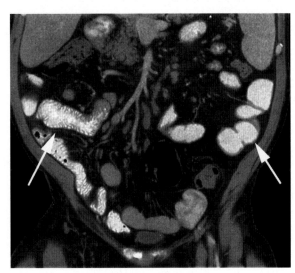

Jejunization of the ileum.

2b **Answer B.** Patients with untreated celiac disease have an **increased risk of developing malignancy**, most commonly lymphoma (T-cell) and less commonly adenocarcinoma or squamous cell carcinoma. Other malignancies that are less commonly associated include oropharyngeal, ovarian, thyroid, breast, and lung cancers.

3 **Answer B.** On the CT, the terminal ileum and to a lesser extent the cecum demonstrate wall thickening. The acute onset of findings and the patient's age do not favor a malignancy. Backwash ileitis in the setting of ulcerative colitis most commonly results in a patulous terminal ileum, not a narrowed lumen as seen in this case. Although Crohn disease may present with the same imaging findings in a young patient, a history of chronic symptoms would be expected.

The relatively acute onset is consistent with an infectious etiology. **In the developed world, *Campylobacter jejuni* is the most common cause of bacterial gastroenteritis, with other pathogens including *Escherichia coli*, *Salmonella* (nontyphoidal), and *Shigella* species**. Viral gastroenteritis pathogens include rotavirus, norovirus, and adenovirus. These diseases are self-limited but may be more serious and even life-threatening in children, older patients, pregnant patients, or people with immunodeficiency.

In this case, the patient was admitted to the hospital due to the severity of his symptoms, and blood cultures were positive for *Salmonella enterica* serotype typhi. Additional history obtained included recent travel to a developing country. The typhoidal type of *Salmonella* infection is usually caused by fecally contaminated food or water causing a systemic illness with little or no diarrhea. Typhoid fever is uncommon in the United States but is still endemic in areas of the world with poor sanitation.

References: Hennedige T, Bindl DS, Bhasin A, et al. Spectrum of imaging findings in Salmonella infections. *AJR Am J Roentgenol* 2012;198(6):W534–W539.

Parry CM, Hien TT, Dougan G, et al. Typhoid fever. *N Engl J Med* 2002;347(22):1770–1782.

4 **Answer D.** The small bowel follow-through demonstrates mild fold thickening of the duodenum and jejunum with the CT demonstrating even more pronounced wall thickening of multiple loops of proximal and mid small bowel. Although such small bowel fold thickening is nonspecific, with the atopic history of this patient, the possibility of eosinophilic enteritis is suggested. Celiac sprue is excluded given the absence of a wheat product intolerance, and the other causes of small bowel fold thickening do not have the same association with allergies.

Eosinophilic enteritis is a rare condition with eosinophilic infiltration of the gastrointestinal tract. It can be primary or associated with other hypereosinophilic conditions such as Churg-Strauss, helminthic infection, hypereosinophilic syndrome, or drugs. The condition has a **high association with atopy**, with peripheral eosinophilia present in 75% to 100% of patients. Increased production of interleukin-5 and activated eosinophils are present. It can involve many segments of the gastrointestinal tract from the esophagus to the rectum but is most common in the stomach and small bowel. It can involve variable layers of the gut wall from the mucosa to the serosa; with the more severe serosal involvement, ascites and pleural effusions may be seen. Treatment is with corticosteroids or other immunosuppressives and dietary restriction.

References: Shanbhogue AK, Prasad SR, Jagirdar J, et al. Comprehensive update on select immune-mediated gastroenterocolitis syndromes: implications for diagnosis and management. *Radiographics* 2010;30(6):1465–1487.

Triantafillidis JK, Parasi A, Cherakakis P, et al. Eosinophilic gastroenteritis: current aspects on etiology, pathogenesis, diagnosis and treatment. *Ann Gastroenterol* 2005;15(2):106–115.

5 **Answer D.** The CT demonstrates diffuse wall thickening of multiple loops of bowel in the pelvis with sparing of bowel loops in the upper abdomen. This patient with node-positive cervical cancer is likely to have had adjuvant radiation (brachytherapy or combined external beam radiation and brachytherapy). **Chronic radiation enteritis** develops between 6 months and 7 years after radiotherapy. This condition may develop in 20% or more of patients who undergo abdominopelvic radiotherapy. Increased risk for development of radiation enteritis is seen in patients with a history of prior surgery or peritonitis, which may cause fixation of bowel loops and with superimposed small vessel disease such as with diabetes.

The gastrointestinal tract is sensitive to radiation, and most patients will develop some diarrhea in the acute phase of radiation enteritis. The bowel segments that are most susceptible are those that are fixed, typically the terminal ileum and rectosigmoid in cases of pelvic radiation.

On a small bowel follow-through, radiation changes manifest as **fold thickening or effacement with tethering and fixed angulation of bowel loops** best appreciated with directed palpation.

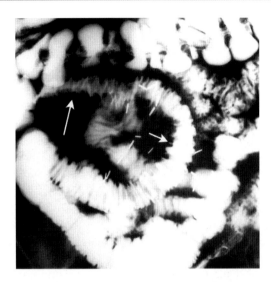

Graft versus host disease is typically seen in the setting of bone marrow transplantation for leukemia. Chemotherapy-related enteritis would be seen in the acute setting and would be diffuse, not isolated to the pelvis. Likewise, while recurrent tumor from carcinomatosis may cause bowel wall thickening from serosal implants, it would be unlikely to be so extensive in the pelvis without some involvement of the upper abdominal bowel loops.

References: Addley HC, Vargas HA, Moyle PL, et al. Pelvic imaging following chemotherapy and radiation therapy for gynecologic malignancies. *Radiographics* 2010;30(7):1843–1856.

Rha SE, Ha HK, Lee SH, et al. CT and MR imaging findings of bowel ischemia from various primary causes. *Radiographics* 2000;20(1):29–42.

6 **Answer D.** The initial CT demonstrates dilatation of a loop of jejunum with a fold that appears to extend significantly into the lumen. This is confirmed on the small bowel follow-through as a smooth circumferential web with a narrow aperture ("**diaphragm disease**"). Webs may be due to congenital atresia, but these present in the pediatric age group. The web is too short and smooth to be associated with a neoplasm or a Crohn stricture.

Nonsteroidal anti-inflammatory drugs (NSAIDs) are associated with small bowel injuries in up to two-thirds of all patients who have used the drugs on a long-term basis. These injuries include erosions and ulcers, which may bleed or rarely perforate. They can also cause thin, diaphragm-like strictures, which are thought to be due to local ischemic effects caused by the prostaglandin inhibitory properties of the NSAIDs. These webs may be difficult to diagnose on imaging if they are nonobstructive due to their resemblance to normal plicae. Although the increased use of capsule endoscopy has been instrumental in documenting the high prevalence of small bowel injuries from NSAIDs, a capsule endoscopy should not be performed in this patient due to likelihood of capsular retention.

References: Fortun PJ, Hawkey CJ. Nonsteroidal antiinflammatory drugs and the small intestine. *Curr Opin Gastroenterol* 2007;23(2):134–141.

Higuchi K, Umegaki E, Watanabe T, et al. Present status and strategy of NSAIDs-induced small bowel injury. *J Gastroenterol* 2009;44(9):879–888.

7 **Answer C.** Findings on the CT are of marked wall thickening of loops of small bowel without evidence of luminal dilatation to suggest obstruction. These findings are described with **angioedema of the intestine. Angioedema is a rare side effect reported with the use of angiotensin-converting-enzyme inhibitors (ACEI), a commonly used antihypertensive medication.** Up to 0.5% of patients receiving these ACEI medications may experience angioedema episodes. This condition is thought to be due to elevated levels of bradykinin, a potent vasodilator and cause of increased capillary permeability. ACEI cause delayed breakdown of bradykinin. There may be a single or recurrent episodes of edema involving the skin, upper airways, or the gastrointestinal tract. The onset of the initial angioedema episode may be within several days of initiation of the medication or may occur years after the initiation of therapy.

The clinical presentation is with abdominal pain, nausea, vomiting, and diarrhea. Both the severe pain and the CT appearance may be mistaken for bowel ischemia. The episodes are self-limited and improvement is not related to cessation of the medication. Serum measurements of C4 and C1-esterase inhibitor may be helpful in confirming the diagnosis.

On CT, bowel wall edema is seen which may lead to a target appearance. Due to the edema, the bowel may be straightened in appearance. There is no obstruction or delay in transit time. A small amount of ascites is often seen. These findings overlap with those that may be seen with intestinal ischemia, Crohn disease, and severe enteritis. Due to the severity of the pain and concern for ischemia, a number of patients with this condition have been taken for emergency exploratory laparotomy. History of ACEI medication, absence of patient risk factors for occlusive vascular disease, as well as a possible history of prior episodes with abrupt onset and remission, may help lead to this diagnosis.

References: De Backer AI, De Schepper AM, Vandevenne JE, et al. CT of angioedema of the small bowel. *AJR Am J Roentgenol* 2001;176(3):649–652.

Scheirey CD, Scholz FJ, Shortsleeve MJ, et al. Angiotensin-converting enzyme inhibitor-induced small-bowel angioedema: clinical and imaging findings in 20 patients. *AJR Am J Roentgenol* 2011;197(2):393–398.

8 **Answer B.** The finding shows a tubular filling defect in the small bowel with a central tract also containing barium. All of the listed parasites are nematodes (roundworms). This example illustrates a large roundworm consistent with an ascarid.

Soil-transmitted helminth infections infect >1.5 billion people worldwide or about 24% of the world's population. Infections occur in the tropical and subtropical regions of the world. In the United States, infections are most commonly seen in the southeastern region. These infections are transmitted by eggs present in human feces which contaminate soil in areas with poor sanitation. The main species that infect people are the roundworm (*Ascaris lumbricoides*), the whipworm (*Trichuris trichiura*), and the hookworms (*Necator americanus and Ancylostoma duodenale*).

Ascaris lumbricoides is the largest nematode involving the human GI tract. In the United States, ascariasis is the third most frequent helminthic infection, following hookworm and *Trichuris* (whipworm). *Ascaris* infection may be asymptomatic, but a large worm burden can cause bowel obstruction. The ascarid may obstruct the biliary and pancreatic ducts causing cholangitis and pancreatitis. The worm's intestinal tract may be visible when it ingests the barium.

References: Khuroo MS. Ascariasis. *Gastroenterol Clin North Am* 1996;25(3):553–577.

Ortega CD, Ogawa NY, Rocha MS, et al. Helminthic diseases in the abdomen: an epidemiologic and radiologic overview. *Radiographics* 2010;30(1):253–267.

9 **Answer B.** The abdominal film a week (Day 7) post ingestion of a capsule for video capsule endoscopy (VCE) demonstrates the capsule in the right abdomen. Another 2 weeks later (Day 21), the capsule has not changed in position. With the development of obstructive symptoms, further urgent definitive imaging is indicated, and a standard CT is the most appropriate choice. Ingestion of large volume of contrast with an enterography is likely to be poorly tolerated given her obstructive symptoms, and the CT is more expeditious than a small bowel follow-through. In addition, MR is contraindicated for theoretical risk of causing capsule movement that might result in bowel obstruction or perforation. The following CT images were obtained, located just adjacent to the level of the retained capsule, demonstrating a long distal ileal stricture consistent with Crohn disease.

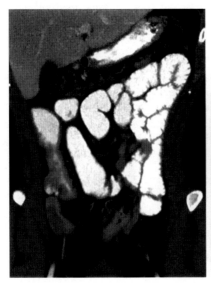 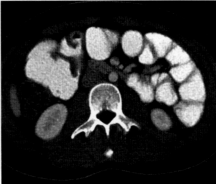

With double-balloon enteroscopy, the stricture was dilated and the capsule recovered.

VCE is useful for direct visualization of segments of bowel (especially small bowel) that cannot be reached with standard endoscopic techniques. Most capsules will reach the colon within 8 hours of ingestion, but reduced motility may significantly delay passage of the capsule. Capsular retention is suspected if not excreted within 15 days of ingestion in an asymptomatic patient, or in patients with symptoms of obstruction or perforation, regardless of time since capsule ingestion. Capsule retention is reported in approximately 2% of patients undergoing VCE.

The most common causes of capsule retention are strictures associated with Crohn disease, nonsteroidal anti-inflammatory drugs (NSAIDS), small bowel tumors, radiation enteritis, or surgical anastomoses. Relative contraindications to VCE include known obstructive causes of any kind, small bowel diverticula, fistulae, and severe motility disorders. If strictures are suspected, a self-dissolving patency capsule may be administered to assess for the presence of strictures that may limit the passage of the video capsule.

References: Bandorski D, Kurniawan N, Baltes P, et al. Contraindications for video capsule endoscopy. *World J Gastroenterol* 2016;22(45):9898–9908.

Pasha SF, Pennazio M, Rondonotti E, et al. Capsule retention in Crohn's disease: a meta-analysis. *Inflamm Bowel Dis* 2020;26(1):33-42.

Rondonotti E. Capsule retention: prevention, diagnosis and management. *Ann Transl Med* 2017;5(9):198.

10a **Answer C.** A partially calcified mesenteric mass in close vicinity to an ileal mass would be most compatible with a **carcinoid tumor with nodal metastases**. This diagnosis is supported by the patient's symptomatology. Tuberculosis is highly unlikely in this patient with no travel history, and this described symptomatology and a single mass with single nodal enlargement on CT examination. Calcifications are rare in lymphoma, unless it has been at least partially treated. The patient's clinical presentation and presence of calcifications in the nodal mass with normal appearance of remaining bowel wall is less suggestive Crohn disease.

Carcinoids are neuroendocrine tumors in the category of APUD (amine precursor uptake decarboxylase) tumors. The majority (70%) of all carcinoids occur in the gastrointestinal tract, although they can occur in any organ. The most common site for gastrointestinal involvement is the rectum (34%), followed by the small bowel (26%), stomach (12%), and appendix (6%). Tumors are submucosal and tend to be well-circumscribed. The diagnosis and management hinge on a combination of biochemical analysis, imaging, and endoscopy.

Of the small bowel sites for carcinoid tumor, the ileum is the most common. On CT, **the classic appearance of a mesenteric metastasis is of a soft tissue mass-like process with radiating projections extending toward the small bowel, often causing angulation and tethering of the bowe**l. This desmoplastic reaction occurs due to the effect of serotonin and other vasoactive peptides produced by the tumor on the local vasculature. The mesenteric mass commonly calcifies.

Unlike this case, the detection of the primary tumor may be challenging in patients presenting with metastatic disease, as the tumors tend to be small. Standard CT and somatostatin receptor scintigraphy (formerly [111]I octreotide scan and now Ga-68 DOTATATE) have relatively low sensitivity for detection of the primary tumors (up to 6% and 23%, respectively). CT or MR enterography may increase the sensitivity for detection of the primary intestinal tumor when good bowel distention is achieved.

10b   **Answer A.** Carcinoid syndrome is characterized by a constellation of symptoms which may include flushing, diarrhea, abdominal pain, wheezing, and palpitations. **Most patients with carcinoid syndrome have extensive liver metastases**, and the symptoms occur when the monoamine oxidase in the liver and lung are unable to metabolize serotonin. Uncommonly, an extraintestinal carcinoid may have the syndrome when the enterohepatic circulation is bypassed.

Metastatic disease is relatively common at the time of diagnosis, with 19% of patients having nodal disease and 21% distant metastases. Liver metastases tend to be hypervascular, and multiphase imaging should be performed as 15% of masses may only be present on the arterial phase. MRI is probably slightly more sensitive than the CT or [111]I octreotide scan for detection of liver metastases.

References: Ganeshan D, Bhosale P, Yang T, et al. Imaging features of carcinoid tumors of the gastrointestinal tract. *AJR Am J Roentgenol* 2013;201(4):773–786.

Levy AD, Sobin LH. From the archives of the AFIP: gastrointestinal carcinoids: imaging features with clinicopathologic comparison. *Radiographics* 2007;27(1):237–257.

11   **Answer C.** The CT demonstrates a large mass in the abdomen with a central cavity containing oral contrast. Adjacent small bowel loops are not dilated, indicating no significant obstruction. This pattern of bowel wall involvement by tumor and expansion of the lumen is known as **aneurysmal dilatation**. Although it can be seen in other tumors including gastrointestinal stromal tumor, metastases, and rarely adenocarcinoma, the **most common cause is non-Hodgkin lymphoma**. Aneurysmal dilatation of the bowel is caused by invasion of the muscularis propria and damage to autonomic nerve plexus.

The gastrointestinal tract is the most frequent extranodal site of involvement by lymphoma. Risk factors include *Helicobacter pylori* infection, immunosuppression due to HIV infection or with organ transplantation, inflammatory bowel disease, or celiac disease. Lymphoma is the most common primary malignancy of the small intestine. Primary non-Hodgkin lymphoma (B-cell and T-cell type), Burkitt lymphoma, MALT lymphoma, and very rarely Hodgkin lymphoma have been described in the small bowel.

Lymphoma has many morphologic variants including focal polypoid masses without wall thickening, multiple polypoid lesions, long segmental infiltrating lesion, ulcerative segmental lesions, and tumor locally infiltrative into adjacent tissue. The tumor does not commonly cause obstruction. Associated bulky lymphadenopathy can suggest the diagnosis.

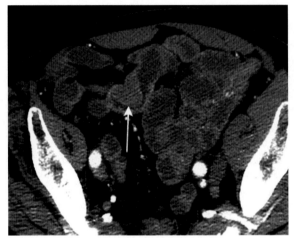 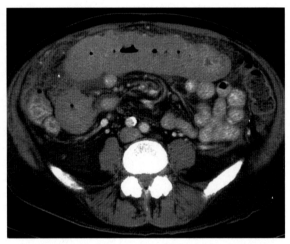

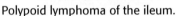

Polypoid lymphoma of the ileum.   Long segment of jejunal involvement by lymphoma.

References: Buckley JA, Fishman EK. CT evaluation of small bowel neoplasms: spectrum of disease. *Radiographics* 1998;18(2):379–392.

Ghai S, Pattison J, Ghai S, et al. Primary gastrointestinal lymphoma: spectrum of imaging findings with pathologic correlation. *Radiographics* 2007;27(5):1371–1388.

12 **Answer B.** There is an annular mass in the distal duodenum with luminal narrowing and obstruction of the stomach and duodenum. Duodenal adenocarcinoma typically presents as a napkin-ring lesion or a polypoid mass. Adenocarcinoma distribution in the duodenum are as follows: 45% horizontal and distal (D3 and D4); 40% descending (D2); and 15% in the bulb (D1). Duodenal carcinoma is rare, accounting for 0.3% of all GI malignancies. Of all small bowel adenocarcinomas however, the duodenum is the most common location accounting for 50% to 75%. Presentation may be secondary to obstruction, bleeding, or abdominal pain. **Increased incidence of duodenal adenocarcinomas are found in patients with familial adenomatosis polyposis syndrome or Gardner syndrome.**

Congenital duodenal atresia is usually found in the descending segment, just distal to the ampulla of Vater. The diagnosis is typically made in the antenatal or neonatal period due to obstructive presentation ("double bubble" seen on ultrasound).

Duodenal lymphoma tends to have longer segment involvement and may demonstrate aneurysmal dilatation (which would be rare for adenocarcinoma). Because fibroblastic reaction is less pronounced in lymphoma and duodenal cells are spared, obstruction in lymphoma is rare.

Nonsteroidal anti-inflammatory agents (NSAIDs) may be associated with obstruction of the small bowel, but the appearance is typically a thin web-like abnormality.

References: Barat M, Dohan A, Dautry R, et al. Mass-forming lesions of the duodenum: a pictorial review. *Diagn Interv Imaging* 2017;98(10):663–675.

Liu Z, Zheng G, Liu J, et al. Clinicopathological features, surgical strategy and prognosis of duodenal gastrointestinal stromal tumors: a series of 300 patients. *BMC Cancer* 2018;18(1):563.

Traubici J. The double bubble sign. *Radiology* 2001;220(2):463–464.

13 **Answer B.** There is a large **polypoid mass** in the jejunum causing a partial obstruction of the small bowel. Although a noncontrast phase is not included with this study, the hyperdensity of the mass suggests enhancement. Appearance of the mass is nonspecific.

Differential for a benign polypoid mass includes an adenoma (although these are considered premalignant), hamartoma (isolated or associated with polyposis syndrome such as Peutz-Jeghers), and other tumors of mesenchymal origin such as a lipoma or leiomyoma. Possibilities for a malignant polypoid mass of the small bowel includes carcinoma (more commonly annular), carcinoid, lymphoma, sarcoma, or a metastasis. Gastrointestinal stromal tumors demonstrate a range of malignant potential and may be polypoid.

In this case, this mass was found to be a gastrointestinal stromal tumor, also called a gut stromal tumor (GST). A GST is the most common gastrointestinal tumor of mesenchymal origin. It is defined by the presence of a tyrosine growth factor receptor (KIT receptor or CD117), which differentiates it from other mesenchymal tumors. The tumor arises from the muscularis propria of the intestinal wall and often has an exophytic growth pattern with masses extending out of the involved organ. This polypoid manifestation is less common.

References: Levy AD, Remotti HE, Thompson WM, et al. Gastrointestinal stromal tumors: radiologic features with pathologic correlation. *Radiographics* 2003;23(2):283–304, 456; quiz 532.

Sandrasegaran K, Rajesh A, Rydberg J, et al. Gastrointestinal stromal tumors: clinical, radiologic, and pathologic features. *AJR Am J Roentgenol* 2005;184(3):803–811.

14 **Answers.**
1. **B**
2. **C**
3. **D**
4. **A**

1. **Heterotopic gastric mucosa** represents congenital gastric rests. These are present at the base of the duodenal bulb (juxtapyloric), have a characteristic polygonal shape, and are 1 to 5 mm in size. These are differentiated from lymphoid hyperplasia, which nodules similar in size but round and distributed throughout the bulb.

2. When the angle of the postbulbar duodenum with the apex of the bulb is acute, redundant folds may mimic a mass, known as a **duodenal flexural pseudotumor**. This changes in shape with peristalsis and does not persist with filling.

3. **Prolapsing gastric mucosa** represents redundant gastric antral mucosa that extends into the base of the duodenal bulb. It has a characteristic mushroom shape and changes during different phases of gastric peristalsis. It is likely of no clinical significance.

4. Brunner glands are mucosal and submucosal alkaline-secreting glands most common in the first part of the duodenum. **Brunner gland hyperplasia** may present as smooth submucosal nodules 5 mm or smaller. When larger than 5 mm (more commonly solitary, although multiple in this case), this may be referred to as a hamartoma. A "Swiss cheese" appearance has been described when nodules are multiple. These may be seen in symptomatic patients or as incidental findings.

References: Eisenberg RL. *Gastrointestinal radiology: a pattern approach,* 2nd ed. Philadelphia, PA: Lippincott, 1990.

Patel ND, Levy AD, Mehrotra AK, et al. Brunner's gland hyperplasia and hamartoma: imaging features with clinicopathologic correlation. *AJR Am J Roentgenol* 2006;187(3):715–722.

An MRI is an acceptable alternate choice for evaluation in a patient who is not recently postoperative and for whom minimizing radiation exposure is a priority. Disadvantages of MRI include the longer scan time and lower spatial resolution.

17b **Answer A.** Adhesions account for up to 70% of small bowel obstructions (SBO) in the developed countries. Most patients will have a history of prior surgery; prior episodes of peritonitis may also result in adhesions. Adhesions are usually not directly visualized on imaging but are implied by a sharp transition in bowel caliber from dilated to nondilated without a mass or other cause for obstruction identified.

Hernias were formerly the most common cause of SBO in the United States and remain so in many foreign countries. As more cross-sectional imaging is being performed, more hernias are being identified and electively repaired.

When neoplasm causes an SBO, it is most commonly due to metastatic disease and peritoneal carcinomatosis.

Crohn disease may present acutely as an SBO due to transmural inflammation and extrinsic serosal disease causing obstruction, or may be due to chronic cicatricial fibrosing strictures.

References: Mullan CP, Siewert B, Eisenberg RL. Small bowel obstruction. *AJR Am J Roentgenol* 2012;198(2):W105–W117.

Silva AC, Pimenta M, Guimaraes LS. Small bowel obstruction: what to look for. *Radiographics* 2009;29(2):423–439.

18a **Answer B.**

18b **Answer A.**

The small bowel follow-through demonstrates a segment of small bowel with folds that are thickened in a uniform fashion and closely spaced together. Normal small bowel fold thickness is 2 to 3 mm in the jejunum and 1 to 2 mm in the ileum, and the number of folds is 4 to 7 per inch in the jejunum. This pattern has been called a "**stacked coin**" or "**picket fence**" appearance. **This pattern typically results from edema or hemorrhage from ischemia, anticoagulant therapy, radiation, or vasculitis.** Crohn disease tends to produce irregular thickening. Eosinophilic enteritis may have straight or irregular fold thickening but tends to be more diffuse. Progressive systemic sclerosis (scleroderma) demonstrates normal or thinned folds.

Many entities are known to cause small bowel fold abnormalities. Clinical information is paramount in forming the differential. While a specific diagnosis may be elusive, radiographic studies (small bowel follow-through and CT or MR enterography) indicate presence and location of disease for directed endoscopic evaluation and biopsy.

A suggested approach to small bowel fold pattern analysis is offered below.

Small Bowel Fold Patterns	
Small Bowel Fold Pattern	**Disease Process**
Straight segmental ("stack of coins")	• Ischemia • Hemorrhage • Vasculitis • Radiation
Straight diffuse	• Edema due to hypoproteinemia • Eosinophilic enteritis • Amyloidosis • Abetalipoproteinemia

(Continued)

Small Bowel Fold Patterns *(Continued)*	
Small Bowel Fold Pattern	**Disease Process**
Irregular segmental	• Crohn's • Lymphoma • Tuberculosis • Yersiniosis • Giardiasis • Strongyloides
Irregular diffuse	• Whipple disease • Intestinal lymphangiectasia • Eosinophilic enteritis • Mastocytosis • Waldenström macroglobulinemia • Amyloidosis • *Mycobacterium avium intracellulare*
Tubular (effaced folds)	• Graft versus host disease • Advanced Crohn's • Advanced radiation • Severe ischemia • Strongyloidiasis

References: Eisenberg RL. Thickening of small bowel folds. *AJR Am J Roentgenol* 2009;193(1):W1–W6.

Levine MS, Rubesin SE, Laufer I. Pattern approach for diseases of mesenteric small bowel on barium studies. *Radiology* 2008;249(2):445–460.

19 | **Answer G.** Establishing the diagnosis of mesenteric ischemia may be extremely challenging for radiologists and clinicians. Bowel ischemia can have a number of different appearances, several of which are illustrated in the images A-F. Due to the highly variable radiographic manifestations of mesenteric ischemia, the clinical presentation must factor heavily when making the diagnosis.

Case A illustrates a target appearance of the ischemic small bowel wall with wall thickening, enhancing mucosa and edematous submucosa. This appearance is nonspecific and may be seen in other enteritides.

Case B demonstrates hypoenhancing bowel wall in the left abdomen (short arrows) and mild mesenteric edema in this case of vascular obstruction due to an omental band. This sign is highly specific for ischemia but uncommon.

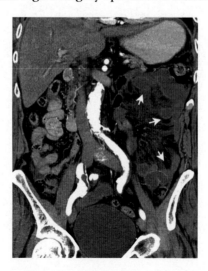

Case C shows bowel wall thickening and free fluid in a patient with paraneoplastic hypercoagulability and superior mesenteric vein thrombus. Wall thickening is most pronounced with venous occlusion.

Case D demonstrates small bowel distention and ileus with normal wall thickness and an infarcted right kidney. This patient had embolization of cardiac thrombus to the right renal artery and superior mesenteric artery. In a pure arterial occlusion, the bowel wall is often normal or may be paper-thin.

Case E demonstrates extensive pneumatosis intestinalis and portal venous gas, which is consistent with transmural infarction in the setting of clinically suspected mesenteric ischemia.

References: Furukawa A, Kanasaki S, Kono N, et al. CT diagnosis of acute mesenteric ischemia from various causes. *AJR Am J Roentgenol* 2009;192(2):408–416.

Wiesner W, Khurana B, Ji H, et al. CT of acute bowel ischemia. *Radiology* 2003;226(3): 635–650.

20a **Answer: D.** The CT images show **Rigler's triad** with **pneumobilia, small bowel obstruction, and ectopic gallstone** (in this case in the distal ileum), diagnostic for gallstone ileus. Gallstone ileus represents a bowel obstruction related to fistulization of a gallstone from the biliary tract into the gastrointestinal tract, typically in elderly women. Mortality has been reported as high as 33% in the past, although it has more recently decreased, possibly due to the development of nonsurgical endoscopic interventions.

In one large series, gallstone ileus accounted for 1% to 4% of all cases of small bowel obstruction but up to 25% of nonstrangulated small bowel obstructions in patients over 65. CT is helpful for finding the point of obstruction, assessing the size of the stone, and for the presence of multiple stones. In most cases, the ectopic stone obstructs at the level of the ileocecal valve, which is the narrowest part of the gastrointestinal tract, but it can be seen in the stomach, duodenum, elsewhere in the small bowel, or the colon.

20b **Answer: B.** Gallstone ileus implies a biliary enteric fistula. A biliary enteric fistula complicates 2% to 3% of all cases of cholelithiasis with associated cholecystitis. The fistula is most often between the gallbladder and duodenum in the setting of chronic cholecystitis, although any communication between the biliary tree and the gastrointestinal tract can result in a similar presentation. Of note, biliogastric fistulization with obstruction at the pylorus or duodenum is also known as Bouveret syndrome.

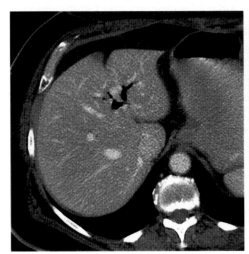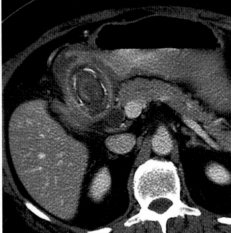

Bouveret syndrome.

References: Brennan GB, Rosenberg RD, Arora S. Bouveret syndrome. *Radiographics* 2004;24(4): 1171–1175.

Lassandro F, Gagliardi N, Scuderi M, et al. Gallstone ileus analysis of radiological findings in 27 patients. *Eur J Radiol* 2004;50(1):23–29.

Lassandro F, Romano S, Ragozzino A, et al. Role of helical CT in diagnosis of gallstone ileus and related conditions. *AJR Am J Roentgenol* 2005;185(5):1159–1165.

Reisner RM, Cohen JR. Gallstone ileus: a review of 1001 reported cases. *Am Surg* 1994;60(6):441–446.

van Hillo M, van der Vliet JA, Wiggers T, et al. Gallstone obstruction of the intestine: an analysis of ten patients and a review of the literature. *Surgery* 1987;101(3):273–276.

21a **Answer B.** Axial and coronal images demonstrate a cluster of small bowel in the right upper quadrant, representing a **right paraduodenal hernia (PDH)**. These occur through the fossa of Waldeyer, a defect in the first part of the jejunal mesentery. The herniated bowel extends behind the superior mesenteric artery, which is displaced anteriorly and inferior to the transverse portion of the duodenum. The hernia contents are located in the right half of the transverse mesocolon and posterior to the ascending mesocolon. This type of hernia occurs more frequently in the setting of nonrotated small bowel. Internal hernias are protrusions of bowel that occur through congenital or acquired defects in the mesentery but remain within the peritoneal cavity in contrast to external hernias. They may be asymptomatic or present with symptoms of bowel obstruction or abdominal pain. Internal hernias may be difficult to diagnose, resulting in significant morbidity and mortality. Paraduodenal hernias extend through congenital defects that occur due to anomalous rotation and fusion of mesentery and peritoneum during embryogenesis.

Classically, paraduodenal hernias (PDHs) were recognized as the most common type of internal hernia accounting for approximately 50% of cases. However, the incidence of transmesenteric hernias is increasing due to the proliferation of abdominal surgery, in particular Roux-en-Y procedures.

21b **Answer A.** Right PDH accounts for 25% of PDHs.

Left PDH accounts for 75% of PDHs. It is more common in men (3:1) and occurs via the fossa of Landzert. The herniated contents lie between the pancreas and stomach to the left of the ligament of Treitz with mass effect on the posterior wall of the stomach and transverse colon. The bowel loops extend into the left portion of the transverse mesocolon and descending mesocolon. The inferior mesenteric vein (IMV) is displaced superiorly and anteriorly.

The foramen of Winslow is the passage between the greater and lesser sacs of the peritoneum, and hernias through this foramen are less common. The mesocolic window is created for a retrocolic Roux limb and can be the site of postoperative obstruction due to constriction or transmesenteric internal hernia.

References: Martin LC, Merkle EM, Thompson WM. Review of internal hernias: radiographic and clinical findings. *AJR Am J Roentgenol* 2006;186(3):703–717.

Takeyama N, Gokan T, Ohgiya Y, et al. CT of internal hernias. *Radiographics* 2005;25(4): 997–1015.

22 **Answer A.** The CT demonstrates an infrarenal fusiform aortic aneurysm, which closely apposes a jejunal loop. The axial image demonstrates that the low-density material adjacent to the opacified aortic lumen is mural thrombus, not a small bowel mass. On the second coronal image, the arrow denotes a small gas bubble located in the periphery of the aneurysm, suggesting a fistulous communication with the bowel.

Aortoenteric fistulas are uncommon causes of gastrointestinal bleeding and are associated nearly 100% mortality if not treated promptly. These fistulas may be primary or secondary. Primary aortoenteric fistulas are almost always associated with an aortic aneurysm, as in this case. Secondary aortoenteric fistulas are complications of aortic reconstruction, either via an open surgical or an endovascular procedure. Secondary aortoenteric fistulas are commonly caused by perigraft infection.

CT angiography is the best single modality for evaluation of a suspected aortoenteric fistula. The CT assesses for the presence of an aneurysm, the location of any prior surgical vascular or endovascular procedures, and the relationship of the aneurysm or surgical site to the bowel. The most common finding in a primary aortoenteric fistula is ectopic gas located adjacent to or within the aorta. The fat plane between the aortal and the involved segment of bowel is obliterated. A retroperitoneal hematoma may be seen.

In the case of a secondary aortoenteric fistula, perigraft infection may occur without fistulization, so the presence of ectopic gas is less specific.

Active extravasation of intravascular contrast into the bowel lumen is diagnostic, but very rarely encountered.

References: Cumpa EA, Stevens R, Hodgson K, et al. Primary aortoenteric fistula. *South Med J* 2002;95(9):1071–1073.

Vu QD, Menias CO, Bhalla S, et al. Aortoenteric fistulas: CT features and potential mimics. *Radiographics* 2009;29(1):197–209.

23 **Answer D.** The CT scan demonstrates herniation of a small bowel loop in the right groin. The small bowel loop extending into the hernia (H) is medial to the inferior epigastric vessels (IEV) (top right). The neck of the hernia is narrow (bottom, arrow) and the right femoral vein is compressed (top left). These findings are compatible with a **femoral hernia**.

Inguinal region hernias can be divided into **inguinal hernias (direct and indirect)** and **femoral hernias**. Direct inguinal hernias pass medial to the inferior epigastric vessels above the inguinal ligament through a defect in Hesselbach triangle (bordered by the inguinal ligament inferiorly, the IEV superolaterally, and the conjoined tendon medially). These have a relatively low risk for incarceration. Indirect hernias are 5× more common than direct hernias, originating at the deep inguinal ring lateral to the IEV and following the inguinal canal inferomedially. In males, these may extend anterior to the spermatic cord into the scrotum. These hernias are at moderate risk for incarceration.

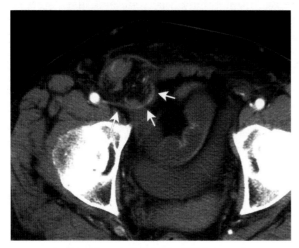

Indirect hernia lateral to IEV (arrows).

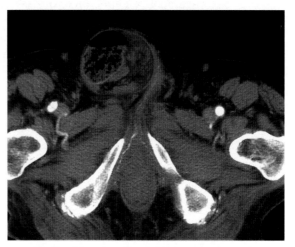

Indirect hernia adjacent to spermatic cord.

Femoral hernias are uncommon, representing 5% of abdominal hernias. They exit below the inguinal ligament into the femoral canal medial to the femoral vein and inferior to the course of the IEV. Venous compression of the femoral vein and collateral vein engorgement may be seen. They typically have a narrow neck; 40% of femoral hernias present with incarceration.

A Spigelian hernia is located in the lower abdominal wall, extending through the spigelian fascia, lateral to the rectus muscle.

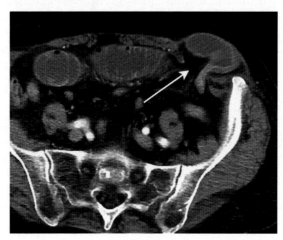

Spigelian hernia.

References: Burkhardt JH, Arshanskiy Y, Munson JL, et al. Diagnosis of inguinal region hernias with axial CT: the lateral crescent sign and other key findings. *Radiographics* 2011;31(2):E1–E12.

Shadbolt CL, Heinze SB, Dietrich RB. Imaging of groin masses: inguinal anatomy and pathologic conditions revisited. *Radiographics* 2001;21 Spec No:S261–S271.

24 **Answer C.** There is a fluid-filled structure, which represents a dilated loop of bowel in the periportal region. The hepaticojejunostomy is well visualized without stricture on the coronal image. **The afferent (pancreaticobiliary) limb is obstructed in this patient leading to the secondary obstruction of the bile duct.** Afferent limb obstruction may be due to adhesions, internal hernias, radiation enteropathy, or recurrent tumor, depending upon the preexisting conditions. The syndrome was first described with Billroth II procedures, which are seldom performed now due to improved medical treatment of peptic ulcer disease. The two most common current clinical settings in which the afferent limb syndrome may be seen are with Roux-en-Y gastric bypass procedures and pancreaticoduodenectomy (Whipple procedures). Complications include perforation of the obstructed afferent limb, bleeding, pancreatitis, or cholangitis. Treatment may be with stenting or surgical correction.

References: Pannala R, Brandabur JJ, Gan SI, et al. Afferent limb syndrome and delayed GI problems after pancreaticoduodenectomy for pancreatic cancer: single-center, 14-year experience. *Gastrointest Endosc* 2011;74(2):295–302.

Sandrasegaran K, Maglinte DD, Rajesh A, et al. CT of acute biliopancreatic limb obstruction. *AJR Am J Roentgenol* 2006;186(1):104–109.

Wise SW. Case 24: afferent loop syndrome. *Radiology* 2000;216(1):142–145.

25 **Answer D.** The duodenum is the most common location in trauma involving the GI tract.

The images demonstrate a **duodenal hematoma**, which initially would be heterogeneous due to active hemorrhage (not shown), becoming more homogenous and hypodense on the follow-up CT. The CT and UGI images show extrinsic compression of the second portion of the duodenum, but oral contrast does pass distal to the level of the hematoma, excluding high-grade obstruction. A stricture similar in location to that seen on the UGI may be caused by an annular pancreas (answer choice C), but the MRI and CT findings do not support that entity. Duodenal hematomas are more common in the pediatric population, and absent signs of perforation can usually be treated conservatively.

References: Kunin JR, Korobkin M, Ellis JH, et al. Duodenal injuries caused by blunt abdominal trauma: value of CT in differentiating perforation from hematoma. *AJR Am J Roentgenol* 1993;160:1221–1223.

Niehues SM, Denecke T, Bassir C, et al. Intramural duodenal hematoma: clinical course and imaging findings. *Acta Radiologica Open* 2019;8:1–8.

26 **Answer B.** Coronal reformatted images from contrast-enhanced CT demonstrate marked distention of the excluded stomach, duodenal C-loop, and proximal small bowel. The dilation extends to a staple line in the left lower quadrant in the figure on the right. The gastric pouch, Roux limb, and distal small bowel are all nondilated, with oral contrast material seen in these segments. The imaging features are compatible with **small bowel obstruction involving the biliopancreatic limb**. Small bowel obstructions (SBO) can affect various segments of the bowel after Roux-en-Y gastric bypass surgery, including the alimentary limb (Roux limb exiting the gastrojejunostomy); the biliopancreatic limb that drains the gastric remnant along with pancreatic and biliary systems; and the common enteric channel downstream from the Roux-en-Y jejunojejunostomy. An SBO with involvement of the biliopancreatic limb is a closed loop obstruction that occurs in close proximity to the jejunojejunostomy. Although the incidence of these types of SBO is low (estimated to be 0.3% to 2.3%), such obstructions are at increased risk for perforation and merit prompt surgical intervention. The diagnosis is more easily made by CT than by fluoroscopy as the biliopancreatic limb will be dilated and fluid filled, contrasting with the normal sized and contrast-opacified alimentary limb and common channel.

References: Levine MS, Carucci LR. Imaging of bariatric surgery: normal anatomy and postoperative complications. *Radiology* 2014;270(2):327–341.

Sandrasegaran K, Maglinte DD, Rajesh A, et al. CT of acute biliopancreatic limb obstruction. *AJR Am J Roentgenol* 2006;186(1):104–109.

27 **Answer D.** Multiple wide-mouthed diverticula are present throughout the small bowel, mostly in the jejunum. **Jejunal diverticulosis** is present in about 1.3% of autopsy and 2.3% of barium small bowel examinations. The diverticula are acquired, and jejunal diverticulosis is more common in the older population, with 80% to 90% affecting patients over 40 years old. A gut motility disorder is present, leading to increased transit time. The subsequent increased intraluminal pressure is felt to be the cause of the diverticula. **The delayed transit time leads to stasis and bacterial overgrowth, which can cause diarrhea and malabsorption**. Treatment of bacterial overgrowth syndrome is with antibiotics (not surgery). Serious complication such as diverticulitis, perforation, bleeding, and intestinal obstruction can occur in 10% to 30% of patients. **CT is less sensitive for detection of jejunal diverticula when compared to small bowel follow-through examinations, as the diverticula can mimic normal bowel loops in cross section**. These diverticula are better appreciated on CT when scrolling through images and observing the relationship to the small bowel loops.

Reference: Fintelmann F, Levine MS, Rubesin SE. Jejunal diverticulosis: findings on CT in 28 patients. *AJR Am J Roentgenol* 2008;190(5):1286–1290.

28 **Answer C.** An ovoid structure associated with the third portion of the duodenum contains solid matter and gas. There is inflammatory stranding in the periduodenal fat. This likely represents the **duodenal diverticulum** seen in the same location on the earlier upper GI study. This diverticulum appears larger and now contains trapped contents, which are not freely draining into the lumen. Duodenal ulcers are more common in the bulb and postbulbar duodenum. Although a walled-off necrotic collection associated with pancreatitis might have a similar appearance, the time course of presenting symptoms does not fit. A gut duplication cyst may become infected, but these are much less common than diverticula.

Duodenal diverticula are very common and are typically asymptomatic incidental findings. The majority are in the second portion of the duodenum, with most of the remainder found in the third portion of the duodenum. Multiple diverticula are common. The diverticula in the second portion of the duodenum are most commonly located in the medial wall around the ampulla. Periampullary diverticula often increase the technical difficulty of cannulating the biliary system for endoscopists. Duodenal diverticula are typically acquired pulsion-type diverticula and are pseudodiverticula, which contain only the mucosal and submucosal layers. Congenital diverticula are rare and may be extraluminal, containing all bowel wall layers, or intraluminal. On CT, the duodenal diverticula often contain large amounts of air and may have air-fluid levels. **When completely fluid filled, they may mimic pancreatic pseudocysts or cystic neoplasms.**

A narrow neck of the diverticulum predisposes to stasis and perforation, as does the presence of foreign bodies such as gallstones or enteroliths. CT findings of duodenal diverticulitis include wall thickening and inflammatory stranding in adjacent tissue. Extraluminal gas may be present but is more commonly contained than free. Although the duodenal diverticula are most commonly asymptomatic, they may become impacted with food and can perforate or hemorrhage. Antibiotic treatment is usually sufficient if perforation is contained, but in some cases, surgery may be indicated.

References: Bittle MM, Gunn ML, Gross JA, et al. Imaging of duodenal diverticula and their complications. *Curr Probl Diagn Radiol* 2012;41(1):20–29.

Pearl MS, Hill MC, Zeman RK. CT findings in duodenal diverticulitis. *AJR Am J Roentgenol* 2006;187(4):W392–W395.

29a **Answer C.** Dose rate to the patient is greatest at the skin where the x-ray beam enters. The entrance exposure limit for standard fluoroscopy is 10 R/min (100 mGy/min). Some fluoroscopic units are capable of a high-output "boost" mode, for which the limit is 20R/min (200 mGy/min).

A typical fluoroscopic entrance exposure rate for a man of average build is approximately 30 mGy/min, and the dose for a standard gastrointestinal fluoroscopy procedure is typically in the 100 mGy range.

Reference: Parry RA, Glaze SA, Archer BR. The AAPM/RSNA physics tutorial for residents. Typical patient radiation doses in diagnostic radiology. *Radiographics* 1999;19(5):1289–1302.

29b **Answer B.** Grids are utilized to improve image contrast by removing scattered radiation, but this is achieved at the cost of an increase in dosage. Removal of the grid will reduce the dose to about one-third to one-half.

The other maneuvers all result in an increase in dosage. Increasing the distance of the image intensifier from the patient (widening the air gap) leads to an increased source-to-image receptor distance and an increased dose.

Utilizing pulsed fluoroscopy instead of continuous fluoroscopy results in a dose reduction. The faster pulse rates result in greater x-ray exposure over a given unit of time, and the slower pulse rates will reduce the x-ray exposure.

Selecting a higher kilovolt peak increases average beam energy (beam hardening) resulting in a greater percentage of x-rays penetrating the patient to reach the image intensifier. This leads to a decrease in tube current and decreased dosage. Conversely, the lower kilovolt peak will result in fewer penetrating beams and an increase in the milliamperage.

References: Hernanz-Schulman M, Goske MJ, Bercha IH, et al. Pause and pulse: ten steps that help manage radiation dose during pediatric fluoroscopy. *AJR Am J Roentgenol* 2011;197(2):475-481.

Mahesh M. Fluoroscopy: patient radiation exposure issues. *Radiographics* 2001;21(4): 1033–1045.

29c **Answer B.** Most current fluoroscopic systems have the pulse fluoroscopy feature, which utilizes short pulses of the x-ray beam rather than continuous emission. Although it may seem that reducing the pulse rate by half should result in a commensurate reduction of dosage by half, most fluoroscopic systems are designed to increase milliamperage with pulse fluoroscopy in order to maintain acceptable image quality without excessive noise. This blunts the dose reduction effect such that changing the frame rate from 30 per second to 15 per second reduces the dosage by about 25%.

References: Aufrichtig R, Xue P, Thomas CW, et al. Perceptual comparison of pulsed and continuous fluoroscopy. *Med Phys* 1994;21(2):245–256.

Mahesh M. Fluoroscopy: patient radiation exposure issues. *Radiographics* 2001;21(4): 1033–1045.

30 **Answer B.** The small bowel follow-through spot image demonstrates multiple well-defined nodules in the terminal ileum, uniform in appearance and measuring 2 to 3 mm in size. These are typical in appearance for **lymphoid nodular hyperplasia**. These may be seen as a normal finding in young adults. When numerous or unusually prominent, they may be associated with infection, food hypersensitivity, or immunodeficiency states.

There is no luminal narrowing to suggest Crohn disease. Carcinoid tumors may be multiple but are typically larger and fewer in number. Lymphoma may manifest as nodular abnormalities, but these would also be larger than seen in this case.

References: Levine MS, Rubesin SE, Laufer I. Pattern approach for diseases of mesenteric small bowel on barium studies. *Radiology* 2008;249(2):445–460.

Mansueto P, Iacono G, Seidita A, et al. Review article: intestinal lymphoid nodular hyperplasia in children—the relationship to food hypersensitivity. *Aliment Pharmacol Ther* 2012;35(9):1000–1009.

31 **Answer B.** Early radiograph obtained during a small bowel follow-through study demonstrates failure of the duodenal C-loop to cross the midline, with multiple jejunal/proximal small bowel segments located in the right abdomen. A radiograph obtained later in the study demonstrates opacification of the cecum which is located in the left pelvis. The imaging features are compatible with **intestinal malrotation**. During embryogenesis, the midgut rotates around a central vascular pedicle before anchoring with the mesentery. Normal rotation and fixation allows the duodenal C-loop to cross the midline and locates the jejunum in left upper quadrant and cecum in the right lower quadrant. A failure of gut rotation can result in abnormal location and poor fixation of the bowel. These congenital anomalies can be clinically significant in infants and children, manifesting as bilious vomiting, duodenal obstruction, or small bowel volvulus. The prevalence in adults is less clear, estimated to occur in 0.2% to 0.5% of the population, with most being asymptomatic. Those with clinically significant symptoms, including postprandial pain or cramping, may benefit from surgery such as the Ladd procedure.

References: Burke MS, Glick PL. Gastrointestinal malrotation with volvulus in an adult. *Am J Surg* 2008;195(4):501–503.

Gamblin TC, Stephens RE Jr, Johnson RK, et al. Adult malrotation: a case report and review of the literature. *Curr Surg* 2003;60(5):517–520.

32a **Answer C.** An ovoid structure containing fluid and layering calculi is seen in the right abdomen associated with the ileum as indicated in this case, which identifies this as a Meckel diverticulum. Meckel diverticulum is the most common congenital anomaly of the gastrointestinal tract, occurring in 2% of the population. This diverticulum is a remnant of the omphalomesenteric (vitelline) duct, which connects the yolk sac to the midgut. This embryologic duct typically closes between the 5th and 8th weeks of gestation. Incomplete duct closure may result in a diverticulum, fistula, cyst, or fibrous band. **A Meckel diverticulum is usually found in the distal small bowel 40 to 100 cm from the ileocecal valve along the antimesenteric side of the ileum.** These diverticula or cysts are lined with heterotopic mucosa, usually gastric and less commonly pancreatic, small bowel, or a combination of different types.

Meckel diverticula may be difficult to distinguish from other small bowel loops on barium studies, especially when similar in diameter to adjacent loops due to problems delineating the ostium and active emptying with peristalsis.

Most patients with a Meckel diverticulum never develop symptoms. Bowel obstruction, bleeding, and diverticulitis account for most cases of symptomatic Meckel diverticula. Bowel obstruction may occur due to trapping of a bowel loop by a meso-diverticular band, volvulus around the band, or intussusception. Heterotopic gastric mucosa within the diverticula may bleed or secrete acid and cause inflammation or perforation. Neoplasms are uncommon (3% of symptomatic diverticula) and include a variety of histologic types, carcinoid being the most common.

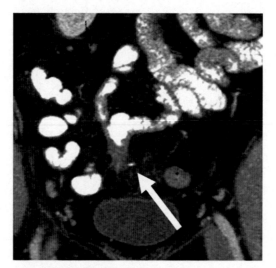

Meckel diverticulitis from perforation due to bone from Cornish game hen.

References: Elsayes KM, Menias CO, Harvin HJ, et al. Imaging manifestations of Meckel's diverticulum. *AJR Am J Roentgenol* 2007;189(1):81–88.

Levy AD, Hobbs CM. From the archives of the AFIP. Meckel diverticulum: radiologic features with pathologic Correlation. *Radiographics* 2004;24(2):565–587.

32b **Answer B.** The ^{99m}Tc RBC scan demonstrated gradual accumulation of radiotracer in the right lower quadrant, which later moves into the right mid abdomen. The CT enteroclysis shows a cystic lesion in the right anterior pelvis with a mural nodule. Findings are consistent with a Meckel diverticulum with ectopic gastric mucosa. Movement of the radiotracer on the later images indicates intraluminal blood.

A gut duplication cyst could contain ectopic gastric mucosa but would not communicate with the lumen and cause GI bleeding in the absence of ulceration or a fistula. The lesion is close to the cecal base and could represent an appendiceal mucocele although the solid nodule that is the presumed bleeding source is at the base of the lesion and would not be the cause of appendiceal orifice obstruction.

A Meckel diverticulum is the most common congenital anomaly of the gastrointestinal tract present in 2% to 3% of the population. The Meckel diverticulum is located within 100 cm of the ileocecal valve. While most are asymptomatic, up to 40% may develop complications including hemorrhage, obstruction, and diverticulitis.

Meckel diverticula are lined with heterotopic tissue in 60% of cases, most commonly gastric mucosa, with pancreatic, duodenal, and Brunner gland foci also found. A 99mTc pertechnetate scan (Meckel scan) can detect the presence of gastric mucosa as the agent behaves in the same manner as halide (e.g., chloride) ions.

Hemorrhage is frequently more severe and common in the pediatric population. Obstruction may be secondary to bowel loops trapped by a fibrous band, volvulus of the diverticulum, or intussusception.

Diverticulitis may be due to elevated acid secretion by the gastric mucosa or to obstruction due to an enterolith or foreign body.

32c **Answer A.** The **omphalomesenteric duct (OMD) or vitelline duct** is the embryonic communication between the yolk sac and the developing midgut. The midgut elongates and herniates into the umbilical cord (6th week of embryogenesis) where it rotates 90 degrees counterclockwise around the axis of the superior mesenteric artery. It returns to the abdomen (by the 10th week) and the OMD regresses. If any portion of the OMD does not atrophy, a number of anomalies may develop including an umbilicoileal fistula (complete persistence), a sinus tract, a cyst, or a fibrous connection from the ileum to the umbilicus.

The other answer choices do not arise from the same embryologic anlage.

References: Elsayes KM, Menias CO, Harvin HJ, et al. Imaging manifestations of Meckel's diverticulum. *AJR Am J Roentgenol* 2007;189(1):81–88.

Levy AD, Hobbs CM. From the archives of the AFIP. Meckel diverticulum: radiologic features with pathologic Correlation. *Radiographics* 2004;24(2):565–587.

33 **Answer D.** The film from the small bowel follow-through demonstrates **dilated loops of small bowel with thin folds that are closely spaced together**. While both gastroesophageal reflux and an ileus are present, the small bowel fold pattern indicates a more specific diagnosis of **scleroderma**. Scleroderma (also known as progressive systemic sclerosis) is an autoimmune disease of unknown etiology in which there is widespread collagen deposition in tissues. It affects multiple organ systems with the skin followed by the GI tract being the most commonly involved. The esophagus is affected in 50% to 90% of cases and the small bowel in 50% of cases.

Smooth muscle fibrosis in the GI tract leads to hypomotility and stasis. This can cause bacterial overgrowth and malabsorption. The fibrosis also leads to small bowel dilatation and a pseudo-obstruction pattern. As the fibrosis tends to involve the circular muscular layer, this leads to valvular packing and fold compression, the "hide-bound" appearance. Significant gastrointestinal involvement with scleroderma has a poor prognosis with a 5-year mortality of over 50%.

Esophageal hypomotility (in the distal 2/3 of the esophagus which has smooth muscle) leads to gastroesophageal reflux and dysphagia, which are the most common gastrointestinal manifestations of the disease. Other visceral manifestations of scleroderma include gastric atony, megaduodenum, and wide-mouthed diverticula (more common in the colon). Absent gastrocolic reflex can lead to constipation.

References: Domsic R, Fasanella K, Bielefeldt K. Gastrointestinal manifestations of systemic sclerosis. *Dig Dis Sci* 2008;53(5):1163–1174.

Pickhardt PJ. The "hide-bound" bowel sign. *Radiology* 1999;213(3):837–838.

34a **Answer B.** The maximum dose in fluoroscopic exposure is delivered to the skin surface at which the x-ray beam enters. Most of the cases of documented radiation-induced skin damage have occurred with cardiac catheterization and interventional procedures, not with diagnostic fluoroscopic procedures. Early transient erythema of the skin may be seen hours following doses of more than **2 Gy**. This occurs due to changes in capillary permeability. The main erythema reaction occurs about 1.5 weeks after exposure and is seen with doses about 6 Gy. Other significant effects include epilation (hair loss), which may be temporary at doses of about 3 Gy, and permanent when the dose exceeds about 7 Gy. Dry and moist desquamation, secondary ulceration, and late erythema occur several weeks after exposure. Late effects to the skin including dermal atrophy and necrosis develop months to years after exposure to 10 to 18 Gy.

34b **Answer C.** With skin entrance exposure rates of between 10 and 50 mGy/min (30 mGy/min for a man of medium build), doses can reach a total of 0.6 to 3 Gy after 1 hour of normal (not high dose) fluoroscopy. As noted above, the threshold dose for erythematous skin changes is 2 Gy.

References: Hall EJ, Giaccia AJ. *Radiobiology for the radiologist,* 6th ed. Philadelphia, PA: Lippincott Williams & Wilkins, 2006.

Parry RA, Glaze SA, Archer BR. The AAPM/RSNA physics tutorial for residents. Typical patient radiation doses in diagnostic radiology. *Radiographics* 1999;19(5):1289–1302.

Wagner LK, Archer BR. *Minimizing risks from fluoroscopic x-rays,* 2nd ed. Houston, TX: Partners in Radiation Management, 1998.

35 **Answer: D.** Fluoroscopic spot image from upper GI study (Figure 14) demonstrates a barium-filled sac within the lumen of the 2nd and 3rd portions of the duodenum, bounded by a thin radiolucent curvilinear line. This is a **duodenal windsock sign** and compatible with **an intraluminal duodenal diverticulum**. An intraluminal duodenal diverticulum is a rare congenital anomaly due to failure of normal recanalization of the duodenal lumen during embryogenesis. As a result, a thin web or diaphragm remains in the lumen and elongates slowly over time with continued intestinal peristalsis. The diverticulum can be eccentrically attached to the duodenal wall or circumferentially attached in which case a small diverticular hole must be present to prevent duodenal obstruction. Patients generally present in 3rd decade of life with epigastric pain and vomiting. Complete duodenal obstruction can occur if the orifice is occluded by food debris. Pancreatitis, cholangitis, and ulcer disease have all been reported as rare complications. Treatment is increasingly performed via endoscopy, although surgical techniques can also be applied.

References: Materne R. The duodenal wind sock sign. *Radiology* 2001;218(3):749–750.

Schroeder TC, Hartman M, Heller M, et al. Duodenal diverticula: potential complications and common imaging pitfalls. *Clin Radiol* 2014;69(10):1072–1076.

36 **Answer D. Peutz-Jeghers syndrome** is characterized by mucocutaneous pigmented lesions and hamartomas of the gastrointestinal tract. There is no gender predominance. Diagnosis is usually made in childhood or early adulthood. Inheritance is autosomal dominant with variable penetrance although some cases may arise from spontaneous mutations to the serine/threonine kinase 11 tumor suppressor gene on chromosome 19p13.

The mucocutaneous pigmentation lesions that are characteristic in Peutz-Jeghers are common in the perioral and periorbital regions. The gastrointestinal polyps of Peutz-Jeghers syndrome are hamartomatous, and the small bowel is the most common site, although they may be found anywhere in the gastrointestinal tract from the stomach to the rectum. Abdominal pain is a common presentation due to small bowel intussusceptions caused by the polyps. Small bowel polyps can ulcerate and bleed.

Although the small bowel polyps are hamartomatous, patients with Peutz-Jeghers syndrome have an increased risk of developing gastrointestinal adenocarcinomas. Most of these carcinomas are found in the stomach, duodenum, and colon, with the small bowel the least common site of malignancy. Although hamartomas are not themselves malignant, possible origins are islands of adenomatous epithelium within the hamartomas or adjacent adenomatous polyps. **Patients with Peutz-Jeghers are also at risk for other malignancies of the pancreas, breast, thyroid, and ovarian and testis.** Overall lifetime risk for intestinal and extraintestinal sources is high, with 1% to 2% risk by age 20 years, over 30% by age 50 years, and more than 80% by age 70 years. Endoscopic surveillance is recommended for malignancy screening, and for polypectomy when possible, to minimize the risk of small bowel obstruction and need for surgical resection.

Neurofibromatosis may be associated with skin lesions, but these are not generally pigmented. Gardner syndrome may involve small bowel polyps and other mesenchymal tumors (e.g., desmoids, osteomas) but do not have pigmented skin lesions. Metastatic melanoma may involve pigmented lesions and small bowel polypoid metastases but would be less common in this age group.

References: Achatz MI, Porter CC, Brugieres L, et al. Cancer screening recommendations and clinical management of inherited gastrointestinal cancer syndromes in childhood. *Clin Cancer Res* 2017;23(13):e107–e114.

Cho GJ, Bergquist K, Schwartz AM. Peutz-Jeghers syndrome and the hamartomatous polyposis syndromes: radiologic-pathologic correlation. *Radiographics* 1997;17(3):785–791.

Rufener SL, Koujok K, McKenna BJ, et al. Small bowel intussusception secondary to Peutz-Jeghers polyp. *Radiographics* 2008;28(1):284–288.

37 **Answer B.** The CT demonstrates marked gastric and duodenal dilatation to the level of the horizontal portion of the duodenum as it crosses over the aorta. Small bowel loops distal to this level are normal in caliber. The aortomesenteric angle (AMA) formed by the superior mesenteric artery (SMA) and the aorta is narrowed with loss of the normal retroperitoneal fat (normal angle is 28 to 65 degrees) and the aortomesenteric distance decreased (normal 10 to 34 mm). This causes **compression of the duodenum as it crosses between the aorta and the SMA** with gastric and proximal duodenal obstruction, known as the **SMA syndrome.** The syndrome is controversial as some degree of compression of the horizontal duodenum may be seen in asymptomatic people. However, in normal individuals, the AMA may be not be as fixed as with patients who have little retroperitoneal fat due to rapid weight loss. Similar compression of the horizontal duodenum between the SMA and aorta may be seen in patients who have had surgical repair of scoliosis.

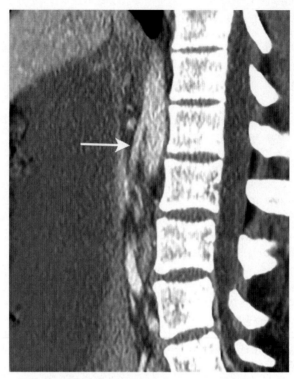

Narrowed aortomesenteric angle (AMA).

The other choices describe variants that are associated with different types of obstruction. The median arcuate ligament causes compression of the celiac artery. Abnormal position of the ligament of Treitz is seen in malrotation with potential for proximal small bowel obstruction due to fibrous bands (Ladd bands). The left renal vein may be compressed if it passes behind the aorta or between the aorta and the SMA.

References: Konen E, Amitai M, Apter S, et al. CT angiography of superior mesenteric artery syndrome. *AJR Am J Roentgenol* 1998;171(5):1279–1281.

Lamba R, Tanner DT, Sekhon S, et al. Multidetector CT of vascular compression syndromes in the abdomen and pelvis. *Radiographics* 2014;34(1):93–115.

QUESTIONS

1 A 34-year-old female presents with 2 days onset of right lower quadrant pain. On examination, the patient has an elevated white blood cell count and a mild fever. A CT performed with intravenous contrast was obtained. What is the most appropriate next step?

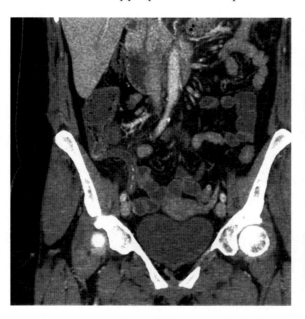 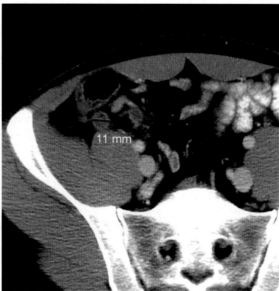

A. Pelvic ultrasound to assess for tuboovarian abscess
B. Repeating the CT study using enteric contrast
C. Surgical consultation
D. No treatment needed for a self-limited condition

2a A 25-year-old previously healthy female presents to the emergency department with right lower quadrant pain of <1-day duration. She is afebrile and laboratory studies show a minimal leukocytosis. What does the CT show?

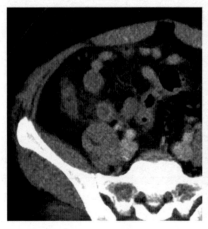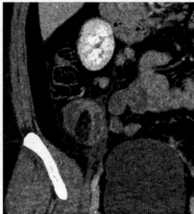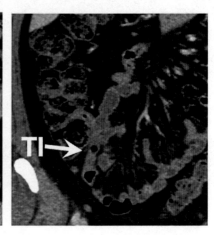

A. Acute appendicitis
B. Crohn ileitis
C. Cecal diverticulitis
D. Normal findings

2b The patient is admitted and started on intravenous antibiotics. The next day her pain and leukocytosis are resolved. What is the appropriate course of action at this point?

A. Appendectomy.
B. Observation on IV antibiotics another 2-3 days and if clinically stable discharge on oral antibiotics and close follow-up.
C. Discharge with no further treatment.
D. Either A or B may be appropriate.

3a A 55-year-old female presents with one week history of left lower abdominal pain. She has a mild leukocytosis and a low-grade fever. What is the next best step in management?

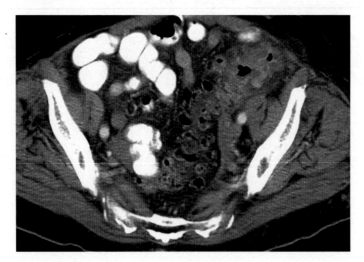

A. No intervention needed, the study is normal
B. Diet modification with course of oral broad-spectrum antibiotics
C. Colonoscopy to evaluate for suspected malignancy
D. Urgent surgical consultation
E. Single-contrast enema to assess for degree of obstruction

3b Regarding colonic diverticula, which of the following statements is TRUE?

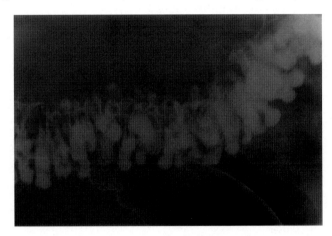

A. Acute diverticulitis is the most common cause of large bowel obstruction.
B. The diverticula are traction-type pseudodiverticula caused by adjacent fibrosis.
C. Diverticula are most common in the rectum and sigmoid colon.
D. Diverticula form at the site of the vasa recta penetration of the bowel wall.

4a A 62-year-old man with a history of left lower quadrant pain and low-grade fever has a CT scan for suspected acute diverticulitis. He was started on an empiric course of antibiotics 3 days before the scan. This case should be interpreted as

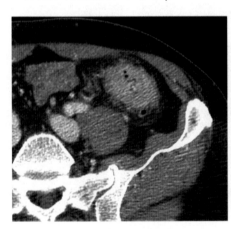 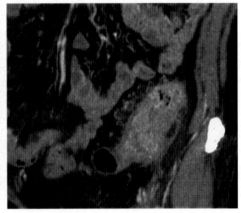

A. Findings consistent with acute uncomplicated diverticulitis
B. Findings of diverticulosis with sigmoid muscular hypertrophy but no diverticulitis
C. Findings could represent acute diverticulitis or colon cancer
D. No abnormalities seen

4b Regarding CT findings distinguishing acute diverticulitis from colon cancer, match the following (choices may be used more than once or not at all):

A. Presence of diverticula
B. Enlarged pericolic lymph nodes
C. Wall thickening over 1 cm
D. Involved segment 10 cm or longer
E. Luminal narrowing with squared shoulder
F. Pericolic fat stranding

1. Favors diverticulitis over colon cancer.
2. Favors colon cancer over diverticulitis.
3. Neither colon cancer nor diverticulitis is strongly favored.

5 A 72-year-old female presents with pneumaturia. A CT scan is obtained. What is the most common cause of the finding below?

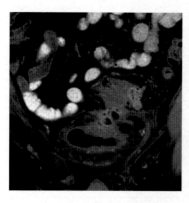
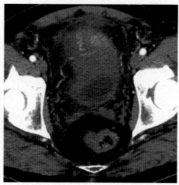
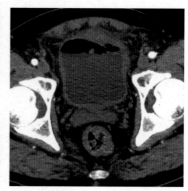

A. Colorectal cancer
B. Crohn disease
C. Diverticulitis
D. Pelvic radiation therapy

6a A 70-year-old female with a history of coronary artery disease and prior myocardial infarcts presents with rectal bleeding and severe abdominal pain. A contrast-enhanced CT scan and follow-up barium enema show a long stricture in the distal transverse colon. What is the most likely etiology?

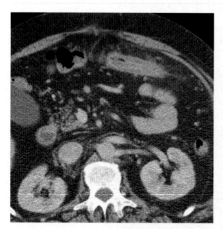
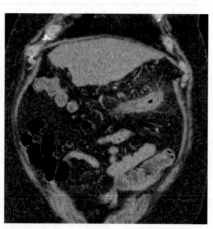
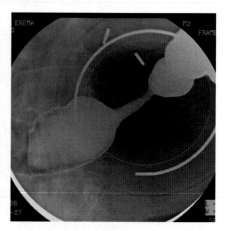

A. Crohn disease
B. Radiation colitis
C. Ischemic colitis
D. Chronic diverticulitis

6b What is the name of the watershed area in the colon between the superior and inferior mesenteric arterial territories?

A. Meyers point
B. Drummond point
C. Sudeck point
D. Griffiths point

7a The colonic arterial branches arise

A. Entirely from the SMA
B. Entirely from the IMA
C. From the SMA, IMA, and internal iliac artery
D. From the SMA, IMA, and external iliac artery
  SMA—superior mesenteric artery
  IMA—inferior mesenteric artery

7b Which of the following arteries or arcades form an important collateral circulation between the SMA and IMA?

A. Arc of Riolan
B. Marginal artery of Drummond
C. Arc of Buhler
D. Both A and B

8 Which portions of the colon are retroperitoneal?

A. Entire colon
B. Ascending, descending, and portion of the rectum
C. Rectum only
D. Cecum and transverse colon

9a An 89-year-old male presents to the emergency room with abdominal pain, and a CT examination was performed. What is the most likely diagnosis?

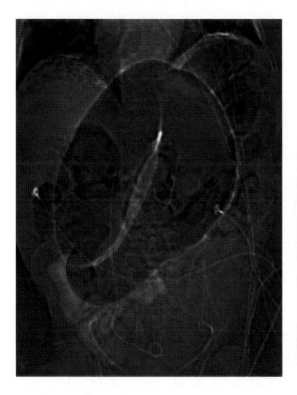
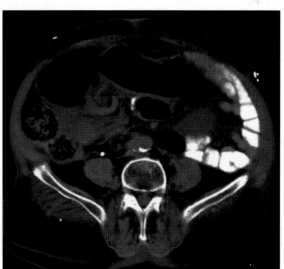

A. Cecal volvulus
B. Cecal bascule
C. Sigmoid volvulus
D. Acute diverticulitis

9b An 88-year-old patient presents with abdominal pain and distention. What is the next most appropriate step regarding management of this patient?

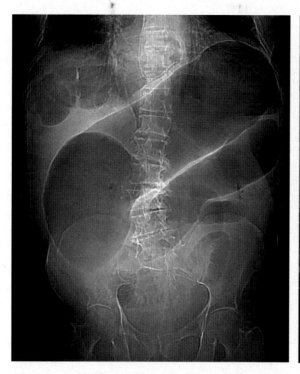
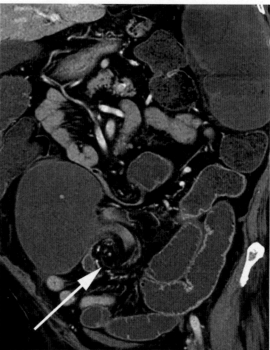

A. Serial observation for a 24-hour period with discharge if hemodynamically stable

B. Emergent surgery.

C. Endoscopic reduction of the torsion.

D. Either B or C may be appropriate depending upon the clinical status of the patient.

10 A 70-year-old male presents for CT colonography following an incomplete colonoscopy. What is the most appropriate next step for this patient?

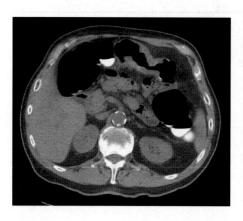
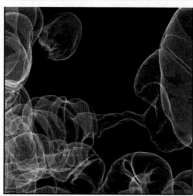
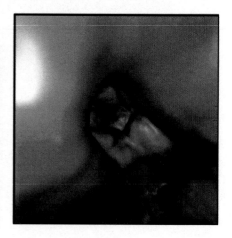

A. Routine screening colonoscopy in 10 years.

B. Routine screening CT colonography in 5 years.

C. Repeat colonoscopy now for biopsy if not already performed versus surgical consultation for resection.

D. Capsule endoscopy to evaluate the proximal small and large bowel.

11a A single-contrast barium enema is performed on a 50-year-old male. A spot film of the sigmoid colon is shown below. What is the appropriate next step?

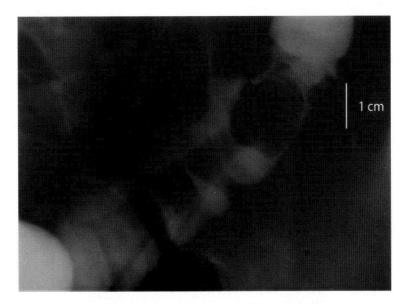

A. Repeat barium examination in 6 months to assess stability
B. Surgical consultation for sigmoid colectomy
C. Colonoscopy with snare polypectomy
D. Flexible sigmoidoscopy with biopsy

11b The risk of a 1.5-cm polyp harboring an invasive cancer is

A. Less than 1%
B. Approximately 10%
C. Approximately 50%
D. Approximately 90%

12a An asymptomatic 69-year-old female with a positive fecal occult blood test undergoes a colonoscopy. A mass at the splenic flexure is found. A CT scan is performed for staging. What is the likely diagnosis?

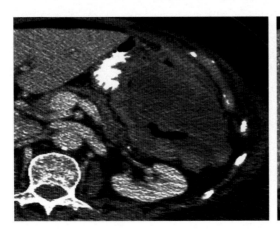
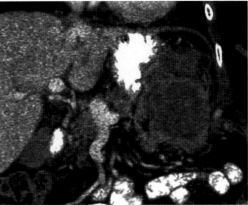

A. Tubulovillous adenoma
B. Gastrointestinal stromal tumor
C. Colonic neuroendocrine tumor
D. Mucinous colon adenocarcinoma

12b What are features of mucinous adenocarcinoma of the colon that distinguish it from the nonmucinous adenocarcinoma?

A. Lower attenuation
B. Marked wall thickening
C. Presence of intratumoral calcifications
D. Worse prognosis
E. All of the above

13 A 57-year-old man with known midrectal adenocarcinoma has a rectal MRI for staging. Based on the displayed image, what is the most likely T stage of disease?

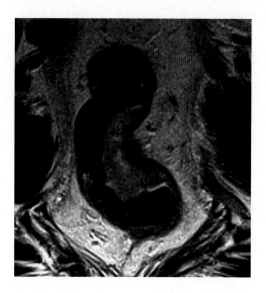

A. T1
B. T2
C. T3
D. T4

14 An 89-year-old female presents with acute-onset abdominal pain and hematochezia. Which clinical scenario best fits the finding?

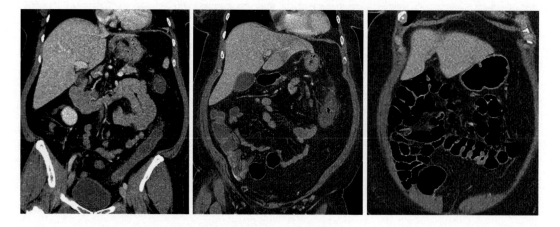

A. History of antibiotic therapy for pneumonia
B. History of cardioversion for cardiac arrhythmia
C. Recent overseas travel
D. History of prior episodes of diverticulitis

15 A 62-year-old female has isolated lung metastases from a colorectal neoplasm. Which of the following is the likely site of her primary tumor?

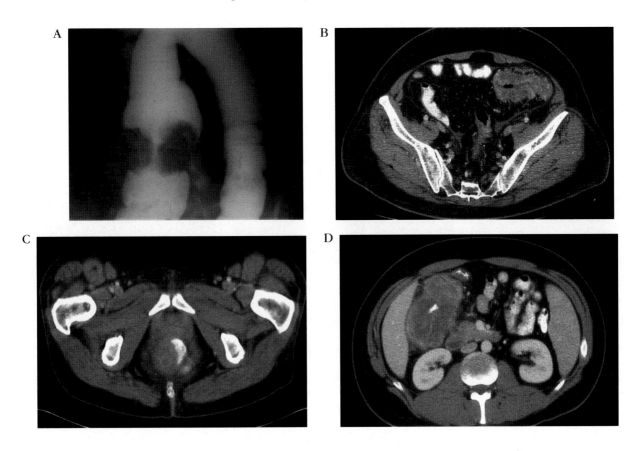

16a A 45-year-old male with a history of pain with defecation is found to have a mass palpable in the left anal canal on digital examination and a left groin mass. MRI of the anal canal region and CT scan are performed.

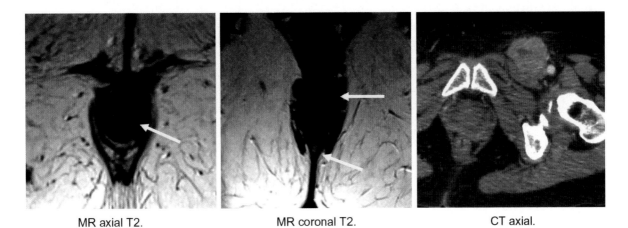

MR axial T2.   MR coronal T2.   CT axial.

The tumor cell type is most likely

A. Adenocarcinoma

B. Squamous cell carcinoma

C. Neuroendocrine tumor

D. Lymphoma

16b Which of the following imaging features is the most important for T staging of the primary tumor?

A. Depth of invasion beyond the external sphincter
B. Extension above the dentate line
C. Tumor signal intensity indicating more aggressive subtype
D. Tumor size

17a An 81-year-old male who has been in the intensive care unit for 2 weeks following a myocardial infarction develops abdominal bloating and diffuse abdominal pain. A CT obtained demonstrates a small bowel and colonic distention with a transition in caliber at the splenic flexure (arrow) without obvious wall thickening or extrinsic abnormality. The most likely diagnosis is

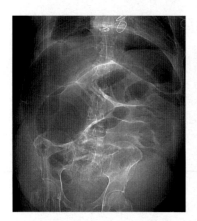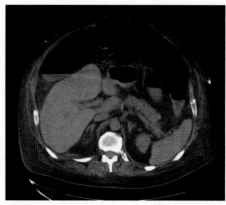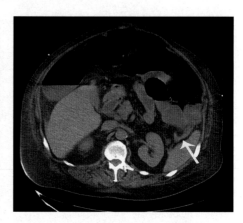

A. Pseudomembranous colitis
B. Acute colonic pseudo-obstruction
C. Mechanical obstruction due to adhesions
D. Mechanical obstruction due to acute diverticulitis

17b In acute colonic pseudo-obstruction, what is the most appropriate next step in management?

A. No change in management needed, as the condition is self-limited.
B. Perform a single-contrast barium enema to exclude an occult neoplasm.
C. Nasogastric decompression.
D. Colonoscopic decompression.

18 The most common site for perforation due to an obstruction from a sigmoid colonic neoplasm is at the

A. Cecum
B. Splenic flexure
C. Sigmoid just proximal to the obstruction
D. At the level of the neoplasm

19 An 85-year-old female with chronic constipation is noted to have abdominal bloating and moderate abdominal discomfort. An abdominal CT is obtained.

No distal obstructing abnormality is found at colonoscopy, and she is treated with rectal tube decompression. She has had multiple repeated admissions for the same presentation, including the scout from a CT 8 months earlier. A biopsy is performed of the bowel. What pathologic changes are most likely?

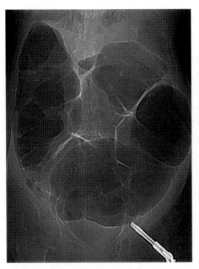 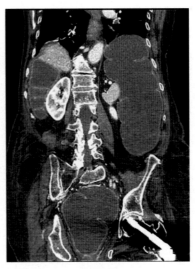

CT scout 8 months prior to the current admission.

A. Fibrosis and amyloid deposition
B. Loss of intramural ganglion cells
C. Muscular hypertrophy
D. No pathologic abnormalities

20a A 25-year-old patient presents with acute abdominal pain. Plain films suggest a small bowel obstruction, and the patient undergoes a single-contrast barium enema. What is the cause of the finding?

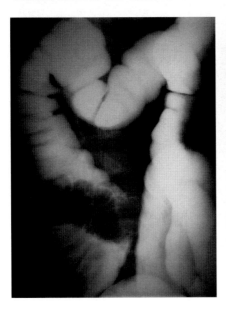 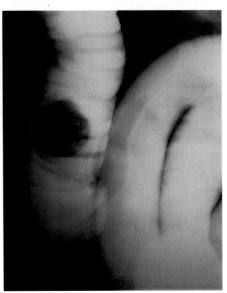

A. Lipomatous ileocecal valve
B. Ileocolic intussusception
C. Appendiceal mucocele
D. Inverted appendiceal stump

20b Regarding the finding above, what are likely associated findings in this 25-year-old patient?

    A. History of perianal fistulae

    B. Mucocutaneous pigmentation perioral region

    C. Gluten sensitivity

    D. Gastroesophageal reflux disease and sclerodactyly

21a A 53-year-old patient presents with right lower quadrant pain. A CT is obtained. What is the likely diagnosis?

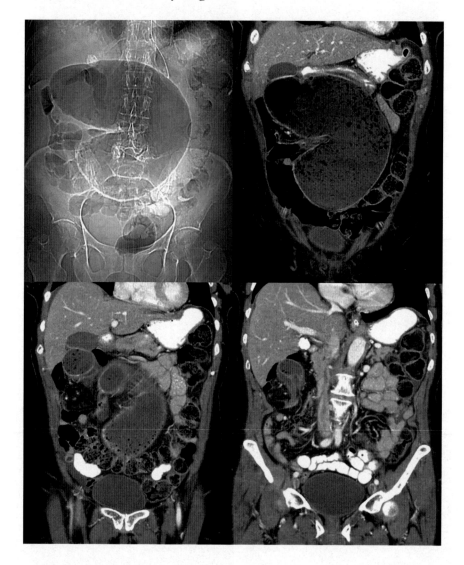

    A. Sigmoid volvulus

    B. Cecal volvulus

    C. Acute appendicitis

    D. Cecal bascule

21b What is the appropriate management for this patient?

    A. Close observation for 24 hours; then discharge if stable

    B. Exploratory laparotomy

    C. Endoscopic decompression

    D. Water-soluble enema reduction

22 An 85-year-old male presents with intermittent bright red blood per rectum and a hematocrit of 28. He receives 2 units of packed red blood cells. Initial colonoscopy fails to detect the site of bleeding. At 11 PM, he becomes hypotensive, develops an episode of ongoing hemorrhage, and has the CT visceral angiogram study below. Following the CT, the bleeding stops, and his blood pressure stabilizes. What is the next step in management?

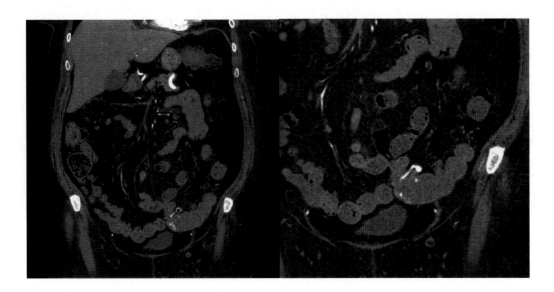

A. Send directly to the angiography suite for catheter embolization.

B. Schedule a repeat emergent colonoscopy within 2 hours.

C. Schedule sigmoid resection within 24 hours.

D. Repeat study with oral contrast to look for an underlying colonic neoplasm.

E. Provide supportive care and observation with reassessment in the morning.

23a A 35-year-old female patient presents to the emergency room with right lower quadrant pain, nausea, and an elevated white blood cell count. The surgery team is concerned about acute appendicitis. She has a positive pregnancy test. What is the next best imaging test for this patient?

A. Low-dose CT without intravenous contrast

B. MRI of the abdomen and pelvis without intravenous contrast

C. Ultrasound of the pelvis, targeted to the right lower quadrant

D. Indium-111 white blood cell scan

23b Ultrasound of the pelvis was performed. Which of the following is true regarding the role of ultrasound imaging in patients with suspected appendicitis?

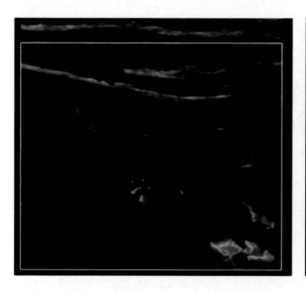 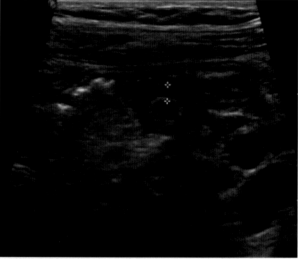

A. Ultrasound examination has high negative predictive value for appendicitis (>95%).

B. Noncompressible blind-ending tubular structure with a diameter >6 mm at the point of maximum tenderness can be considered diagnostic for appendicitis.

C. Presence of periappendiceal fluid on ultrasound examination suggests a diagnosis of ruptured appendicitis.

D. The normal peristalsing small bowel loops in right lower quadrant virtually excludes appendicitis, if the appendix is not visualized.

E. The nonvisualization rate (for a normal appendix) is 10% to 20% on ultrasound.

24a A 45-year-old male presents with acute-onset lower abdominal pain of 2 days' duration. He presents to the emergency department and is found to be afebrile with a normal WBC count. A CT of the abdomen and pelvis is obtained. What is the most likely diagnosis?

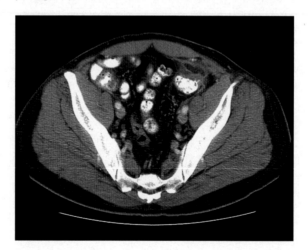

A. Acute appendicitis

B. Diverticulitis

C. Omental infarct

D. Epiploic appendagitis

24b The most appropriate management for the patient would be

    A. Analgesics and outpatient observation
    B. Emergent surgical consultation
    C. Inpatient admission and intravenous antibiotics
    D. Oral antibiotics

25a An asymptomatic 55-year-old male has a screening colonoscopy with findings of an extrinsic bulge at the cecal base. A CT scan is performed the next week. What is the most likely diagnosis?

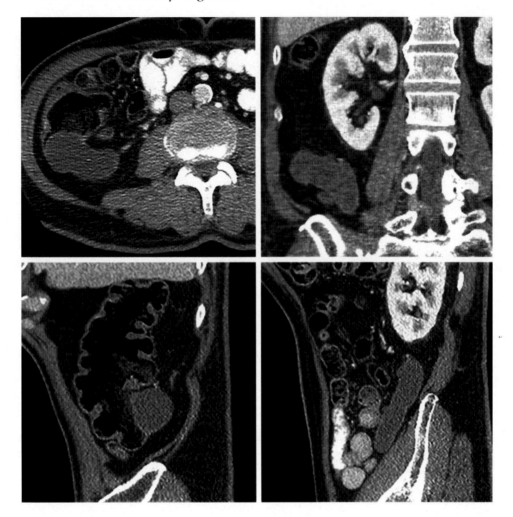

    A. Mucocele
    B. Acute appendicitis
    C. Meckel diverticulum
    D. Epiploic appendagitis

25b What associated feature helps distinguish between a benign versus malignant cause of a mucocele?

    A. Shape
    B. Presence of septations
    C. Calcifications in the wall
    D. Intraperitoneal free fluid
    E. Mural nodularity

26 An 86-year-old male presents with chronic abdominal pain, constipation, and bloating. An abdominal radiograph and a CT are obtained. Approximately what percentage of large bowel obstructions does this finding account for?

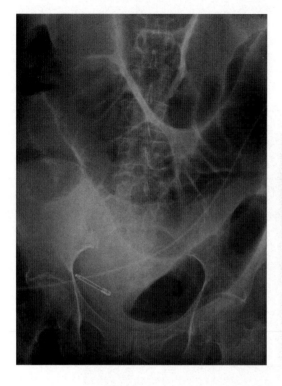

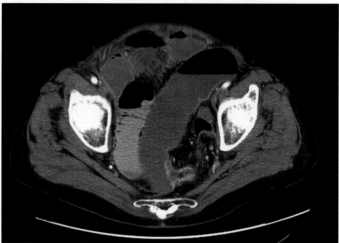

A. 95% or greater
B. 60%
C. 20%
D. Less than 5%

27 A 56-year-old female undergoing chemotherapy for acute myelogenous leukemia presents with abdominal pain and watery diarrhea. The patient is afebrile and has a WBC count of 850 cells/mm³. Regarding neutropenic colitis, which of the following statement is TRUE?

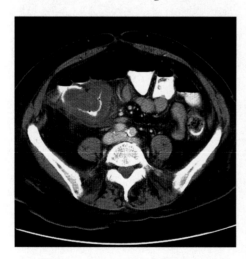

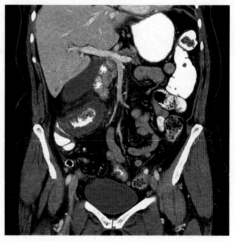

A. The finding more commonly involves the left colon.
B. Pneumatosis intestinalis is an indication for emergent surgery.
C. The radiographic appearance is distinct from that of *C. difficile* colitis.
D. The cause is likely multifactorial with ischemia, hemorrhage, and infection among possible contributing factors

28a A 36-year-old female has a history of intermittent abdominal pain. She undergoes a barium enema. Full abdominal film and spot views of the sigmoid are performed. What are your interpretations of the findings?

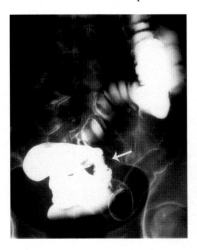 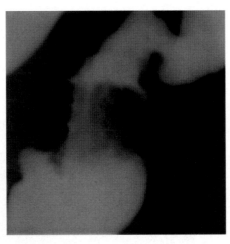 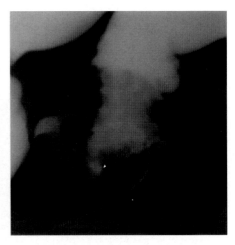

   A. Normal examination
   B. Finding suspicious for a colonic neoplasm
   C. Acute ulcerative colitis changes
   D. Diverticulitis

28b The patient in this case undergoes a colonoscopy, and while luminal narrowing is encountered in the sigmoid, no mucosal abnormality is seen. What is the next best step?

   A. Surgical exploration
   B. CT colonography
   C. MR pelvis with T1-weighted fat-suppressed imaging
   D. Pelvic ultrasound

29 A 28-year-old patient recently completed a course of oral and topical treatment for ulcerative colitis and is currently asymptomatic. What term best describes the polyps seen in the double-contrast barium enema?

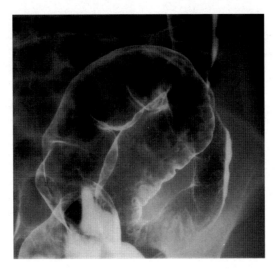

   A. Adenomatous polyps
   B. Acute inflammatory polyps
   C. Postinflammatory polyps
   D. Pseudopolyps with a background of submucosal ulceration

30 In the patients below with inflammatory bowel disease, match the image with the diagnosis with the strongest association. Each answer may be used once, more than once, or not at all.

A. Acute ulcerative colitis
B. Active Crohn enterocolitis
C. Either disease in chronic phase
D. Neither disease

1.

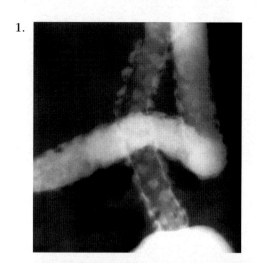

2.

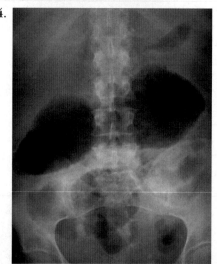

3.

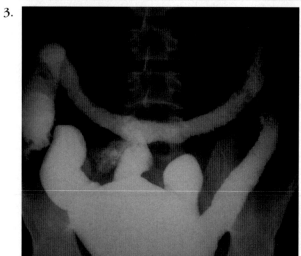

4.

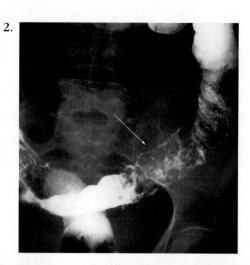

5.

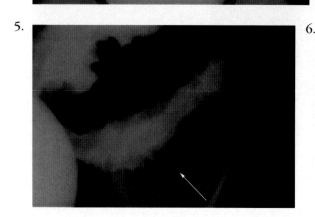

6.

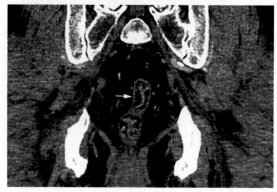

7.
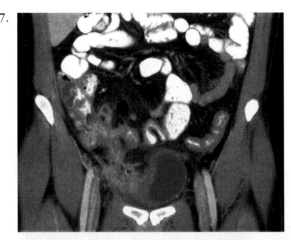

8.
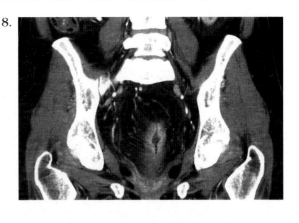

9.
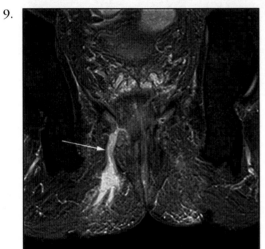
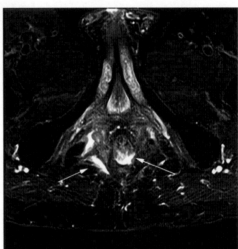

31 A 50-year-old female presents for her first screening CT colonography with the following finding. Before the study could be interpreted, the patient was discharged home in asymptomatic condition. What is the most appropriate next step?

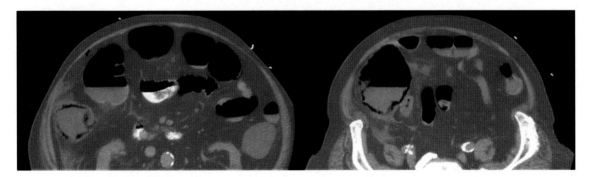

A. Surgical consultation to evaluate for bowel perforation.
B. Surgical consultation to evaluate for bowel ischemia.
C. Gastroenterology consultation to consider colonoscopy.
D. Call the patient and if she is asymptomatic, no treatment is necessary.

32a A 21-year-old female with a 2-year history of intermittent crampy abdominal pain and loose stools presents to the emergency department with fever, worsening abdominal pain over the past week, and bloody diarrhea. What does the CT demonstrate?

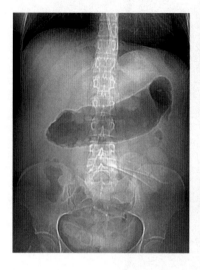
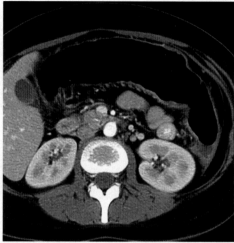
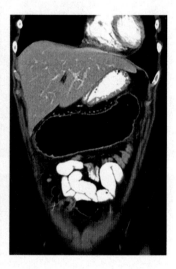

A. Normal bowel gas pattern
B. Dilated stomach
C. Cecal volvulus
D. Toxic colitis

32b What is the most likely etiology?

A. *C. difficile* colitis
B. Ulcerative colitis
C. Ischemic colitis
D. Salmonella colitis

33 An 82-year-old male with a history of intermittent abdominal pain and inability to pass gas or stool had a CT performed. What is the cause of the obstruction?

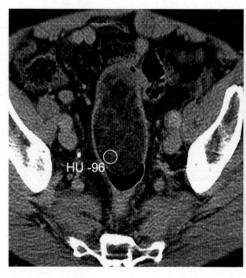
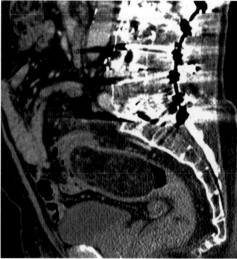

A. Adenocarcinoma
B. Lipoma
C. Stool ball
D. Villous adenoma

34a A 29-year-old female presents with abdominal pain and fullness. The following CT images are obtained. A colonoscopy is performed, and biopsy of the cecal mass reveals adenocarcinoma. The patient's father died at age 48 of colon cancer, and a maternal aunt was recently diagnosed with a large colonic polyp. What is the most likely diagnosis?

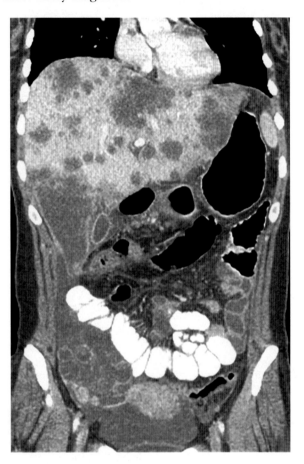

A. Familial adenomatosis polyposis
B. Hereditary nonpolyposis colorectal cancer (Lynch syndrome)
C. Gardner syndrome
D. Cronkhite-Canada syndrome

34b What additional imaging should be considered for this patient?

A. PET scan
B. Octreotide scan
C. Pelvic ultrasound and endometrial sampling
D. Thyroid ultrasound

35a A 20-year-old male presents with a palpable abnormality at the angle of the jaw. What additional study should be considered?

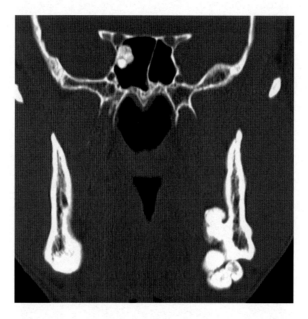

A. Double-contrast barium enema or colonoscopy
B. CT enterography
C. MRCP
D. Brain MRI with contrast

35b A 35-year-old patient presents with the following findings:

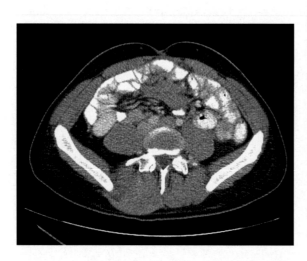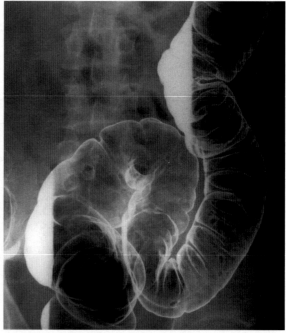

Which of the following genetic abnormality is present?

A. Germ-line mutation in *APC* gene on chromosome 5q21
B. Defect in a DNA mismatch repair gene
C. Mutation in the *PTEN* gene on arm 10q
D. A germ-line mutation of the *STK11/LKB1* tumor suppressor gene

36 A 25-year-old female presents with abdominal pain, fever, and bloody diarrhea of 4 days onset. She has no history of prior similar episodes and is otherwise healthy. The emergency department physician is concerned for acute appendicitis and orders a CT of the abdomen and pelvis. What do you recommend next?

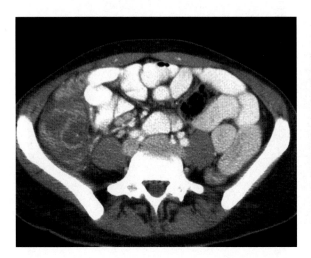 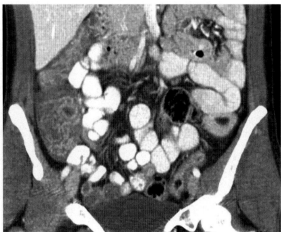

A. Surgical consultation for acute appendicitis

B. Intravenous corticosteroids for acute ulcerative colitis flare

C. Stool cultures and empiric antibiotics

D. CT angiogram for suspected embolic ischemic colitis

37 Match the following type of infections with the typical distribution of the colitis. Each answer may be used once, more than once, or not at all.

A. *Salmonella typhi*

B. *Mycobacterium tuberculosis*

C. *Chlamydia trachomatis* (lymphogranuloma venereum)

D. *Entamoeba histolytica*

E. *Shigella*

F. Cytomegalovirus

G. Shiga toxin–producing *E. coli*

1. More often right sided

2. More often left sided

3. Most commonly diffuse

38 The inpatient below presented with abdominal pain and diarrhea following a course of antibiotic therapy. The cause of this process is thought to be secondary to which of the following organism?

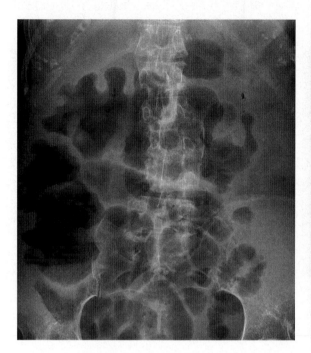 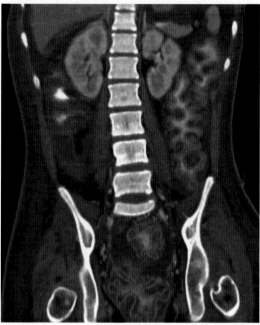

A. Gram-negative anaerobe producing toxin D
B. Gram-positive anaerobe producing toxin B
C. Gram-negative aerobe producing toxin A
D. Gram-positive aerobe producing toxin C

ANSWERS AND EXPLANATIONS

1 **Answer C.** There is a blind-ending tubular structure 11 mm in diameter extending from the cecum with slightly thickened and enhancing walls. Mild stranding of the surrounding fat is noted. Findings are consistent with **acute appendicitis**. There is no localized fluid collection or extraluminal gas collections to indicate perforation or abscess.

Acute appendicitis is a common entity, accounting for up to 14% of all cases of acute abdominal pain presenting to the emergency department. Although ultrasound may be performed instead of CT in a young patient to avoid radiation, CT has the highest accuracy (95% to 98%) for detection of acute appendicitis. It is ideally performed with intravenous contrast. Oral contrast may help distinguish between unopacified bowel loops and abscesses, but lack of enteric contrast has not been shown to alter the diagnostic quality significantly in patients presenting with acute abdominal pain.

The findings of a dilated appendix (>6 mm in diameter) and surrounding fat stranding have a high positive predictive value for diagnosing acute appendicitis. The presence of an appendicolith is less helpful, as these may be seen in patients who do not have active inflammation. **Note also that the diameter of >6 mm may not necessarily indicate appendicitis in the absence of wall thickening and periappendiceal inflammatory fat stranding**. The combined findings in this case are highly specific, and a pelvic ultrasound to assess for an alternate diagnosis is unnecessary. A case of suspected acute appendicitis requires **urgent surgical evaluation**. Untreated appendicitis may lead to perforation, which is associated with a 2 to 10 times increase in mortality rates compared to uncomplicated appendicitis as well as significant increased morbidity.

References: Stoker J, van Randen A, Lameris W, et al. Imaging patients with acute abdominal pain. *Radiology* 2009;253(1):31–46.

Pinto Leite N, Pereira JM, Cunha R, et al. CT evaluation of appendicitis and its complications: imaging techniques and key diagnostic findings. *AJR Am J Roentgenol* 2005;185(2):406–417.

2a **Answer A.** There is a dilated tubular structure in the right lower quadrant with wall thickening and adjacent inflammatory fat stranding consistent with **acute appendicitis**. The terminal ileum is normal, and there is no cecal wall thickening or diverticula demonstrated. No extraluminal gas or abscess is documented.

2b **Answer D.** This patient's symptoms are very mild and responded well to initial intravenous antibiotics. Continued treatment is still warranted to prevent complications of perforation and consequent peritonitis and pelvic abscess. The standard of care for the treatment of acute appendicitis historically has been surgical appendectomy within 12 to 24 hours, performed now most commonly with laparoscopic technique. However, recent clinical trials suggest another option is **antibiotic therapy alone (initially intravenous followed by an oral course) with close follow-up may be sufficient for some cases of uncomplicated appendicitis.** The patient in this case received 1 day of intravenous antibiotics and was discharged on a course of oral antibiotics. A follow-up CT was performed showing complete resolution of inflammatory changes.

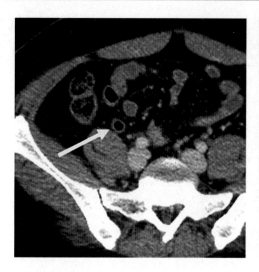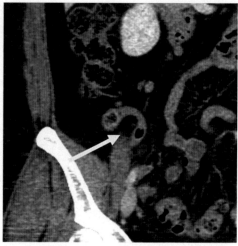

References: Salminen P, Tuominen R, Paajanen H, et al. Five-year follow-up of antibiotic therapy for uncomplicated acute appendicitis in the APPAC Randomized Clinical Trial. *JAMA* 2018;320(12):1259–1265.

Smink D, Soybel D. Management of acute appendicitis in adults. In: Weiser M (ed), *UpToDate*. Waltham, MA: UpToDate. Accessed on June 5, 2020.

3a **Answer B.** The findings on the CT are of sigmoid diverticula, wall thickening, and pericolonic fat infiltration. These findings are consistent with **acute uncomplicated diverticulitis**. No free intraperitoneal gas or associated abscess is seen. Most cases of acute diverticulitis are simple (75%) and can be managed as an outpatient. The remaining 25% are complicated, with associated abscesses, fistula, obstruction, peritonitis, or sepsis. Urgent surgery is necessary in cases of ongoing perforation, which is uncommon. Management of acute uncomplicated diverticulitis includes a 7- to 14-day course of broad-spectrum oral antibiotics and a low-residue diet. Colonoscopy is relatively contraindicated in the acute setting, as insufflation can increase the risk of free perforation. A single-contrast barium enema was formerly performed prior to the widespread use of CT. Classic findings of acute diverticulitis include intramural contrast ("tram-tracking") in a segment of colon with diverticula and luminal narrowing. The enema examination is uncomfortable for the patient due to colonic spasm. CT can assess the degree of proximal obstruction and is superior to the enema in evaluation of the extraluminal tissues for abscess and free perforation. CT can also diagnose other conditions mimicking diverticulitis including inflammatory bowel disease, epiploic appendagitis, malignancy, and adnexal pathology.

3b **Answer D.** Diverticula form in an area of relative weakness in the bowel where the vasa recta penetrate the bowel wall. They are **pulsion-type pseudodiverticula** (not traction-type). Increased intraluminal pressure or trauma from food particles erode the wall and cause a localized microperforation, which is usually walled off by adjacent fat. The diverticula are most commonly found in the sigmoid and descending colon. **They are not seen in the rectum where the longitudinal muscle covers the entire circumference of the bowel.**

Acute diverticulitis may cause partial obstruction but is a relatively uncommon cause of complete obstruction, accounting for 10% of all large bowel obstructions. Diverticular disease is more common in older individuals with a prevalence of 5% by age 40, 30% by age 60, and 65% by age 80.

References: Thoeni RF, Cello JP. CT imaging of colitis. *Radiology* 2006;240(3):623–638.

World Gastroenterology Organisation (WGO). Practice Guidelines. Diverticular disease. 2007. Available at http://www.worldgastroenterology.org/diverticular-disease.html. Accessed on July 4, 2015.

4a **Answer C.** The CT demonstrates a few sigmoid colonic diverticula, sigmoid wall thickening, and some infiltration of the pericolic fat. While the inflammatory changes support the suspicion of diverticulitis, the degree of wall thickening is concerning for a mass.

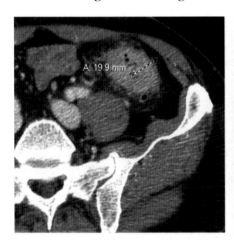 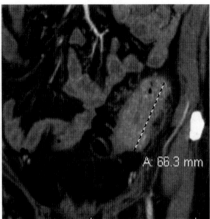

Following completion of the antibiotic therapy, a follow-up colonoscopy was performed, which revealed a colon carcinoma. Pathology showed transmural extension of tumor into the pericolic fat.

4b **Answers: A-3; B-2; C-2; D-1; E-2; F-1.**

Some findings on CT are helpful in the distinction between acute diverticulitis and colon cancer.

CT Features Favoring Acute Diverticulitis or Colon Cancer	
Favors acute diverticulitis	• Involves segment ≥10 cm • Pericolic fat stranding
Favors colon cancer	• Wall thickness >1 cm • Luminal narrowing with squared shoulders • Enlarged pericolic lymph nodes

Note that just the presence of diverticula does not necessarily favor diverticulitis as diverticula are prevalent in both patient groups. The demographics of colon cancer and diverticulitis overlap in that these conditions are both found in older individuals in industrialized countries. Recommendations of treatment for diverticulitis published in 2006 by the American Society of Colon and Rectal Surgery include follow-up colonoscopy 6 to 8 weeks following resolution of acute diverticulitis for differentiation from colon cancer, ischemia, and inflammatory bowel disease. Recent studies have questioned the need for routine colonoscopy following uncomplicated acute diverticulitis due to the low yield in such cases. However, **colonoscopy should still be performed for cases where radiographic features overlap with malignancy or clinical course is protracted.**

References: Ben Yaacoub I, Boulay-Coletta I, Julles MC, et al. CT findings of misleading features of colonic diverticulitis. *Insights Imaging* 2011;2(1):69–84.

Lips LM, Cremers PT, Pickhardt PJ, et al. Sigmoid cancer versus chronic diverticular disease: differentiating features at CT colonography. *Radiology* 2015;275(1):127–135.

5 **Answer C.** Coronal and axial contrast-enhanced CT images demonstrate diffuse sigmoid wall thickening with perisigmoid mesenteric inflammatory changes and free fluid consistent with acute diverticulitis. There is diffuse bladder wall thickening and air within the bladder. Findings are consistent with diverticulitis with **a colovesical fistula**. A colovesical fistula is a communication between the colonic and bladder lumina.

The most common etiologies include

- Diverticulitis (60%)
- Colorectal cancer (20%)
- Crohn disease (10%)
- Radiation therapy for pelvic malignancy
- Appendicitis
- Trauma

The clinical presentation may include pneumaturia, fecaluria, recurrent urinary tract infections, and rectal passage of urine.

Imaging findings include air within the bladder, perivesicular inflammatory changes, demonstration of the actual fistula on fluoroscopy or CT cystogram, and associated findings from the underlying cause (i.e., diverticulitis, Crohn disease, or malignancy). The fistula is located in the dome of the bladder in 60% of cases, in the posterior wall in 30%, or the trigone in 10%.

Reference: Pollard SG, Macfarlane R, Greatorex R, et al. Colovesical fistula. *Ann R Coll Surg Engl* 1987;69(4):163–165.

6a **Answer C.** The CT and barium enema show a segmental fixed stricture in the distal transverse colon with a laminar enhancement pattern (submucosal edema) and adjacent mesenteric fatty stranding. Margins of the stricture are smooth. Colonic narrowing can be related to a wide variety of infectious, inflammatory, and iatrogenic etiologies. In this particular **watershed location near the splenic flexure** in a patient with a history of myocardial infarcts, ischemic colitis with resultant stricture is the most likely etiology. The stricture is shorter than would be expected for radiation colitis. No diverticula are identified to suggest diverticulitis. While a segment of Crohn colitis may have a similar appearance, the clinical presentation is more compatible with ischemia.

6b **Answer D.** **Griffiths critical point** refers to a watershed area in the colon occurring near the splenic flexure. It is formed by an anastomosis between the ascending left colic arteries, a branch of the inferior mesenteric artery (IMA), with the marginal artery of Drummond. This anastomosis is absent in 43% of patients or tenuous in 9%. When this anastomosis is absent or poor, the colon near the splenic flexure is susceptible to ischemia.

Sudeck point is a similar watershed area in the rectosigmoid colon arterial supply at the anastomosis between the superior rectal artery and the last sigmoid branch of the IMA.

References: Meyers MA. Griffiths' point: critical anastomosis at the splenic flexure. Significance in ischemia of the colon. *AJR Am J Roentgenol* 1976;126(1):77–94.

van Tonder JJ, Boon JM, Becker JH, et al. Anatomical considerations on Sudeck's critical point and its relevance to colorectal surgery. *Clin Anat* 2007;20(4):424–427.

Wiesner W, Khurana B, Ji H, et al. CT of acute bowel ischemia. *Radiology* 2003;226(3).

7a **Answer C.** The cecum and appendix are supplied by the ileocolic artery, a superior mesenteric artery (SMA) branch. The ascending colon and hepatic flexure are supplied by the ileocolic and right colic arteries, which are branches of the SMA. The transverse colon is supplied primarily by the middle colic artery, an SMA branch. Some of the transverse colon may also be supplied by anastomotic arcades between the right and left colic arteries. The descending and sigmoid colon are supplied by the left colic and sigmoid arteries, which are inferior mesenteric artery (IMA) branches. The junction of the blood supply from the SMA and IMA in the left transverse colon denotes the embryologic division between the midgut and the hindgut. The rectum and anal canal are supplied by the superior rectal artery, a continuation of the IMA. The lower rectum is supplied by the middle and inferior rectal arteries, branches of the internal iliac arteries.

7b **Answer D.** The **arc of Riolan** is a collateral bordering arcade between the proximal middle colic artery (an SMA branch) or right transverse branch of the right colic artery and a branch of the left colic artery (an IMA branch). This arcade is located near the root of the mesentery in a relatively proximal location. The **marginal artery of Drummond** is also a collateral artery between branches of the SMA and IMA but is located peripherally, forming a continuous arterial circle along the inner border of the colonic wall. The junction between branches of the SMA and IMA territories may be variably discontinuous (this area is known as Griffiths point) and is a watershed zone prone to ischemia.

The arc of Buhler is a persistent anastomosis between branches of embryonic ventral segmental arteries, forming a connection between the celiac and superior mesenteric artery.

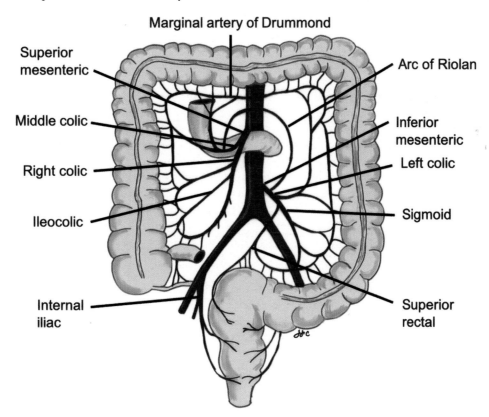

References: DiPoce J, Jimenez G, Weintraub J. Historical perspective: eponyms of vascular radiology. *Radiographics* 2014;34(4):1120–1140.

Meyers MA. Griffiths' point: critical anastomosis at the splenic flexure. Significance in ischemia of the colon. *AJR Am J Roentgenol* 1976;126(1):77–94.

8 **Answer B.** The ascending, descending, and lower two-thirds of the rectum are retroperitoneal. The cecum, transverse, and sigmoid colon have a mesentery and are intraperitoneal.

9a   **Answer C.** There is a dilated loop of bowel on the CT scout with an "upside down U" configuration or "coffee bean" appearance, the cleft of the bean formed by the two apposed walls of the sigmoid. The axial CT image demonstrates a whirlpool sign of twisted compressed sigmoid colonic loops with radiating engorged vessels, which confirms the diagnosis of a sigmoid volvulus. The normal right colon can be seen on both the axial CT and the scout image, which excludes the diagnosis of cecal bascule and cecal volvulus. Acute diverticulitis accounts for 10% of all cases of LBO, and neither colonic diverticula nor the characteristic inflammatory changes are demonstrated on this CT.

Sigmoid volvulus occurs when the sigmoid twists along its mesenteric axis causing a closed loop obstruction. Sigmoid volvulus is three to four times more common than cecal volvulus. It occurs most commonly in the elderly, who are more likely to have an elongated and chronically dilated sigmoid colon. The diagnosis is often obvious on plain film radiography with the previously mentioned signs. CT can confirm the diagnosis and assess for evidence of bowel ischemia or perforation.

A water-soluble enema, performed under low pressure may help distinguish between an obstructed volvulus versus nonobstructed dilated sigmoid colon. When obstruction is present, a "bird's beak" appearance of the contrast column is encountered at the point of obstruction.

References: Jaffe T, Thompson WM. Large-bowel obstruction in the adult: classic radiographic and CT findings, etiology, and mimics. *Radiology* 2015;275(3):651–663.

Osiro SB, Cunningham D, Shoja MM, et al. The twisted colon: a review of sigmoid volvulus. *Am Surg* 2012;78:271–279.

Peterson CM, Anderson JS, Hara AK, et al. Volvulus of the gastrointestinal tract: appearances at multimodality imaging. *Radiographics* 2009;29:1281–1293.

9b   **Answer D.** Surgical consultation is recommended for any patient with suspected sigmoid volvulus. Initial endoscopic reduction may be attempted in stable patients and is successful in 75% to 95% of patients. Emergent surgery is typically indicated in patients with peritonitis, unsuccessful endoscopic decompression, or when there is evidence of bowel ischemia. Sigmoid volvulus is the third most common cause of large bowel obstruction in adults in the United States but is the leading cause in many other parts of the world including Africa and Asia.

References: Hodin RA. Sigmoid volvulus. In: Lamont JT (ed). *UpToDate*. Waltham, MA: UpToDate. Accessed on July 17, 2015.

Osiro SB, Cunningham D, Shoja MM, et al. The twisted colon: a review of sigmoid volvulus. *Am Surg* 2012;78(3):271–279.

10   **Answer C.** Axial, surface-rendered, and endoluminal 3D views from a CT colonography show an annular constricting transverse colonic mass, which is likely the reason for the incomplete colonoscopy. CT colonography is the study of choice over air-contrast barium enema for screening the nonvisualized proximal colon to exclude a synchronous mass or polyp. If performed with IV contrast, CT colonography can also simultaneously stage the remainder of the abdomen and pelvis for operative or oncologic management. This annular constricting mass is highly suspicious for malignancy. The most appropriate next step in management for this C-RADS C4 lesion is histologic correlation. This could be obtained by repeat colonoscopy with biopsy versus surgical consultation for consideration of colonic resection.

Reference: Zalis ME, Barish MA, Choi JR, et al. CT colonography reporting and data system: a consensus proposal. *Radiology* 2005;236(1):3–9.

11a   **Answer C.** The finding on this single-contrast examination is a pedunculated polyp approximately 1.5 cm in size. As this does not appear to be a hyperplastic polyp and is >1 cm in size, the lesion cannot be classified as benign and should be resected. As the lesion is pedunculated, it is amenable to a snare polypectomy performed during a colonoscopy. The risk of invasive malignancy is lower than for a sessile polyp of comparable size and does not justify the increased risk of a sigmoid colectomy over colonoscopic resection. A polypectomy is required to assess for invasion into the stalk, so a limited biopsy is not appropriate. Full colonic preparation is not required for a sigmoidoscopy but would be necessary if electrocautery is to be performed to minimize the rare risk of a colonic explosion due to excess colonic gas. Finally, the presence of a left-sided colonic lesion should prompt investigation of the entire colon for a metachronous proximal lesion.

Reference: Taylor JM, Hosie KB. The malignant polyp: polypectomy or surgical resection? In: Dr. Marco Bustamante (ed). *Colonoscopy and colorectal cancer screening - future directions.* InTech, 2013. ISBN: 978-953-51-0949-5, doi: 10.5772/52865.

11b Answer B. Most colon cancers are thought to develop directly from adenomatous polyps. The risk for a polyp containing an invasive cancer is directly related to size. A polyp below 1 cm in size, which represents the vast majority of polyps, has a <1% risk of containing a malignancy. A polyp between 1 and 2 cm has an approximate 10% risk of containing a malignancy, and a polyp >2 cm has a risk of >25%. Villous adenomas are also much more likely than tubular adenomas to contain malignancy.

References: Gazelle GS, McMahon PM, Scholz FJ. Screening for colorectal cancer. *Radiology* 2000;215(2):327–335.

Lieberman DA, Rex DK, Winawer SJ, et al. Guidelines for colonoscopy surveillance after screening and polypectomy: a consensus update by the US Multi-Society Task Force on Colorectal Cancer. *Gastroenterology* 2012;143(3):844–857.

12a Answer D. Images demonstrate a large circumferential mass at the splenic flexure of the colon. The wall is markedly thickened, and there is no obstruction. This mass is not a polypoid tubulovillous adenoma. The mass is notable for the low attenuation of the wall, suggesting a mucinous neoplasm. The low attenuation would not be atypical for a neuroendocrine tumor. A large gastrointestinal stromal tumor may have low attenuation due to necrosis, but gastrointestinal stromal tumors are rare (<1% of colorectal tumors) compared to the much more common adenocarcinomas (95% to 97% of colorectal tumors).

12b Answer E. Mucinous colorectal carcinomas are a subtype of adenocarcinoma that produce a large amount of extracellular mucin (≥50% of the tumor mass). This mucin results in a lower attenuation on CT compared to the nonmucinous type of adenocarcinoma. The extracellular mucin tends to dissect through the colonic wall, and bowel wall thickening is often more severe (>2 cm) and eccentric with mucinous tumors. Mucinous tumors have a greater tendency for intratumoral calcifications and demonstrate more heterogeneous contrast enhancement than nonmucinous tumors. **Mucinous carcinomas are noted for their higher incidence of lymphatic invasion, local recurrence, and distant metastases leading to an overall worse prognosis than the nonmucinous variety**.

References: Green JB, Timmcke AE, Mitchell WT, et al. Mucinous carcinoma—just another colon cancer? *Dis Colon Rectum* 1993;36(1):49–54.

Horton KM, Abrams RA, Fishman EK. Spiral CT of colon cancer: imaging features and role in management. *Radiographics* 2000;20(2):419–430.

Ko EY, Ha HK, Kim AY, et al. CT differentiation of mucinous and nonmucinous colorectal carcinoma. *AJR Am J Roentgenol* 2007;188(3):785–791.

13 **Answer C.** Axial T2-weighted image shows a sessile polypoid mass along the left rectal wall with intermediate signal consistent with rectal cancer. Disruption of the low signal intensity muscularis propria layer is seen at the central portion of the mass, which is the invasive margin. The intermediate tumor signal extends into the adjacent fat (and not into any pelvic organ or peritoneum) consistent with T3 stage disease.

Colorectal cancer is the third most common cancer in the United States. Rectal cancer is prone to local recurrence and systemic metastatic disease. The use of total mesorectal excision (TME) and neoadjuvant chemoradiotherapy for locally advanced cancer has significantly improved local disease control. Rectal MRI using a phased-array coil and fast spin-echo T2-weighted sequences provides high spatial resolution images for accurate primary tumor (T) staging. This allows for **assessment of mesorectal fascial involvement for determination of the circumferential resection margin**. Rectal MRI is also useful for regional lymph nodes (N), local metastasis (M) staging (with additional distant metastatic staging completed with larger field abdominopelvic MR and/or CT), and for extramural vascular invasion.

Tumor limited to the submucosa indicates T1 stage disease and is implied by the presence of lower signal intensity tumor within the relatively high signal intensity submucosa but with preservation of the relatively low signal intensity outer muscularis propria layer of the rectal wall. Extension of higher signal intensity tumor within the relatively low signal intensity muscularis propria without extramural extension represents T2 stage disease. Visualization of lower signal intensity tumor extension from the rectal wall into the high signal intensity perirectal fat indicates at least T3 stage disease. This tumor extension may be broad-based, nodular, or spiculated, although in some cases low signal intensity desmoplastic tissue may mimic tumor, potentially leading to overstaging. Lastly, visualization of tumor invasion directly into adjacent organs such as the prostate gland, seminal vesicles, bladder, uterus, or vagina, or through a peritoneal reflection indicates T4 stage disease.

At some institutions, endoscopic ultrasound is performed for T staging of rectal cancer. This is a more operator-dependent technique.

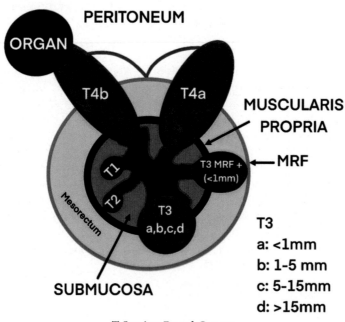

T Staging Rectal Cancer.

References: Horvat N, Carlos Tavares Rocha C, Clemente Oliveira B, et al. MRI of rectal cancer: tumor staging, imaging techniques, and management. *Radiographics* 2019;39(2): 367–387.

Kaur H, Choi H, You YN, et al. MR imaging for preoperative evaluation of primary rectal cancer: practical considerations. *Radiographics* 2012;32(2):389–409.

14 **Answer B.** The CT scan shows diffuse wall thickening of the colon from the splenic flexure to the distal descending colon with sparing of the right and transverse colon. This follows the vascular distribution supplied by the inferior mesenteric artery. Given the long segment of involvement, an embolic source (cardioversion in this case) is the most likely cause of this ischemic colitis, in the setting of poor collateral circulation. The segmental nature of the colitis would be unusual for both pseudomembranous and infectious colitis (conditions implied by the scenarios in answers A and C). While diverticulitis is common in the elderly population, the segment of involvement is much longer than expected, and hematochezia is not a common finding at presentation.

References: Thoeni RF, Cello JP. CT imaging of colitis. *Radiology* 2006;240(3):623–638.

Washington C, Carmichael JC. Management of ischemic colitis. *Clin Colon Rectal Surg* 2012;25(4):228–235.

15 **Answer C.** The venous drainage of the colon and upper rectum is to the portal vein. Thus, tumors of the colon and upper rectum (transverse, distal descending, right colon in answers A, B, and D) will most commonly metastasize to the liver initially. The lower rectum has dual drainage. The superior hemorrhoidal vein drains into the inferior mesenteric drain and then into the portal vein. The middle and inferior hemorrhoidal veins drain into iliac veins and then the inferior vena cava. Thus, a lower rectal tumor may present with pulmonary metastases bypassing the liver. Isolated lung metastases are twice as more likely in rectal CA than colon CA.

References: Horton KM, Abrams RA, Fishman EK. Spiral CT of colon cancer: imaging features and role in management. *Radiographics* 2000;20(2):419–430.

Tan KK, Lopes Gde L Jr, Sim R. How uncommon are isolated lung metastases in colorectal cancer? A review from database of 754 patients over 4 years. *J Gastrointest Surg* 2009;13(4):642–648.

16a **Answer B.** The MRI demonstrates an intermediate signal intensity mass in the mid to lower anal canal extending to the anal verge favoring an anal primary tumor. Rectal cancers of the anorectal region are much more common than anal cancers, and their territories may overlap when the tumors are extensive, rendering identification of the primary origin ambiguous. Histology is central to the distinction between anal and rectal cancers. **The majority (80% to 85%) of anal cancers are a squamous histologic subtype, in distinction to rectal cancers, which are almost all adenocarcinomas.** Anal cancers are strongly associated with human papilloma virus (HPV), with increased risk in patients with human immunodeficiency virus (HIV) infection.

Identification of the primary tumor origin is important because anal cancers and low rectal cancers have different patterns of nodal and systemic spread and are staged and treated differently.

Anal carcinoma is relatively uncommon, accounting for 1.5% of gastrointestinal tract cancers. Imaging with pelvic MRI, with its high contrast resolution, provides important information for primary locoregional staging and assessment of treatment response. Transanal ultrasound may be more accurate than MRI for detection of small superficial tumors but does not include important lymph node stations higher in the pelvis or the groin. FDG PET/CT is also used for assessment of primary tumor size, lymph node involvement, and distant metastases.

16b **Answer D. Primary anal cancers are staged entirely on the basis of size and not the depth of invasion**. The sphincter complex is the structure most commonly infiltrated, followed by the rectum. Tumors that invade the vagina, bladder, urethra, and prostate are T4 tumors, but involvement of the anal sphincter muscles, rectal wall, perianal, skin or subcutaneous tissues does not constitute T4 disease.

The dentate line is an important landmark that may be seen macroscopically but is not delineated on MRI; it is estimated to be near the junction of the upper two-thirds and the lower third of the anal canal. Anal canal tumors with epicenter below the dentate line drain to the inguinal and femoral lymph nodes, while those with epicenter above the dentate line drain to the perirectal, internal iliac, and retroperitoneal nodes.

Inguinal lymph node involvement in patients with anal cancers as in this case is an important independent prognostic factor (for treatment response and overall mortality).

References: Kochhar R, Plumb AA, Carrington BM, et al. Imaging of anal carcinoma. *AJR Am J Roentgenol* 2012;199(3):W335–344.

Matalon SA, Mamon HJ, Fuchs CS, et al. Anorectal cancer: critical anatomic and staging distinctions that affect use of radiation therapy. *Radiographics* 2015;35(7):2090–2107.

Surabhi VR, Menias CO, Amer AM, et al. Tumors and tumorlike conditions of the anal canal and perianal region: MR imaging findings. *Radiographics* 2016;36(5):1339–1353.

17a **Answer B.** No bowel wall thickening to suggest an underlying colitis is seen. Adhesions are a very rare cause of acute colonic obstruction in distinction to small bowel obstruction. There are no inflammatory changes at the transition of caliber to suggest an acute diverticulitis.

The imaging findings and clinical setting are consistent with an **acute colonic pseudoobstruction (ACPO)**. ACPO, also known as Ogilvie syndrome, involves the development of markedly dilated colon in the absence of a mechanical obstruction. The condition is usually seen in hospitalized debilitated patients with serious underlying conditions such as myocardial infarction, trauma, sepsis, recent surgery, and neurologic abnormalities. The onset may be rapid or insidious (over 3–5 days). **The dilatation usually involves the proximal colon including the ascending and transverse colon, typically with a transition to decompressed bowel at the splenic flexure.** Occasionally, the transition point may be more distal or absent. The greatest dilatation is at the cecum, due to the inverse relationship between the intraluminal pressure needed to distend a viscus and the diameter (Laplace law). In this patient with an incompetent ileocecal valve, there is also small bowel dilatation. The pathophysiology of ACPO is not fully understood, but an imbalance of the autonomic innervation to the colon with excess sympathetic tone and/or diminished parasympathetic tone is felt to be contributory.

17b **Answer D.** In acute colonic pseudoobstruction (ACPO), the increased intraluminal pressure in the bowel in the setting of a competent ileocecal valve elevates the risk of bowel perforation, so early intervention is important. If a mechanical obstruction at the transition is still considered a possibility after the CT, a water-soluble iodinated contrast enema may be performed, but barium is contraindicated due to the risk of perforation and barium peritonitis. Nasogastric tube placement is recommended but may not be as helpful in the setting of a competent ileocecal valve. Distal decompression is optimal, and colonoscopic decompression is the most effective treatment. This may need to be repeated if the distention recurs, or a rectal tube may be left in place. Pharmacologic agents that stimulate colonic motility also may be considered, such as neostigmine.

References: Choi JS, Lim JS, Kim H, et al. Colonic pseudoobstruction: CT findings. *AJR Am J Roentgenol* 2008;190(6):1521–1526.

De Giorgio R, Knowles CH. Acute colonic pseudo-obstruction. *Br J Surg* 2009;96(3):229–239.

18 **Answer A.** With a competent ileocecal valve, an obstructing colonic lesion results in a closed-loop obstruction. In the small bowel, the most common site for perforation is just proximal to the point of obstruction. In the colon, **the most common site for perforation is the cecum**, regardless of where the downstream obstruction is located. Laplace law states that the intraluminal pressure needed to distend a hollow viscus is inversely proportional to the diameter. As the cecum has the greatest diameter of any segment of the colon, the tension on the wall is greatest placing it at the highest risk for ischemia, necrosis, and perforation. Cutoff values for maximal normal colonic diameter are reported to be in the range of >6 cm for the transverse colon and >9 cm for the cecum. Risk of cecal perforation increases at a diameter of 10 cm, but the acuity of the onset of obstruction is equally important, with rapid onset of dilatation posing a higher risk for perforation.

Reference: Krajewski K, Siewert B, Eisenberg RL. Colonic dilation. *AJR Am J Roentgenol* 2009;193(5):W363–W372.

19 **Answer B.** The CT scout from the current study demonstrates diffuse colonic dilatation, with the corresponding coronal reconstruction from that examination showing involvement including the distal rectum. The scout from a CT performed 8 months earlier demonstrates an almost identical pattern.

Colonic pseudoobstruction may be acute or chronic. The chronic form presents with a history of recurrent obstructive symptoms such as chronic constipation and absence of a history of major surgery or illness, as is typical with the acute form. **As with any cause of colonic dilatation, decompression is indicated when the cecal diameter exceeds about 12 cm, although perforation is rare in chronic pseudoobstruction compared to the acute form.** The chronic form is difficult to treat and does not respond to parasympathetomimetic agents. Although surgery has not found to be effective, in cases where surgery has been performed or a full-thickness biopsy of the colonic wall has been obtained, atrophic changes with decreased number of intramural ganglion cells have been described. In some cases, inflammatory or neoplastic causes for ganglion dysfunction have been documented.

References: Choi JS, Lim JS, Kim H, et al. Colonic pseudoobstruction: CT findings. *AJR Am J Roentgenol* 2008;190(6):1521–1526.

De Giorgio R, Sarnelli G, Corinaldesi R, et al. Advances in our understanding of the pathology of chronic intestinal pseudo-obstruction. *Gut* 2004;53(11):1549–1552.

20a **Answer B.** The finding on the barium enema is of a mass in the colon with a "**coiled-spring**" appearance consistent with an ileocolic **intussusception**. On CT, as in this example from another patient, the diagnosis of intussusception is readily apparent with a target appearance with central mesenteric fat and vessels associated with the intussusceptum telescoping into the adjacent bowel, the intussuscipiens.

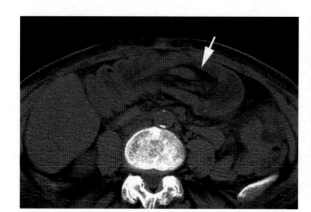
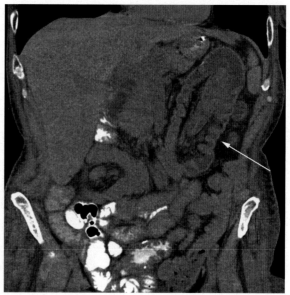

The lesion is not at the cecal tip and therefore not associated with the appendix. While in the region of the ileocecal valve, a lipomatous ileocecal valve has a morphology resembling lips, not concentric rings.

20b **Answer B.** Intussusceptions are much more common in the pediatric population, in which they are most commonly idiopathic. **In adults, 70% to 90% of intussusceptions are caused by a lead point.** Small bowel intussusceptions may occur without a lead point in adult patients with celiac sprue (answer C), bowel motility disorders such as progressive systemic sclerosis (answer D), or Crohn disease (answer A), but these intussusceptions are transient and nonobstructive. These patients may have mild intermittent pain or be asymptomatic. Such intussusceptions have been recognized more frequently with widespread use of CT.

In this case, the intussusceptum is large and was responsible for bowel obstruction, indicating a likely lead point in an adult patient. Among the options, mucocutaneous pigmentation in the perioral region is seen with Peutz-Jeghers, which would be associated with a mass acting as a potential lead point. Peutz-Jeghers syndrome is an autosomal dominant condition associated with multiple hamartomas, which may be found in the stomach, small bowel, and colon. The small bowel hamartomatous polyps frequently lead to intussusceptions as in this case. **Although these polyps are not premalignant, Peutz-Jeghers is associated with a higher rate of adenomas and adenocarcinomas, which can occur anywhere in the GI tract**.

References: Buck JL, Harned RK, Lichtenstein JE, et al. Peutz-Jeghers syndrome. *Radiographics* 1992;12(2):365–378.

Kim YH, Blake MA, Harisinghani MG, et al. Adult intestinal intussusception: CT appearances and identification of a causative lead point. *Radiographics* 2006;26(3):733–744.

21a **Answer B.** The CT demonstrates a markedly dilated loop of colon in the central abdomen with decompressed transverse, descending, and rectosigmoid colon. A transition to narrowed bowel on posterior slices with a bird's beak appearance is seen.

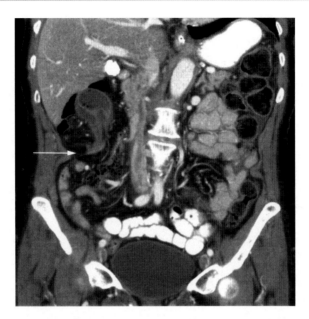

Findings are consistent with a **cecal volvulus**. Cecal volvulus involves axial torsion of the cecum around its own mesentery. Incomplete peritoneal fixation of the cecum is a common anatomic variant (present in 11% to 25% of the population) that increases cecal mobility and predisposes the cecum to torsion. Acquired adhesions from prior surgery or inflammatory disease may contribute to fixation of a portion of the bowel and increase the risk for volvulus.

Cecal volvulus is uncommon, accounting for about 1% of all intestinal obstructions. Clinical presentation is variable and can be insidious or acute, with colicky abdominal pain usually present, but occasionally with nausea and vomiting that may mimic the much more common small bowel obstruction.

Abdominal plain films may be suggestive, but CT is the imaging technique of choice. CT is very sensitive, confirming the diagnosis in 90% of volvulus patients. CT findings include a dilated cecum, decompressed distal colon, and displacement of the cecum often into the left upper quadrant. A "whirl" sign associated with the dilated cecum is highly specific for a volvulus.

21b **Answer B.** There is a 20% to 25% risk of concurrent cecal necrosis. Surgery is the primary treatment option. Unlike for sigmoid volvulus, endoscopic reduction is not as useful, being technically more difficult to perform and with high recurrence rates of volvulus. For the same reason, enema reduction is not suggested. Surgical options range from cecopexy and cecostomy to resection of the cecum, right hemicolectomy, or ileocolectomy.

References: Moore CJ, Corl FM, Fishman EK. CT of cecal volvulus: unraveling the image. *AJR Am J Roentgenol* 2001;177(1):95–98.

Rosenblat JM, Rozenblit AM, Wolf EL, et al. Findings of cecal volvulus at CT. *Radiology* 2010;256(1):169–175.

22 **Answer E.** The images obtained during the arterial phase of a CT angiography study demonstrate findings of contrast extravasation in the sigmoid colon from a diverticulum. **Diverticular bleeding is the most common cause of lower GI bleeding in the older patient population** (33% in one series). In most cases (86%), the bleeding will stop without intervention, and the patient may be observed with supportive care. While colonoscopy may be considered for prophylactic treatment (e.g., epinephrine and electrocoagulation) after a significant bleed, this may wait for an elective procedure in the morning if the patient remains stable. Urgent surgery is reserved for recurrent refractory bleeding and carries with it a significant morbidity and mortality risk in this elderly patient. The diagnosis is definitive on the CT angiogram with no evidence of a mass lesion, despite lack of oral contrast.

CT angiography has become a very useful diagnostic tool in the setting of acute GI bleeding and is supplanting technetium-99m–tagged red blood cell (RBC) scanning in some centers. Advantages include its widespread availability and ability to pinpoint the exact location of the bleed, which will be useful in any choice of interventional therapy. Disadvantages include the inability to reimage without a repeat injection for intermittent bleeding, risk of contrast allergic reaction and nephrotoxicity in patients with renal insufficiency, and interpretive difficulty if any preexisting positive oral contrast is present.

References: Adams JB, Margolin DA. Management of diverticular hemorrhage. *Clin Colon Rectal Surg* 2009;22(3):181–185.

Geffroy Y, Rodallec MH, Boulay-Coletta I, et al. Multidetector CT angiography in acute gastrointestinal bleeding: why, when, and how. *Radiographics* 2011;31(3):E35–E46.

23a **Answer C.** The radiation dose and cost of the examination are primary considerations when choosing the optimal imaging for a pregnant patient. As the patient's history strongly suggests the possibility of acute appendicitis, **the most appropriate initial examination is an ultrasound of the right lower quadrant**. Ultrasound is lower in cost, is easily available compared to MRI, and can be readily performed without significant delay. An MRI without contrast would be an acceptable subsequent test if the ultrasound fails to identify the appendix or is equivocal. Gadolinium-based contrast agents should be avoided as they cross the placenta, and the long-term effects of gadolinium on the fetus are unclear. CT presents a radiation risk to the fetus, although it can be performed in pregnant patients with an acute abdomen if the benefit outweighs the risk. An indium-111 white blood cell scan has a very high radiation dose and also is not routinely indicated in the workup of suspected appendicitis even in nonpregnant patients.

23b **Answer B.** **Ultrasound** is the initial imaging modality of choice in children and pregnant patients with suspected appendicitis. The classic finding for acute appendicitis on ultrasound is a **noncompressible blind-ending tubular structure >6 mm in diameter**, located at the point of maximum tenderness and is considered diagnostic for appendicitis.

On a recent meta-analysis by Van Randen et al., the sensitivity and specificity of ultrasound were found to be at 78% and 83%, respectively. In practice, however, ultrasound is operator dependent, and the diagnostic accuracy is variable. The visualization of a normal appendix can be achieved only in 2% to 6% of cases.

Periappendiceal fluid can be appreciated as a result of inflammation and does not necessarily indicate rupture of the appendix. Small bowel loops can demonstrate normal peristalsis in the presence of acute appendicitis, in particular in the early stages. An appendicolith can also be seen as a secondary finding.

References: Karul M, Berliner C, Keller S, et al. Imaging of appendicitis in adults. *Rofo* 2014;186(6):551–558.

Parks NA, Schroeppel TJ. Update on imaging for acute appendicitis. *Surg Clin North Am* 2011;91:141–154.

24a **Answer D.** The CT findings are of a sausage-shaped fatty mass abutting the anterior wall of the sigmoid colon with surrounding inflammation consistent with **acute epiploic appendagitis**. Epiploic appendages are pedunculated projections of subserosal fat arising from the surface of the colon. They contain a vascular pedicle with two paired arteries and a single draining vein. They may have a length of 0.5 to 5 cm, with the average length 3 cm.

These are present throughout the colon but are largest and most numerous in the sigmoid colon with the descending and right colon the next most common sites. Torsion of the appendage may lead to vascular occlusion with inflammation and is the most common cause of epiploic appendagitis. Much less commonly, epiploic appendagitis may be caused by an incarcerated hernia, intestinal obstruction, or intussusception. Rarely, they may become intraperitoneal loose bodies.

On CT, acute epiploic appendagitis presents as a <5-cm ovoid fat density mass adjacent to the colon with surrounding inflammatory changes. There may be a **central dot representing a thrombosed vein and a ring sign of thickened peritoneal lining** (although these characteristic findings are not universally present).

The clinical presentation may mimic acute appendicitis or diverticulitis, but in distinction, patients with epiploic appendagitis are usually afebrile without a leukocytosis. Omental infarction is another less common condition that may have a similar clinical presentation to epiploic appendagitis. On CT, the omental infarct may be larger, and the central thrombosed vein is absent. It is most commonly seen in anterior to the transverse colon or anteromedial to the ascending colon.

24b **Answer A.** Epiploic appendagitis is typically a **self-limited condition** not requiring surgery. Anti-inflammatory agents for pain and observation are the most appropriate therapy. Antibiotics are not routinely indicated. Patients typically recover within 10 days.

References: Rajesh A. The ring sign. *Radiology* 2005;237(1):301–302.

Singh AK, Gervais DA, Hahn PF, et al. Acute epiploic appendagitis and its mimics. *Radiographics* 2005;25(6):1521–1534.

25a **Answer A.** The CT scan demonstrates a fluid-density tubular mass with a thin wall indenting the cecal base. There is no adjacent fat stranding to indicate acute appendicitis or epiploic appendagitis, and the patient is asymptomatic. The mass is not associated with small bowel, as would be expected with a Meckel diverticulum. This represents an **appendiceal mucocele**, which is a descriptive term for a dilated, mucin-filled appendix. An appendiceal mucocele may be caused by nonmalignant luminal obstruction (mucous retention cyst) or by a mucin-secreting neoplasm. When rupture or invasion of a mucin-secreting appendiceal tumor occurs, intraperitoneal spread of mucinous deposits may occur, called pseudomyxoma peritonei.

An appendiceal mucocele may mimic the dilated appendix seen with appendicitis and may actually present with clinical acute appendicitis due to obstruction (absent in this case). **The presence of mural calcification and a diameter greater than expected for appendicitis (>13 mm) may favor a mucocele.**

25b **Answer E.** Shape, septations, wall calcifications, and the presence of intraperitoneal free fluid do not distinguish between benign and malignant forms. **Mural nodularity or irregular wall thickening has been associated with malignant mucoceles due to an adenocarcinoma.** In addition to nodal and metastatic involvement, histologic grade is important in staging. The biologic behavior of appendiceal mucinous tumors does not follow conventional definitions of benign or malignant patterns, and these neoplasms may be classified as low grade or high grade. Staging and prognosis differs from colorectal adenocarcinoma. Intraperitoneal extension of tumor confined to the periappendiceal region is considered T4 disease, while extension beyond is considered metastatic.

References: Bennett GL, Tanpitukpongse TP, Macari M, et al. CT diagnosis of mucocele of the appendix in patients with acute appendicitis. *AJR Am J Roentgenol* 2009;192(3):W103–W110.

Leonards LM, Pahwa A, Patel MK, et al. Neoplasms of the appendix: pictorial review with clinical and pathologic correlation. *Radiographics* 2017;37(4):1059–1083.

26 **Answer B.** The findings demonstrate an apple-core sigmoid mass with abrupt shelf-like margins causing high-grade obstruction of the proximal bowel. Large bowel obstruction (LBO) is 5 times less common than a small bowel obstruction. **Neoplasm is the most common cause of all large bowel obstructions**.

Common Causes of Large Bowel Obstruction	Percentage
Neoplasm	60%–80%
Volvulus (sigmoid, cecal, transverse)	11%–15%
Diverticulitis	4%–10%

Uncommon causes of LBO (accounting for <5% total) include hernias, inflammatory bowel disease, extrinsic compression from abscess or other mass, fecal impaction, and intraluminal foreign bodies.

Large bowel obstruction is an abdominal emergency. CT is the most accurate and useful modality for imaging. A contrast enema (water soluble) may help distinguish between a true obstruction and a pseudoobstruction such as is commonly seen at the splenic flexure in both acute and chronic pseudoobstructions.

Reference: Jaffe T, Thompson WM. Large-bowel obstruction in the adult: classic radiographic and CT findings, etiology, and mimics. *Radiology* 2015;275(3):651–663.

27 **Answer D.** **Neutropenic colitis** is a poorly understood entity that is probably multifactorial, with ischemia, infection, hemorrhage, and possible neoplastic cellular infiltration potential contributing factors. Although the pathologic abnormality can involve any segment of the bowel in neutropenic colitis, **the cecum is the most common site**. While surgery was felt to be indicated in most cases in the past, the current trend favors conservative supportive nonsurgical care, even in the presence of pneumatosis.

C. difficile infection is a common case of colitis in the neutropenic patient occurring after chemotherapy or antibiotic therapy. *C. difficile* colitis tends to have diffuse involvement but can be focal and involve the right colon only. Likewise, neutropenic colitis may be diffuse, so the radiographic appearances of neutropenic colitis and *C. difficile* colitis have considerable overlap. The mural thickening and wall nodularity does tend to be more pronounced in *C. difficile* colitis.

Reference: Kirkpatrick ID, Greenberg HM. Gastrointestinal complications in the neutropenic patient: characterization and differentiation with abdominal CT. *Radiology* 2003;226(3): 668–674.

28a **Answer B.** There is a short segment of circumferential narrowing in the sigmoid colon that is persistent on multiple views and cannot be attributed to transient spasm. The abnormal segment has shelf-like margins and spiculated contours. Appearance is concerning for primary colonic neoplasm, and endoscopy is warranted.

Although images of the sigmoid are performed with single-contrast technique, there are no mucosal changes or contour abnormalities of the remainder of the colon on the overhead image to suggest ulcerative colitis. No diverticula are identified on this examination, although edema may obscure the perforated diverticulum. Diverticulitis is commonly associated with luminal narrowing due to edema and spasm, but the involved segment of narrowing is typically long, and the stricture is relatively short in this case.

28b **Answer C.** As the patient is a young female, the possibility of an endometrioma should be considered. An MR of the pelvis with T1-weighted fat-suppressed series can best demonstrate the characteristic high signal of the **endometrioma**, as seen in this case from a different patient.

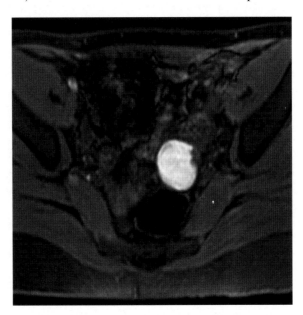

Up to a third of patients with endometriosis will have endometrial implants on the gastrointestinal tract. The most commonly affected segments of the bowel are in the dependent portion of the pelvis, with the rectosigmoid the most frequently involved segment. Appearance of an endometrial implant on the colon is variable. If asymmetric, puckering of the wall may be seen; if circumferential, as in this case, the stricture may resemble a primary colon carcinoma. The implants are serosal but can erode through the subserosal layer and cause thickening of the muscularis propria. The overlying mucosa is almost always intact.

Reference: Woodward PJ, Sohaey R, Mezzetti TP Jr. Endometriosis: radiologic-pathologic correlation. *Radiographics* 2001;21(1):193–216; questionnaire 288–194.

29 **Answer C.** There are multiple filling defects in the colon seen on this double-contrast barium enema. The background mucosa is smooth and normal in appearance, indicating absence of active inflammatory disease. These are consistent with **postinflammatory polyps**. Although these may resemble a polyposis syndrome, they are not adenomatous, and their characteristic morphology with the appropriate clinical history should suggest the correct diagnosis.

A variety of terms are used to describe the fixed filling defects that can be seen in the colon on imaging studies in the setting of inflammatory bowel disease. The terminology, which can be confusing, reflects the different stages of the inflammation that are associated with the disease throughout its course. The following are the main terms encountered and their definitions:

- *Polyp*: A generic term used to describe a mass that projects into the lumen of the bowel above the level of the surrounding mucosa. It usually arises from the mucosa but may derive from deeper layers. It can be neoplastic (benign or malignant) or inflammatory, and distinguishing between these possibilities on a radiographic basis may be difficult.

- *Pseudopolyp*: A term used to describe a residual mucosal island between areas of ulceration. The ulceration may be so extensive as to simulate the baseline mucosa with the islands of relatively normal or slightly inflamed mucosa appearing to project above the baseline. As the mass-like defect does not truly project beyond the mucosal level, it is termed a pseudopolyp. These may be seen in late stages of ulcerative colitis where the ulcerations of the submucosa have become confluent leaving isolated islands of mucosa. This term may also be applied to Crohn disease with cobblestoning, where the deep longitudinal and transverse fissures between the inflamed mucosa cause them to appear as polyps.

- *Postinflammatory polyps*: These are true polyps (not pseudopolyps as they are *sometimes erroneously* called). These have been previously thought to form from regenerating epithelium in the healing phase of an inflammatory colitis. Newer studies suggest that they may be hamartomatous rather than regenerative. They can often be filiform or bridging. They are more common in ulcerative colitis but may be seen in other conditions including Crohn disease, ischemia, and infectious colitis.

References: Buck JL, Dachman AH, Sobin LH. Polypoid and pseudopolypoid manifestations of inflammatory bowel disease. *Radiographics* 1991;11(2):293–304.

Lim YJ, Choi JH, Yang CH. What is the clinical relevance of filiform polyposis? *Gut Liver* 2012;6(4):524–526.

Spark RP. Filiform polyposis of the colon. First report in a case of transmural colitis (Crohn's disease). *Am J Dig Dis* 1976;21(9):809–814.

30 **Answers:**

Ulcerative colitis and Crohn's are inflammatory bowel diseases with distinct pathologic features. Radiographic findings reflecting these pathologic characteristics have been described extensively in the literature. While colonoscopy for surveillance has supplanted barium enemas to a large extent, CT and MR play a critical role in evaluation of extraintestinal tissues. Colonoscopy may be contraindicated in some patients, and recognition of classic findings on barium studies remains important.

Comparison of Major Features of Ulcerative Colitis and Crohn disease:

Ulcerative Colitis (UC)	Crohn Disease (CD)
Involves colon (terminal ileum occasionally involved with backwash ileitis)	Involves entire digestive tract (terminal ileum and cecal involvement common)
Continuous involvement	Discontinuous involvement
Rectal disease common (95%)	Perianal disease common
Symmetric involvement bowel wall	Asymmetric involvement bowel wall
Generally superficial (except fulminant form that can involve muscularis)	Transmural (fissures, fistulae, abscesses)
Wall thickening, but less than Crohn disease	Pronounced wall thickening
Increased risk of colorectal CA	Increased risk of colorectal CA

30.1 **Answer A.** The findings on this single-contrast barium enema demonstrate narrowing of the colonic caliber and multiple rounded outpouchings, which are typical "collar button" ulcers. The continuous colonic involvement and ahaustral appearance support the diagnosis of acute ulcerative colitis in this case. These represent ulcers of crypt abscesses with undermining of the submucosa and are seen in the advanced stages of acute disease. The deep extent of the ulcer is limited by the relatively resistant muscle layer. These are most commonly associated with ulcerative colitis but may be seen less commonly in Crohn disease and in other colitides including amebiasis, shigellosis, and ischemia.

30.2 **Answer B.** On this barium enema, there is a segment of left colon with polypoid filling defects and intramural fissures in longitudinal and transverse directions. This "cobblestoning" appearance is seen in active Crohn colitis when deep ulcerations traverse the bowel wall between islands of heaped-up inflammatory mucosa leading to pseudopolyp formation. Note the skip involvement of the colon, typical for Crohn disease.

30.3 **Answer A.** This barium enema demonstrates the typical ahaustral "lead pipe" appearance of acute ulcerative colitis. The entire colon is involved in a continuous fashion, a hallmark of acute ulcerative colitis in distinction to Crohn disease. Involvement may be partial, but the disease proceeds from the rectum, and the left colon is invariably involved in acute ulcerative colitis. Note that chronic ulcerative colitis may heal in an irregular fashion, with skip areas mimicking Crohn colitis.

30.4 **Answer A.** On this plain film of the abdomen, the transverse colon is dilated with ill-defined polypoid contours of the walls. These radiographic findings are seen in patients who are significantly ill (whose symptoms may include fever, leukocytosis, tachycardia, and hypotension) leading to the clinical term "toxic megacolon." As the colon wall may also be abnormal without dilatation, the more generalized term would be "toxic colon." The findings were first described in the setting of acute ulcerative colitis and are most commonly seen in this entity. Crohn disease may rarely present with toxic megacolon. Since the early description, the same findings have been observed in other severe inflammatory colitides, including pseudomembranous, other infectious, ischemic, and radiation colitis.

30.5 **Answer B.** The single-contrast barium enema demonstrates luminal narrowing of the sigmoid colon with transverse fissures and ulcerations. These deep fissuring ulcers, linear or "rose thorn" shaped, highlight the transmural penetrating nature of acute Crohn disease.

30.6 **Answer C.** The CT demonstrates a target appearance to the segment of the colon with a layer of intramural fat. This fat halo sign is associated with chronic inflammatory disease and can be seen in both ulcerative colitis and Crohn disease, although more common in the former. In Crohn disease, the intramural fat tends to involve the terminal ileum and the right colon. It has been described in patients with graft versus host disease and in patients undergoing cytoreductive therapy. It may also be seen as an incidental finding in asymptomatic patients, potentially related to obesity. With the increased utilization of noncontrast CT for evaluation of kidney stones (CT KUB), there has been increasing detection of intramural intestinal fat often without a clear antecedent history of inflammatory bowel disease.

30.7 **Answer B.** On this CT, there is wall thickening of the cecum and terminal ileum with extensive inflammatory fat stranding in the surrounding fat and abnormal soft tissue tracts between multiple bowel loops consistent with fistulae. There is also extension into the right bladder wall with wall thickening. These changes highlight the penetrating nature of acute Crohn enterocolitis.

30.8 **Answer B.** The CT shows wall thickening of the rectosigmoid. The adjacent vasa recta are dilated and separated by prominent pericolic fat. This leads to a striped pattern known as the "comb" sign, a finding of active Crohn disease.

30.9 **Answer B.** This MRI demonstrates a perirectal/perianal fistula involving the intersphincteric space and extending into the right ischiorectal fat. Perianal abnormalities in active Crohn disease are common and can manifest as fistulae, fissures, and abscesses. There may be anal canal or distal rectal strictures associated as well. Patients with perianal disease are likely to have ileocolitis or other sites of colitis, not just disease involving the small bowel. MRI provides the best anatomic detail due to its superior contrast resolution.

References: Buck JL, Dachman AH, Sobin LH. Polypoid and pseudopolypoid manifestations of inflammatory bowel disease. *Radiographics* 1991;11(2):293–304.

Deepak P, Bruining DH. Radiographical evaluation of ulcerative colitis. *Gastroenterol Rep (Oxf)* 2014;2(3):169–177.

Gore RM, Balthazar EJ, Ghahremani GG, et al. CT features of ulcerative colitis and Crohn's disease. *AJR Am J Roentgenol* 1996;167(1):3–15.

Harisinghani MG, Wittenberg J, Lee W, Chen S, Gutierrez AL, Mueller PR. Bowel wall fat halo sign in patients without intestinal disease. *AJR Am J Roentgenol* 2003;181(3):781–784.

Lichtenstein JE, Madewell JE, Feigin DS. The collar button ulcer. A radiologic-pathologic correlation. *Gastrointest Radiol* 1979;4(1):79–84.

Meyers MA, McGuire PV. Spiral CT demonstration of hypervascularity in Crohn disease: "vascular jejunization of the ileum" or the "comb sign". *Abdom Imaging* 1995;20(4):327–332.

Roggeveen MJ, Tismenetsky M, Shapiro R. Best cases from the AFIP: ulcerative colitis. *Radiographics* 2006;26(3):947–951.

Schaffler A, Herfarth H. Creeping fat in Crohn's disease: travelling in a creeper lane of research? *Gut* 2005;54(6):742–744.

Thoeni RF, Cello JP. CT imaging of colitis. *Radiology* 2006;240(3):623–638.

31 **Answer D.** The CT colonography images show colonic pneumatosis, which is a radiographic finding, not a clinical diagnosis. The prognosis of this finding depends on the cause of the pneumatosis and not the extent of findings on imaging (even in the presence of portal venous gas or pneumoperitoneum). Pneumatosis may be an ominous finding in a patient presenting with signs and symptoms of bowel ischemia. As an incidental finding in an asymptomatic patient, possible etiologies of benign pneumatosis include medications (such as steroids), recent endoscopy or surgery, emphysema, barotrauma, lupus, or, as in this patient's case, colonic insufflation for CT colonography. Further evaluation or treatment is rarely necessary.

References: Feczko PJ, Mezwa DG, Farah MC, et al. Clinical significance of pneumatosis of the bowel wall. *Radiographics* 1992;12(6):1069–1078.

Pickhardt PJ, Kim DH, Taylor AJ. Asymptomatic pneumatosis at CT colonography: a benign self-limited imaging finding distinct from perforation. *AJR Am J Roentgenol* 2008;190(2):W112–W117.

32a **Answer D.** The scout film demonstrates an abnormally dilated loop of bowel in the upper abdomen with nodular contours of the wall. The CT images show the dilated loop is the transverse colon with loss of haustral folds and irregular thickening of the wall. With the clinical presentation, this entity is consistent with toxic colitis.

32b **Answer B. Toxic colitis** is a complication of a severe colitis in which the enervation of the colon is compromised by the severe inflammation, leading to poor muscular tone and dilatation. This entity has often been called toxic megacolon, but as the degree of dilatation may not be severe, toxic colitis is the more appropriate term. Despite the nodular contours suggesting wall thickening, with toxic colitis, the colonic wall is friable and more prone to perforation. For this reason, **contrast enema studies and colonoscopy are contraindicated when toxic colitis is suspected.** Toxic colitis is most commonly due to inflammatory bowel disease (ulcerative colitis more frequently than Crohn disease). It may also be seen with infectious agents (especially *C. difficile*) or ischemic colitis. In this case, the provided history suggests an underlying chronic condition, and the patient's age does not fall into the typical demographic group at risk for ischemic colitis.

References: Barral M, Boudiaf M, Dohan A, et al. MDCT of acute colitis in adults: an update in current imaging features. *Diagn Interv Imaging* 2015;96(2):133–149.

Maddu KK, Mittal P, Arepalli CD, et al. Colorectal emergencies and related complications: a comprehensive imaging review—noninfectious and noninflammatory emergencies of colon. *AJR Am J Roentgenol* 2014;203(6):1217–1229.

Thoeni RF, Cello JP. CT imaging of colitis. *Radiology* 2006;240(3):623–638.

33 **Answer B.** The CT demonstrates a large mass with mixed internal fat density, including macroscopic fat consistent with a lipoma. Lipomas are the most common submucosal lesion of the gastrointestinal tract. Most gastrointestinal lipomas arise in the colon. Although submucosal, lipomas may develop a pedicle and appear intraluminal. Most lipomas are asymptomatic, but when large, they may ulcerate and bleed or intussuscept, with or without obstruction. Lipomas may be diagnosed when they contain material with Hounsfield units between −120 and −80, but **some lipomas (especially when they intussuscept) may contain soft tissue higher in attenuation and can be mistaken for malignancy.**

References: Chang CC, Liu KL. Colonic lipoma with intussusception. *Mayo Clin Proc* 2007;82(1):10.

Thompson WM. Imaging and findings of lipomas of the gastrointestinal tract. *AJR Am J Roentgenol* 2005;184(4):1163–1171.

34a **Answer B. Hereditary nonpolyposis colorectal cancer (HNPCC)** also known as **Lynch syndrome** is the most common of the hereditary colorectal cancer syndromes. This syndrome accounts for about 2% to 6% of all colorectal cancers. Familial adenomatous polyposis (FAP) accounts for <1% of colorectal cancers. Gardner syndrome is considered a variant of FAP with associated lesions including osteomas, desmoid, and other benign extracolonic lesions. Cronkhite-Canada is extremely rare and not familial. Gastrointestinal polyps (mostly inflammatory) are present associated with other ectodermal abnormalities of the skin, hair, and nails.

34b **Answer C.** Hereditary nonpolyposis colorectal cancer (HNPCC) is caused by a germ-line defect in DNA mismatch repair genes. It has an autosomal dominant inheritance pattern, although most cases are sporadic. Patients are at risk for early-onset colon cancer and metachronous and synchronous colon cancers. There is an elevated risk for other types of cancer, with endometrial cancer being the most common extracolonic tumor. Current gynecologic screening recommendation for women with Lynch syndrome is for annual endometrial sampling and transvaginal ultrasound beginning at age 30 to 35 years. The lifetime cumulative risk of endometrial cancer for women with Lynch syndrome is 40% to 60%, which equals or exceeds their risk of colorectal cancer. Increased risk for tumors of the ovary, stomach, small intestine, hepatobiliary tract, upper urinary tract, brain, and skin has been described. A PET scan, while useful for screening does not provide as specific information for the other organs at risk.

References: Ahnen DJ, Axell L. Lynch syndrome (hereditary nonpolyposis colorectal cancer): clinical manifestations and diagnosis. In: Lamont JT (ed). *UpToDate.* Waltham, MA: UpToDate. Accessed on July 19, 2015.

Umar A, Boland CR, Terdiman JP, et al. Revised Bethesda Guidelines for hereditary nonpolyposis colorectal cancer (Lynch syndrome) and microsatellite instability. *J Natl Cancer Inst* 2004;96(4):261–268.

35a **Answer A.** Osteomas of the skull and mandible, especially if multiple, and dental abnormalities including odontomas and supernumerary or unerupted teeth should raise the question of Gardner syndrome (familial adenomatous polyps, multiple osteomas, and mesenchymal tumors of the skin and soft tissues including epidermoid cysts and desmoids). The extracolonic findings can precede the colonic abnormalities. As the colonic polyps are adenomatous and there is a 100% malignant transformation rate, colonic screening is important.

Reference: Panjwani S, Bagewadi A, Keluskar V, et al. Gardner's syndrome. *J Clin Imaging Sci* 2011;1:65.

35b **Answer A.** The CT demonstrates a mesenteric mass consistent with a desmoid tumor, and the double-contrast barium enema demonstrates multiple small colonic polyps in this patient with Gardner syndrome. Gardner syndrome is a subtype of familial polyposis coli characterized by multiple osteomas of the skull and mandible, colonic polyposis, and mesenchymal tumors of the skin and soft tissues. It is caused by a mutation in the *adenomatous polyposis coli (APC)* gene located on chromosome 5q21. Syndromes with a germ-line mutation in the *APC* gene include FAP, Gardner syndrome, some families with Turcot syndrome, and attenuated adenomatous polyposis coli (AAPC).

Other colonic polyposis syndromes are associated with genetic mutations. HNPCC (hereditary nonpolyposis colorectal cancer) is associated with a defect in a DNA mismatch repair. Cowden disease (multiple hamartoma syndrome), an autosomal dominant condition with variable expression, can be associated with a mutation in the *PTEN* gene on arm 10q. Peutz-Jeghers is an autosomal dominant condition associated with germ-line mutation of the *STK11/LKB1* (serine/threonine kinase 11) tumor suppressor gene, located on band 19p13.3.

Reference: Syngal S, Brand RE, Church JM, et al. ACG clinical guideline: genetic testing and management of hereditary gastrointestinal cancer syndromes. *Am J Gastroenterol* 2015;110(2):223–262; quiz 263.

36a **Answer C.** Given the patient's age, **infectious colitis** is a primary consideration. Inflammatory bowel disease may be considered, but infection should be excluded before the patient receives empiric steroid treatment. Ischemic colitis is unlikely given the patient's young age. The appendix is not included in these images, but the abnormality involves a significant segment of the right colon, not just the cecum; bloody diarrhea is also not a common finding with acute appendicitis.

Cases of bacterial colitis from food-borne enteropathogens are increasing in number due to increased consumption of fresh vegetables and fruits. In the United States, the major causes of bloody diarrhea from infectious sources in decreasing order of occurrence are *Shigella, Campylobacter*, nontyphoid *Salmonella*, and Shiga toxin–producing *E. coli*.

References: DuPont HL. Clinical practice. Bacterial diarrhea. *N Engl J Med* 2009;361(16):1560–1569.

Thoeni RF, Cello JP. CT imaging of colitis. *Radiology* 2006;240(3):623–638.

37 **Answers**

    A. 1

    B. 1

    C. 2

    D. 1

    E. 2

    F. 3

    G. 3

The appearance of acute infectious colitis on CT is commonly nonspecific, with wall thickening, pericolonic stranding, and variable amounts of ascites. While most cases of colitis can have diffuse involvement, there are predominant patterns of distribution.

Typical Location Colonic Infections		
Right-Sided	Left-Sided	Diffuse
Salmonella	Shigella	E. coli
Yersinia	Lymphogranuloma venereum	Cytomegalovirus
Tuberculosis	Gonorrhea	
Amebiasis	Schistosomiasis	

References: DuPont HL. Clinical practice. Bacterial diarrhea. *N Engl J Med* 2009;361(16):1560–1569.

Thoeni RF, Cello JP. CT imaging of colitis. *Radiology* 2006;240(3):623–638.

38 **Answer B.** Images include a plain radiograph of the abdomen showing bowel dilatation and nodular, markedly thickened haustral folds, known as thumbprinting. The coronal CT demonstrates a pancolitis with severe wall thickening. While the colitis is not pathognomonic in appearance, the clinical history is suggestive of pseudomembranous colitis. *Clostridium difficile* colitis (pseudomembranous colitis) is a common cause of diarrhea seen in sick hospitalized patients. Clinical presentation is typically with diarrhea, fever, elevated white cell count, and abdominal pain with distension.

Clostridium difficile is a **gram-positive anaerobe**, which colonizes the colon after normal colonic flora has been disrupted, typically due to antibiotic use or chemotherapy within 6 weeks of presentation. *C. difficile* produces two toxins (A and B), which have both cytotoxic and enterotoxic effects on the bowel. The clinical manifestations are thought to be predominantly due to **toxin B**. An exudate composed of fibrin, white cells, and cellular debris forms a pseudomembrane on the mucosa of the colon, which is characteristic. Definitive diagnosis is made by isolating *C. difficile* toxin in a stool sample.

Abdominal films show bowel dilatation, mural thickening, and thumbprinting from thickened haustral folds. Advanced cases may have free intraperitoneal air from perforation. The CT demonstrates marked bowel wall thickening with a shaggy mucosal outline and may demonstrate pericolic stranding and free fluid. Involvement is usually pancolonic, but it may be segmental. Rectal involvement is seen in 90% to 95% of the cases.

References: Boland GW, Lee MJ, Cats AM, et al. Antibiotic-induced diarrhea: specificity of abdominal CT for the diagnosis of Clostridium difficile disease. *Radiology* 1994;191(1):103–106.

Kirkpatrick ID, Greenberg HM. Evaluating the CT diagnosis of Clostridium difficile colitis: should CT guide therapy? *AJR Am J Roentgenol* 2001;176(3):635–639.

Kirkpatrick ID, Greenberg HM. Gastrointestinal complications in the neutropenic patient: characterization and differentiation with abdominal CT. *Radiology* 2003;226(3):668–674.

1a A 63-year-old man presents with epigastric pain. Based on the findings on the T2W MR image, what is the most likely diagnosis?

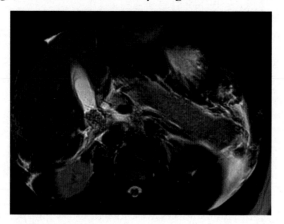

A. Pancreatitis
B. Cholecystitis
C. Diverticulitis of the descending colon
D. Perforated gastric ulcer

1b A contrast-enhanced CT was performed 4 days later. What finding is demonstrated?

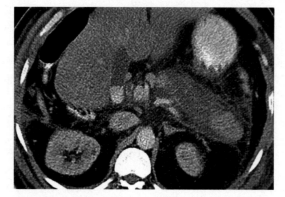

A. Biliary ductal obstruction
B. Pancreatic ductal obstruction
C. Pancreatic necrosis
D. Gallbladder hemorrhage

1c Another CT was obtained 2 weeks after onset of initial symptoms. Based on the findings in the image below, which statement is most likely correct?

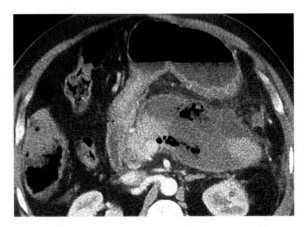

A. There is a collection drained by a percutaneous catheter.
B. There is a collection with a fistula to the stomach.
C. There is an infected collection.
D. There is a collection with acute hemorrhage.

2 A patient presenting with epigastric pain is clinically suspected to have acute pancreatitis. What is the most sensitive and appropriate test in making the initial diagnosis?

A. CT
B. Serum insulin level
C. MRI
D. Serum lipase level

3 A 73-year-old woman presents with jaundice. An MRI was performed. What is the most likely diagnosis?

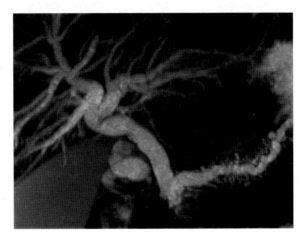

A. Ampullary stenosis
B. Chronic pancreatitis
C. Pancreatic ductal carcinoma
D. Duodenal carcinoma

4 A 34-year-old woman with right upper quadrant pain was imaged with CT scan to evaluate a finding on ultrasound. Part of the pancreatic head and body are shown, with the tail of the pancreas not included in the imaging plane. What is the most likely diagnosis?

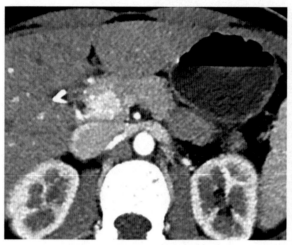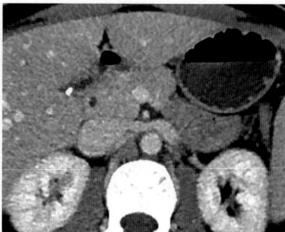

A. Aneurysm of the gastroduodenal artery
B. Neuroendocrine tumor
C. Pancreatic ductal adenocarcinoma
D. Lymphoma

5 A 42-year-old woman presents with abdominal pain and the CT shown below. What is the most likely cause of this diagnosis?

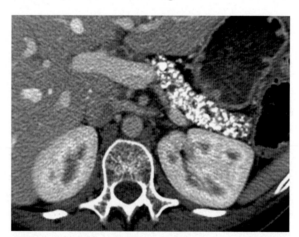

A. Hyperlipidemia
B. Gallstones
C. Heavy alcohol consumption
D. Cystic fibrosis

6a Two days following an assault, this 31-year-old man developed abdominal pain and underwent CT. Which of the following is the most appropriate next step in management?

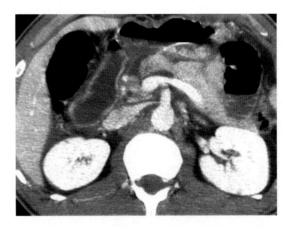

A. Serum amylase and lipase levels with serial abdominal examinations
B. Diagnostic peritoneal lavage with amylase level on collected fluid
C. Emergent reconstruction with Whipple procedure
D. Endoscopic retrograde cholangiopancreatography

6b Following surgical exploration and placement of surgical drains, the patient underwent an ERCP. What is the finding?

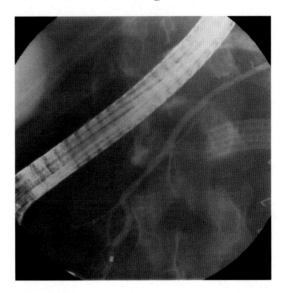

A. Acinarization of contrast
B. Pancreatic duct injury
C. Bile leak
D. Pseudoaneurysm

7 A 60-year-old man presents with left upper quadrant pain. Based on the MR images shown, what is the most likely diagnosis?

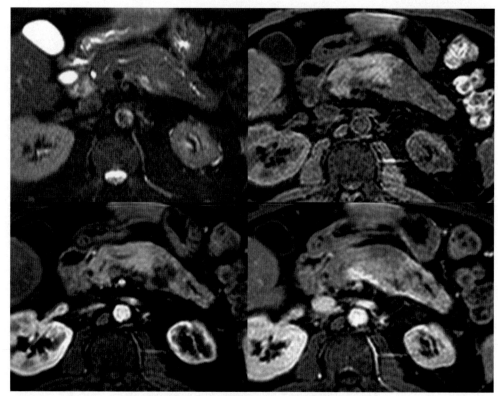

Top row: FS T2W and FS T1W images. **Bottom row:** Arterial and venous phase FS T1W+gad.

    A. Mucinous cystadenocarcinoma
    B. Intraductal papillary mucinous neoplasm
    C. Neuroendocrine neoplasm
    D. Pancreatic ductal adenocarcinoma

8 A 39-year-old man presents with symptoms of epigastric pain and vomiting. Based on the CT images shown below, what is the most likely diagnosis?

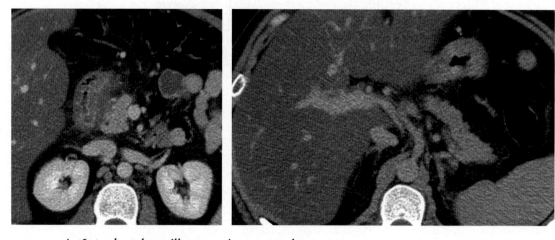

    A. Intraductal papillary mucinous neoplasm
    B. Groove pancreatitis
    C. Ampullary carcinoma
    D. Duodenal diverticulitis

For each patient in questions 9 to 15, select the most likely diagnosis (A to J). Each option may be used once or not at all.

A. Intraductal papillary mucinous neoplasm—branch type
B. Intraductal papillary mucinous neoplasm—mixed main duct and branch type
C. Duodenal diverticulum
D. Serous microcystic cystadenoma
E. Mucinous cystic neoplasm (cystadenoma/cystadenocarcinoma)
F. Solid pseudopapillary tumor
G. Cystic fibrosis
H. Mature teratoma
I. Choledochocele

9 A 64-year-old man.

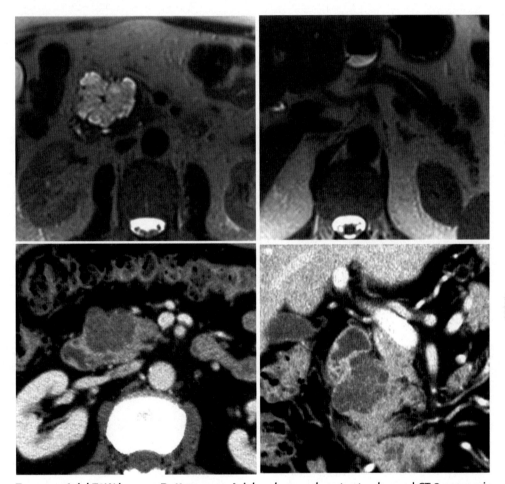

Top row: Axial T2W images. **Bottom row:** Axial and coronal contrast-enhanced CT 2 years prior.

10 A 66-year-old woman.

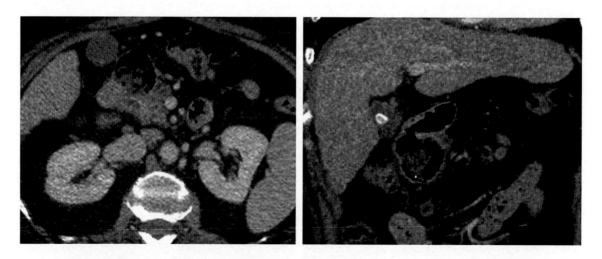

11 A 67-year-old woman.

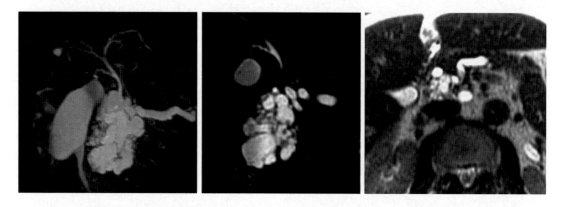

12 A 56-year-old woman.

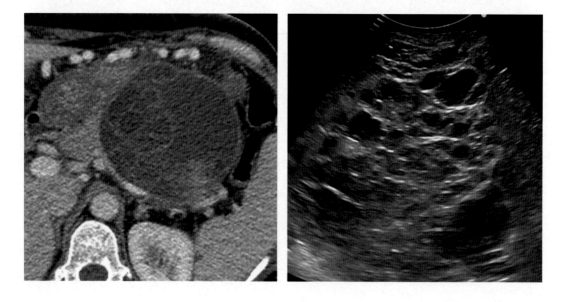

13 A 26-year-old man.

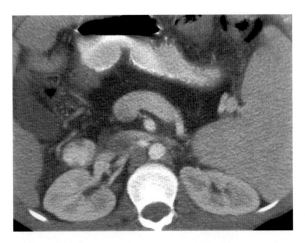

14 A 68-year-old woman.

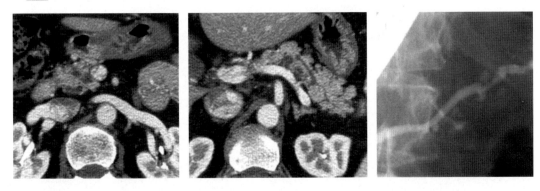

15 A 31-year-old woman.

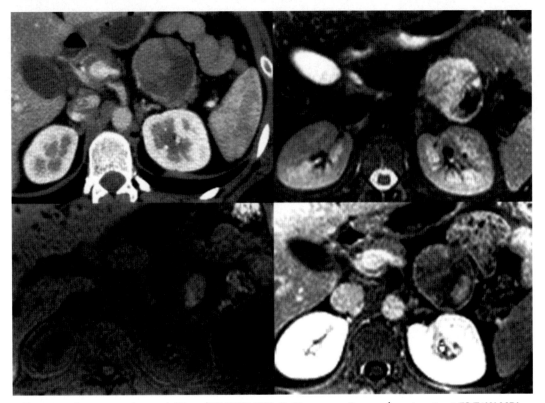

Top row: Contrast-enhanced CT and FS T2W MRI. **Bottom row:** Pre- and postcontrast FS T1W MRI.

16   A 60-year-old woman presents with abdominal pain. What abnormality is
demonstrated on these axial and coronal CT images?

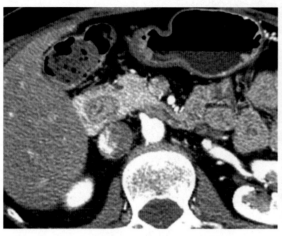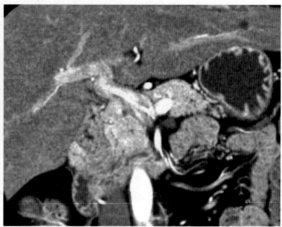

A. Annular pancreas
B. Ampullary carcinoma
C. Papillitis
D. Ectopic pancreatic rest

17a   A 58-year-old woman presents to the emergency department with dyspnea.
Multiple images from an abdominal CT are shown from superior to inferior.
What is the most likely etiology of the findings?

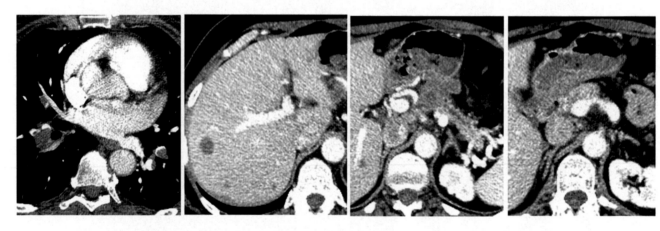

A. Sarcoidosis
B. Septic emboli
C. Lung carcinoma
D. Pancreatic carcinoma

17b   What is the most appropriate treatment for the underlying disease?

A. Chemotherapy
B. Surgical resection
C. Antibiotics
D. Steroids

18 A 30-year-old woman presents with increase in abdominal pain. What is the most likely diagnosis?

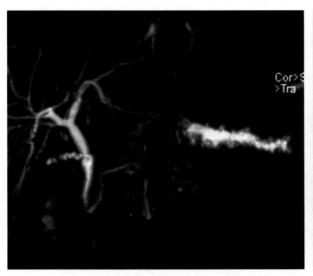
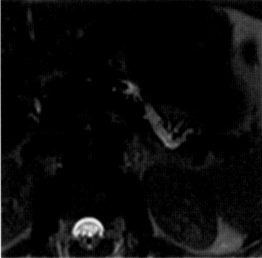

    A. Autoimmune pancreatitis
    B. Chronic pancreatitis with ductal stone
    C. Intraductal papillary mucinous neoplasm
    D. Serous microcystic cystadenoma

19a A 39-year-old woman with diarrhea and abdominal discomfort was evaluated with CT and MRI. Based on the images shown below, which statement is TRUE regarding the appearance of the pancreatic head?

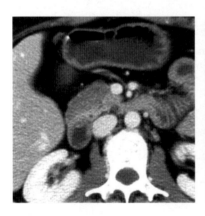
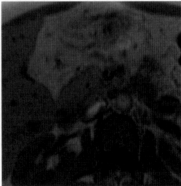
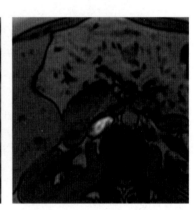

    A. There is signal loss on the fat-saturated MR image compared to the non–fat-saturated image.
    B. There is signal loss on the out-of-phase MR image compared to the in-phase image.
    C. Enhancement on the venous phase is greater than on the arterial phase.
    D. Enhancement on the arterial phase is greater than on the venous phase.

19b What is the diagnosis based on the images in the previous question?
    A. Lipoma
    B. Pancreatic ductal adenocarcinoma
    C. Neuroendocrine tumor
    D. Focal fatty infiltration

20 Pancreatic neuroendocrine neoplasms are associated with which of the following syndromes?

A. Multiple endocrine neoplasia type 1
B. Multiple endocrine neoplasia type 2a
C. Multiple endocrine neoplasia type 2b

21 A 50-year-old woman with intermittent abdominal pain was evaluated with MRI. What is the most likely diagnosis?

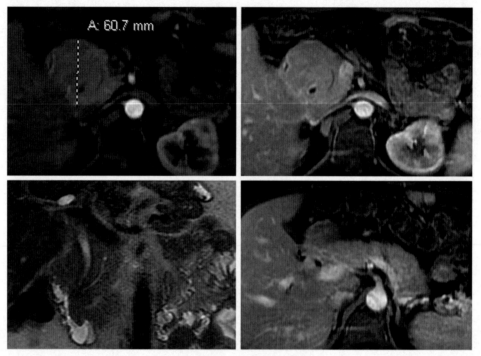

Top row: Axial arterial and venous phase FS T1W MRI. **Bottom row:** Coronal T2W and axial venous phase FS T1W MRI.

A. Pancreatic ductal adenocarcinoma
B. Neuroendocrine tumor
C. Lymphoma
D. Leiomyosarcoma

22 What ductal anatomy is demonstrated on this MRCP?

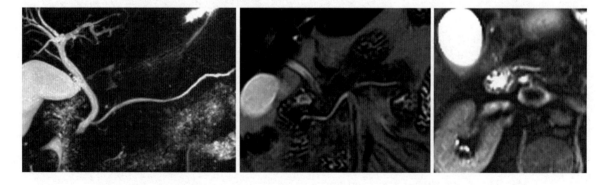

A. Ansa pancreatica
B. Pancreas divisum
C. Long common channel of pancreatic and biliary ducts
D. Annular pancreas

23 A 77-year-old woman patient has a distant history of a surgical procedure. What is the structure labeled with arrows on the CT?

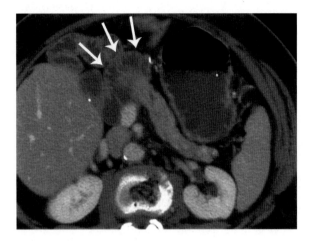

A. Normal afferent limb
B. Recurrent cystic pancreatic neoplasm
C. Gallbladder
D. Abscess

24 Which hormone may be administered intravenously during MRCP to improve visualization of the pancreatic duct?

A. Cholecystokinin
B. Secretin
C. Glucagon
D. Insulin

25 A 49-year-old woman with back pain is evaluated with CT scan for a pancreatic finding partially imaged on a lumbar MRI. She is subsequently referred to your institution for further management of a presumed pancreatic pseudocyst. What is the most appropriate treatment strategy?

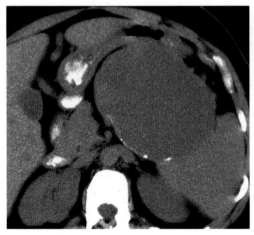 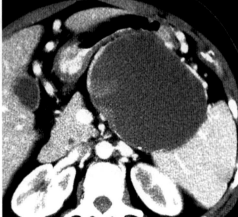

A. Antibiotics
B. Percutaneous drainage
C. Transgastric endoscopic drainage
D. Tumor resection

26a What is the likely diagnosis on this abdominal CT?

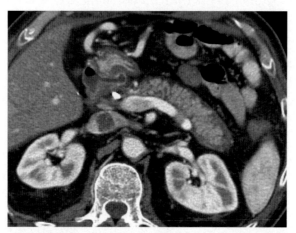

Image courtesy of Dr. Priya Bhosale, Department of Diagnostic Radiology, The University of Texas, MD Anderson Cancer Center, Houston, Texas.

A. Pancreatic necrosis
B. Metastasis
C. Lymphoma
D. Autoimmune pancreatitis

26b Elevation of which serum marker is most specific for autoimmune pancreatitis?

A. IgG4
B. CRP
C. CA19-9
D. Chromogranin A

27 A 70-year-old man with a history of extrapancreatic malignancy underwent surveillance CT. Arterial and venous phase images are shown. Which of the following primary malignancy is the most likely etiology of this pancreatic mass?

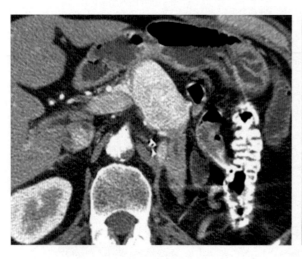 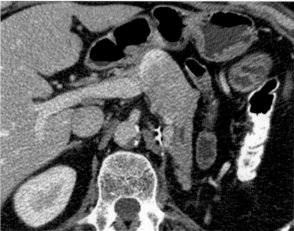

A. Lymphoma
B. Melanoma
C. Renal cell carcinoma
D. Lung carcinoma

28a A 54-year-old woman with a 4-month history of necrotizing pancreatitis with walled-off necrosis undergoes a CT scan. What finding is demonstrated?

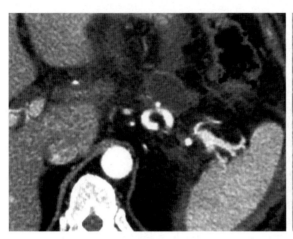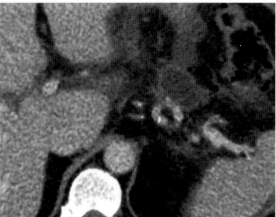

A. Pancreatic ductal adenocarcinoma
B. Pancreatic ductal stone
C. Splenic artery active hemorrhage
D. Splenic artery pseudoaneurysm

28b The CT finding was not recognized, and the patient presents 6 weeks later with worsening abdominal pain and anemia. A routine venous phase CT scan was performed with axial and sagittal images shown. She is hemodynamically stable. What is the most appropriate next step in management?

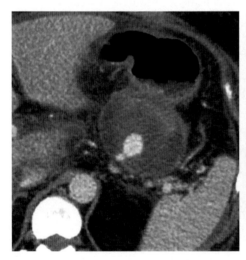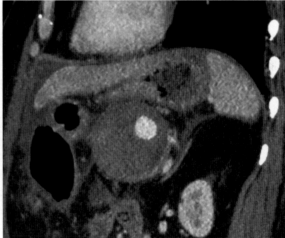

A. Angiography with embolization
B. Open surgery with debridement
C. Intravenous fluids and pain medication
D. Percutaneous drainage with catheter placement

ANSWERS AND EXPLANATIONS

1a **Answer A.** Findings are consistent with **acute pancreatitis, most likely related to gallstones.** There is diffuse edema around the pancreas. The gland is also diffusely enlarged and edematous with T2W hyperintensity and effacement of the normal acinar architecture. Multiple small stones are visible in the gallbladder. **Cholelithiasis and heavy alcohol consumption together account for about 90% of cases of acute pancreatitis in developed countries.** The other answer choices do not cause edema around the entire pancreas.

1b **Answer C.** Part of the pancreatic body and tail are not enhancing, consistent with **necrotizing pancreatitis.** Density of <30 HU in the gland during the pancreatic phase (40 to 45 seconds after contrast injection) is suggestive of parenchymal necrosis. **Most patients with necrotizing pancreatitis have combined necrosis involving both the pancreatic parenchyma and peripancreatic fat**, rather than one type of necrosis alone.

The revised Atlanta classification recognizes **two types of acute pancreatitis: (1) interstitial edematous pancreatitis** (IEP), which is much more common, and **(2) necrotizing pancreatitis** (NP), which accounts for 5% to 10% of cases. CT after 72 hours is more accurate in detecting necrosis than CT performed earlier. Necrosis can be difficult to diagnose early because mild hypodensity within the gland may represent either edema or early gland necrosis. Peripancreatic fat stranding may be seen in interstitial edematous pancreatitis (IEP) or early peripancreatic fat necrosis. Peripancreatic fat necrosis may manifest as heterogeneous peripancreatic collections interspersed in the fat.

Regarding the other answer choices, the high density in the gallbladder represents dependent calcified gallstones visible on CT. There is no biliary or pancreatic ductal dilation to indicate obstruction.

The revised Atlanta criteria for acute pancreatitis redefined collections by time after onset and the presence or absence of necrosis. **Any of the following collections could be sterile or infected.**

Revised Atlanta Classification of Fluid Collections in Acute Pancreatitis*		
	Type of Acute Pancreatitis	
Time After Onset	Interstitial Edematous Pancreatitis (IEP)	Necrotizing Pancreatitis (NP)
<4 weeks	Acute peripancreatic fluid collection (APFC)	Acute necrotic collection (ANC) • Parenchymal necrosis alone • Peripancreatic necrosis alone • Pancreatic and peripancreatic necrosis combined (most common)
≥4 weeks	Pancreatic pseudocyst	Walled-off necrosis (WON)

*Any collection may be either sterile or infected.

1c **Answer C.** There is a collection representing **combined pancreatic and peripancreatic necrosis** that is becoming organized with an enhancing rim. Since it is within 4 weeks from onset of symptoms, it is considered an acute necrotic collection (ANC) and not yet walled-off necrosis (WON) according to the revised Atlanta classification. **Gas is present within the collection,**

which is highly suspicious for infection. There is no fistula to bowel or a percutaneous drain demonstrated that would account for gas otherwise. **Rim enhancement not a reliable indicator of infection** because it invariably develops as a collection matures. The foci of gas are scattered in the collection due to the complex viscous nature of the contents. CT cannot reliably distinguish sterile from infected collections, since **fewer than 25% of infected collections contain gas**. Infection may be suspected based and clinical decompensation and laboratory values, and aspiration may be required for diagnosis. **A collection may become infected at any time requiring drainage**, while asymptomatic sterile collections may not require intervention. There is no high density in the collection that would suggest acute hemorrhage.

References: Foster BR, Jensen KK, Bakis G, et al. Revised Atlanta Classification for acute pancreatitis: a pictorial essay. *Radiographics* 2016;36(3):675–687.

Shyu JY, Sainani NI, Sahni VA, et al. Necrotizing pancreatitis: diagnosis, imaging, and intervention. *Radiographics* 2014;34(5):1218–1239.

2 **Answer D.** Most patients with **acute pancreatitis (AP) are diagnosed without imaging** based on clinical presentation and laboratory values. **Serum lipase level elevation is more sensitive** than imaging in the diagnosis of acute pancreatitis. The pancreas may appear normal on imaging. Serum insulin levels have no role in diagnosis of AP.

The role of imaging in the setting of uncomplicated AP is primarily to identify cholelithiasis as a treatable cause. Ultrasound is the most appropriate imaging study for this purpose. If the diagnosis of AP is equivocal or if worsening symptoms suggest a complication, imaging with contrast-enhanced CT scan or MRI (with/without contrast with MRCP) would be considered appropriate for diagnosis or further evaluation.

References: ACR Appropriateness Criteria: Acute pancreatitis. American College of Radiology website. https://acsearch.acr.org/docs/69468/Narrative. Published 1998. Updated 2019. Accessed August 16, 2020.

Shinagare AB, Ip IK, Raja AS, et al. Use of CT and MRI in emergency department patients with acute pancreatitis. *Abdom Imaging* 2015;40(2):272–277.

3 **Answer C.** Coronal image from MR cholangiopancreatography (MRCP) demonstrates dilation of the pancreatic and biliary ducts consistent with the "double-duct" sign. The most common cause is obstruction by **pancreatic ductal adenocarcinoma**. Other neoplasms of the ampulla, pancreas, and periampullary region such as duodenal carcinoma can also produce the double-duct sign. Benign causes include chronic pancreatitis and ampullary stenosis, but these are diagnoses of exclusion. Dilation of multiple side branches in addition to the main pancreatic duct, as seen in this case, may or may not be evident.

References: Ahualli J. The double duct sign. *Radiology* 2007;244(1):314–315.

Lopez Hänninen E, Amthauer H, Hosten N, et al. Prospective evaluation of pancreatic tumors: accuracy of MR imaging with MR cholangiopancreatography and MR angiography. *Radiology* 2002;224(1):34–41.

4 **Answer B.** There is a mass in the pancreatic head with hyperenhancement on arterial phase and isoenhancement on venous phase compared to surrounding pancreas, most likely a **pancreatic neuroendocrine tumor** (PNET). There is **no pancreatic or biliary ductal dilation** to suggest ductal obstruction by the mass. This is also a common feature of PNET.

An aneurysm of the gastroduodenal artery (GDA) may mimic a hypervascular neoplasm in the region of the pancreatic head. However, this mass is not as bright as the aorta on the arterial phase and is more posterior than expected for the GDA. A metastasis from renal cell carcinoma (not an answer choice) is also hypervascular and can be considered in the appropriate clinical setting. Lymphoma is typically hypovascular without arterial enhancement.

PNETs may be **functioning or nonfunctioning**. Patients with functioning PNETs may manifest symptoms of hormonal overproduction, allowing earlier diagnosis when the tumor is small. The **most common functioning subtype is insulinoma**, accounting for nearly half of functioning pancreatic NETs. Other subtypes include gastrinoma, glucagonoma, VIPoma (producing vasoactive intestinal peptide), and somatostatinoma.

Nonfunctioning tumors are more common than functioning tumors, accounting for up to 80% of tumors. They may be asymptomatic or present when large with **symptoms of mass effect**. Large tumors are more likely to be **heterogeneous with cystic, necrotic, or calcified components.** The large PNET below in a different patient is heterogeneous and shows calcification (black arrow) and compression of the splenic vein. **About 15% of pancreatic NETs are cystic** and may be difficult to differentiate from other cystic pancreatic lesions. A clue to a cystic NET is a **hypervascular rim** (white arrow) on the arterial phase image in another patient on the right.

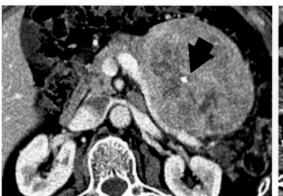 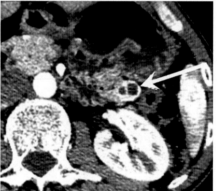

PNETs typically behave indolently. Curative surgical resection or enucleation is the preferred treatment. ^{68}Ga-DOTATATE PET/CT has evolved to become the functional imaging study of choice over ^{111}In-octreotide scan for tumors expressing somatostatin receptors (SSRs). Metastatic disease to the liver may be treated with radiofrequency ablation or chemoembolization. Other treatment options include somatostatin analogues (such as octreotide) and chemotherapy.

The World Health Organization classifies pancreatic neuroendocrine *tumor* (PNET) as one of two major types of pancreatic neuroendocrine *neoplasm* (PNEN). The other type of PNEN is pancreatic neuroendocrine *carcinoma* (PNEC), which is poorly differentiated with aggressive features and worse prognosis compared to PNET. PNECs can resemble pancreatic ductal adenocarcinoma in imaging features and behavior, appearing hypovascular with ductal obstruction and vascular invasion. PNECs may have low expression of SSRs, and functional imaging with ^{18}F-FDG PET/CT may be more sensitive than ^{68}Ga-DOTATATE PET/CT.

References: Khanna L, Prasad SR, Sunnapwar A, et al. Pancreatic neuroendocrine neoplasms: 2020 update on pathologic and imaging findings and classification. *Radiographics* 2020;40(5):1240–1262.

Raman SP, Hruban RH, Cameron JL, et al. Pancreatic imaging mimics: part 2, pancreatic neuroendocrine tumors and their mimics. *AJR Am J Roentgenol* 2012;199(2):309–318.

5 **Answer C.** Calcifications diffusely involving the pancreas are specific for **chronic pancreatitis**. Chronic **alcohol consumption** accounts for 70% to 90% of cases of chronic pancreatitis in developed countries. Less common causes are chronic biliary tract disease, hereditary pancreatitis, cystic fibrosis, hyperlipidemia, hypercalcemia (most commonly hyperparathyroidism), medications, and pancreas divisum. Chronic pancreatitis, thought to be an entity distinct from acute pancreatitis, is a disease of prolonged inflammation leading to fibrosis and gland dysfunction. **Focal or diffuse pancreatic calcifications are present in half of patients**, visible on CT and occasionally on radiographs as shown in the following image from a different patient (arrows).

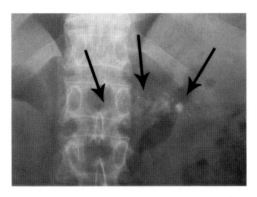

References: Javadi S, Menias CO, Korivi BR, et al. Pancreatic calcifications and calcified pancreatic masses: pattern recognition approach on CT. *AJR Am J Roentgenol* 2017;209(1):77–87.

Wolske KM, Ponnatapura J, Kolokythas O, et al. Chronic pancreatitis or pancreatic tumor? A problem-solving approach. *Radiographics* 2019;39(7):1965–1982.

6a **Answer D. Endoscopic retrograde cholangiopancreatography**

6b **Answer B.** This patient has a **pancreatic laceration with duct injury**. There is direct CT evidence of laceration (white arrow) at the head–neck junction of the pancreas. There are indirect signs including fluid tracking between the splenic vein and pancreas as well as fluid in the right anterior pararenal space. The next question is whether the main pancreatic duct is intact or injured, as this will determine the appropriate treatment. On CT, the pancreatic duct is not well evaluated. **ERCP can help identify ductal injury** and can be performed before, during, or after surgical exploration. Complex surgery such as Whipple procedure is considered only when severe parenchymal and ductal disruption is found. ERCP in this case reveals contrast extravasation (black arrow) from the duct consistent with pancreatic duct injury.

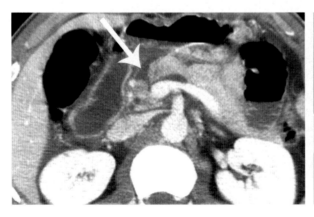
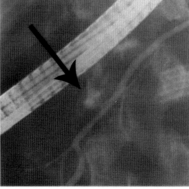

While the other answer choices could result in contrast collections on ERCP, they are not correct. Acinarization from overpressurization during injection is more diffuse and ill defined. The bile ducts and vessels are not opacified on ERCP, so the image is not diagnostic for a bile leak or pseudoaneurysm.

When the main pancreatic duct is disrupted, surgery is almost always indicated. Rarely is stenting alone successful. External or percutaneous surgical drainage is usually adequate for side-branch ductal injury. Pancreatic injury is typically caused by **blunt trauma compressing the pancreas against the vertebral column**, especially motor vehicle accidents in adults and bicycle handlebar accidents in children. The pancreatic body is the portion of the pancreas injured in two-thirds of cases. Pancreatic trauma can be difficult to detect, and the injured **pancreas may appear normal on CT** in 20% to 40% of patients imaged within 12 hours of trauma. Serum amylase is often elevated after blunt pancreatic trauma but is nonspecific and may also be elevated in salivary gland, duodenal, and hepatic injuries. It is a more reliable indicator of pancreatic injury if persistently elevated or rising.

References: Debi U, Kaur R, Prasad KK, et al. Pancreatic trauma: a concise review. *World J Gastroenterol* 2013;19:9003–9011.

Dreizin D, Bordegaray M, Tirada N, et al. Evaluating blunt pancreatic trauma at whole body CT: current practices and future directions. *Emerg Radiol* 2013;20:517–527.

7 **Answer D.** Imaging findings are consistent with **pancreatic ductal adenocarcinoma** (PDA). There is a mass (arrows) at the junction of the body and the tail of the pancreas causing mild upstream ductal dilation. Duct obstruction may be subtle prominence with abrupt transition as in this case. There is classic **hypoenhancement on the late arterial phase** (image on the bottom left), which can resemble a cystic, mucinous, or necrotic component. However, **enhancement progressively increases as expected with desmoplastic (fibrosing) tumors** such that the entire lesion appears solid and nearly isodense to surrounding pancreas on later phase. On the T2W image, there is no marked hyperintensity that would indicate fluid, and the other answer choices of cystic neoplasm are incorrect. The other answer choice of neuroendocrine tumor is typically hyperenhancing, not hypoenhancing, on arterial phase. The tail has abnormal signal intensity due to postobstructive change and may appear atrophic. Since PDA may be isoenhancing and difficult to identify on imaging, **pancreatic ductal dilation may require further investigation with endoscopy and tissue sampling even if no definite mass is visible.**

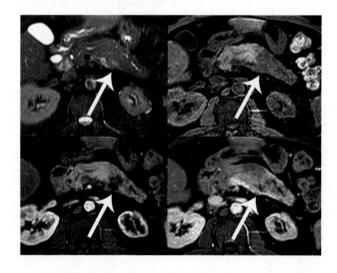

PDA is a highly aggressive malignancy arising from the ductal epithelium and accounts for 90% of all pancreatic malignancies. Two-thirds are located in the pancreatic head, which can result in the double-duct sign of both pancreatic and biliary ductal dilation. Prognosis is poor, with 75% of patients unresectable at diagnosis and a 5-year survival rate of 5% for all stages combined. Serum CA19-9 level in some cases may be elevated and helpful in assessing response to treatment.

References: Low G, Panu A, Millo N, et al. Multimodality imaging of neoplastic and nonneoplastic solid lesions of the pancreas. *Radiographics* 2011;31(4):993–1015.

Schawkat K, Manning MA, Glickman JN, et al. Pancreatic ductal adenocarcinoma and its variants: pearls and perils. *Radiographics* 2020;40(5):1–20.

8 **Answer B.** The findings in this case are characteristic for **groove (paraduodenal) pancreatitis**. There is inflammatory fat stranding (long arrow) identified in the groove between the pancreatic head and duodenum. The pancreatic parenchyma in this case appears normal, and there is also no evidence of inflammation of the body or tail. No ductal dilation is identified. The duodenum is thickened (short arrows) with submucosal edema. In some cases of groove pancreatitis, **there may be cyst formation in the groove or in the thickened duodenal wall**. There is little to no retroperitoneal fluid around the rest of the pancreas, in contradistinction to interstitial edematous pancreatitis (IEP).

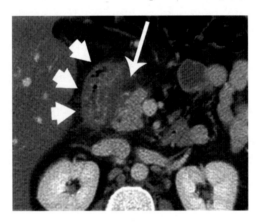

Groove pancreatitis is an **uncommon form of chronic pancreatitis**. This patient's groove pancreatitis, as well as the diffuse hepatic steatosis visible on these images, were thought to be alcohol related. **Definitive diagnosis may be difficult due to variable clinical, laboratory, and imaging features.** Serum lipase level can be normal or only slightly elevated. In the segmental form, there is involvement of the pancreatic head, and features can overlap with pancreatic or ampullary neoplasms. Enlargement of the pancreatic head may be seen in these cases, causing pancreaticobiliary ductal dilation. Groove pancreatitis is **strongly associated with heavy alcohol use, but underlying pathophysiology is unclear**. Treatment is generally conservative.

There is no diverticulum in the vicinity to indicate duodenal diverticulitis. No ampullary mass or ductal dilation is shown to suggest ampullary carcinoma. Intraductal papillary mucinous neoplasm would be a cystic lesion with or without a dilated main pancreatic duct. Duodenitis (not an answer choice) with or without ulcer may be the cause of wall thickening and fat stranding, but **duodenal ulcers are uncommonly postbulbar** unless there is hyperacidity such as in the setting of Zollinger-Ellison syndrome.

References: Perez-Johnston R, Sainani NI, Sahani DV. Imaging of chronic pancreatitis (including groove and autoimmune pancreatitis). *Radiol Clin North Am* 2012;50(3):447–466.

Raman SP, Salaria SN, Hruban RH, et al. Groove pancreatitis: spectrum of imaging findings and radiology-pathology correlation. *AJR Am J Roentgenol* 2013;201:W29–W39.

9 **Answer D.** This **serous microcystic cystadenoma** is a **lobulated cluster of numerous (>6) small cysts (<2 cm) separated by fibrous septae.** There is a small noncalcified **stellate central scar** better demonstrated on the MRI. **Calcification of the scar** (not present in this case) would be best appreciated on CT. Despite the lesion occupying the pancreatic head, there is **no upstream ductal dilation**, favoring a benign or indolent nonaggressive process. There is no growth compared to the CT 2 years prior. A **honeycomb pattern** of microcysts may be better depicted on T2W MR images, because the conglomerate of enhancing walls of the tiny cysts **on CT can mimic a solid mass**.

Serous microcystic cystadenomas are typically seen in the **elderly**, women more than men. They are benign cystic tumors that are usually incidentally discovered and managed conservatively. However, lesions that are symptomatic due to large size or rapid growth may be surgically resected.

References: Choi JY, Kim MJ, Lee JY, et al. Typical and atypical manifestations of serous cystadenoma of the pancreas: imaging findings with pathologic correlation. *AJR Am J Roentgenol* 2009;193(1):136–142.

Dewhurst CE, Mortele KJ. Cystic tumors of the pancreas: imaging and management. *Radiol Clin North Am* 2012;50(3):467–486.

10 **Answer C.** Periampullary **duodenal diverticula are common**, with identifying features of gas, debris, as well as continuity with the duodenal lumen. They often invaginate into the pancreatic head like this one does and **can mimic a pancreatic cystic lesion**. They change in shape, size, and contents from study to study. They are a **significant source of ERCP failure**, interfering with cannulation of the ampulla. Duodenal diverticula are **usually incidental and rarely symptomatic**, but complications may include perforation, hemorrhage, stone formation, and diverticulitis. A choledochocele can present as a small cystic structure in the ampullary region, and it represents a focal cystic dilation of the common bile duct that can protrude at the ampulla. It should not contain gas if sphincterotomy has not been performed.

References: Macari M, Lazarus D, Israel G, et al. Duodenal diverticula mimicking cystic neoplasms of the pancreas: CT and MR imaging findings in seven patients. *AJR Am J Roentgenol* 2003;180(1):195–199.

Nikolaidis P, Hammond NA, Day K, et al. Imaging features of benign and malignant ampullary and periampullary lesions. *Radiographics* 2014;34(3):624–641.

11 **Answer B.** This complex cystic mass communicating with a dilated main pancreatic duct is consistent with a **mixed main duct and branch type of intraductal papillary mucinous neoplasm** (IPMN). When manifesting as a complex cystic mass, IPMNs characteristically appear as an **unencapsulated conglomerate of pleomorphic round and tubular cysts** as demonstrated in this case. Large size >3 cm, main ductal dilation, and soft tissue nodularity are features associated with a greater risk of malignancy. At endoscopy, mucin may be directly visualized extruding from the papilla. Duct dilation of >5 mm is worrisome, with dilation of ≥10 mm considered high risk. **The risk of malignancy IPMNs with main duct component is high.** IPMNs communicate with the pancreatic duct as do pseudocysts (not an answer choice), so aspirates from both lesions can contain amylase.

References: Cunningham SC, Hruban RH, Schulick RD. Differentiating intraductal papillary mucinous neoplasms from other pancreatic cystic lesions. *World J Gastrointest Surg* 2010;2(10):331–336.

Megibow AJ, Baker ME, Morgan DE, et al. Management of incidental pancreatic cysts: a white paper of the ACR Incidental Findings Committee. *J Am Coll Radiol* 2017;14(7):911–923. doi: 10.1016/j.jacr.2017.03.010

12 **Answer E.** This **mucinous cystic neoplasm** (MCN) is a large **encapsulated** complex cystic lesion with **thick irregular internal septations and mural nodularity**. Contrast this with the morphology of the serous microcystic cystadenoma, which has numerous small cysts clustered together to form an unencapsulated lesion with multilobulated margins. In differentiating the two entities, fewer internal cystic components of a larger size (≥2 cm) favor MCN, while more numerous cysts of a smaller size (<2 cm) favor serous microcystic cystadenoma. Calcifications may be present in both, but the calcification in serous microcystic cystadenoma is usually within the stellate central scar. Complexity of cystic lesions may be underestimated on CT but better appreciated on ultrasound (as shown) and MRI. MCNs are **malignant (cystadenocarcinoma) or have malignant potential (cystadenoma)** and should be resected. The greater the cyst complexity, the higher the risk of malignancy. **Margins of cystadenocarcinomas may appear invasive** with focal irregularities. **The majority (90%) occur in the body or tail** of the pancreas and in **women** much more often than men. **Ovarian stroma** is typical at pathology, even in male patients.

References: Dewhurst CE, Mortele KJ. Cystic tumors of the pancreas: imaging and management. *Radiol Clin North Am* 2012;50(3):467–486.

Sahani DV, Kambadakone A, Macari M, et al. Diagnosis and management of cystic pancreatic lesions. *AJR Am J Roentgenol* 2013;200(2):343–354.

13 **Answer G.** The abdominal organ most commonly involved in **cystic fibrosis** (CF) is the pancreas. **Complete fatty replacement** is end-stage and seen at a mean age of 17 years. The fatty gland is seen anterior to the splenic vein. Fatty replacement is also seen with obesity, diabetes, and chronic pancreatitis.

In CF, inspissated secretions chronically obstructing the pancreatic duct lead to complete parenchymal replacement by fat and fibrosis, resulting in pancreatic insufficiency. Other pancreatic imaging findings may include **pancreatitis, calcifications, and cysts**. Due to effective management of lung disease, median life expectancy of CF patients is now over 40 years. **Abdominal manifestations increase with age and can significantly contribute to morbidity and mortality.** CF may involve the liver (steatosis, cirrhosis, portal hypertension), biliary tree (gallstones, sclerosing cholangitis, microgallbladder), bowel (distal ileal obstruction syndrome, intussusception, appendicitis, constipation, pneumatosis, fibrosing colopathy), and kidneys (nephrolithiasis, amyloid). Bowel, pancreatic, and biliary malignancies are being increasingly diagnosed in patients with CF as the patient population ages.

References: Averill S, Lubner MG, Menias CO, et al. Multisystem imaging findings of cystic fibrosis in adults: recognizing typical and atypical patterns of disease. *AJR Am J Roentgenol* 2017;209(1):3–18.

Lavelle LP, McEvoy SH, Ni Mhurchu E, et al. Cystic fibrosis below the diaphragm: abdominal findings in adult patients. *Radiographics* 2015;35(3):680–695.

14 **Answer A.** On the CT, multiple small cystic lesions are scattered throughout the pancreas. The main pancreatic duct is not significantly dilated. At ERCP, contrast opacification of these lesions confirms communication with the main duct. Findings are consistent with **multiple branch type intraductal papillary mucinous neoplasms** (IPMNs). These lesions are characteristically pleomorphic, with some appearing round and others tubular. At upper endoscopy, mucin may be observed extruding from the papilla. **Small branch type IPMNs carry a lower risk of malignancy** than main duct and mixed type IPMNs. Management of small IPMNs or other small nonspecific cysts <3 cm is often conservative, with follow-up imaging to monitor for size increase, main duct dilation, or nodularity. Multiple small pancreatic cysts can be seen in von Hippel-Lindau disease (not among the answer choices). Less commonly, pancreatic cysts have also been identified in autosomal-dominant polycystic kidney disease, tuberous sclerosis, and cystic fibrosis. Cysts in these diseases do not communicate with the main duct. Among the answer choices, a choledochocele can present as a small cystic structure, but it represents focal distal biliary dilation located at the ampulla.

References: Megibow AJ, Baker ME, Morgan DE, et al. Management of incidental pancreatic cysts: a white paper of the ACR Incidental Findings Committee. *J Am Coll Radiol* 2017;14(7):911–923.

Raman SP, Kawamoto S, Blackford A, et al. Histopathologic findings of multifocal pancreatic intraductal papillary mucinous neoplasms on CT. *AJR Am J Roentgenol* 2013;200(3):563–569.

15 **Answer F.** An encapsulated cystic mass with solid enhancing components and hemorrhage in a young woman is most likely a solid pseudopapillary tumor (SPT), which is also known as solid pseudopapillary epithelial neoplasm (SPEN) and Frantz tumor. A heterogeneous mass requires careful correlation of pre- and postcontrast images for accurate interpretation. Anteriorly (short arrows), there is increase in signal intensity from pre- to postcontrast MR images in the bottom row, consistent with enhancing soft tissue. This corresponds to an area of internal nodularity on CT. On the postcontrast FS T1W MRI image on the bottom right, a nodular area of high signal intensity (long arrow) could potentially be misinterpreted as enhancing soft tissue. However, precontrast high T1 and low T2 signal intensity is most likely hemorrhage, with no enhancement.

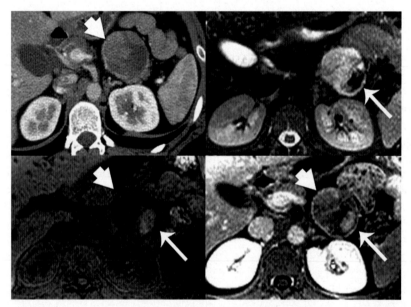

Top row: Contrast-enhanced CT and FS T2W MRI. **Bottom row:** Pre- and postcontrast FS T1W MRI showing enhancing component (*short arrows*) and nonenhancing hemorrhagic component (*long arrows*).

The main differential diagnosis in this patient demographic would be a cystic neuroendocrine tumor (not an answer choice). There is no evidence of fat in this cystic mass in this young patient that would be diagnostic for a mature teratoma. A mature teratoma (dermoid cyst) is a germ cell tumor found in children and young adults that rarely arises in the pancreas. There is fat in >90% of cases and calcium in >50%. On CT, fat within the lesion would be very low in density at <−20 HU and visually similar to the density of fat elsewhere, such as in the mesentery. On MRI, fat would appear dark on any fat-saturated sequence.

The widespread utilization of CT and MR imaging has increased the number of pancreatic cysts detected. The key features of four important pancreatic cystic neoplasms are summarized in the following table. **Not included here are collections related to pancreatitis (pseudocysts and walled-off necrosis)**

and neuroendocrine tumors with cystic/necrotic components, which should also be considered in the differential diagnosis of a cystic pancreatic lesion. Endoscopic ultrasound with FNA and fluid analysis in some cases can help differentiate cystic tumors and assess risk of malignancy.

Features of Cystic Pancreatic Neoplasms*

Neoplasm	Demographics	Morphology	Calcification	Prognosis and Management
Serous microcystic adenoma	"Grandmother lesion" • Age > 60 • Mostly women • Also in von Hippel-Lindau	• Cluster of small thin-walled cysts (<2 cm each), >6 in number • Lobulated margins • Honeycomb or sponge-like appearance in 20% • Central stellate scar	30% centrally	Benign. Usually no treatment.
Mucinous cystic neoplasm	"Mother lesion" • Age ~ 50 • Almost all women	• Larger cysts (≥2 cm each), ≤6 in number • Dominant encapsulated round or oval cyst • Thick wall, septations or mural nodularity • 90% in body or tail • ↑ CEA in aspirate • Main differential diagnosis is pseudocyst (↓ CEA)	15% marginal or septal	Malignant or premalignant. Resect.
Intraductal papillary mucinous neoplasm (IPMN)	"Grandfather lesion" • Age > 60 • Mostly men	• Pleomorphic (tubular, ovoid, round, branching) • Communicate with duct, by definition • Single or multiple lesions • Types: Side-branch, main duct, or combined • Higher risk of malignancy when main duct involved • Mucin seen extruding from papilla at endoscopy • ↑ CEA in aspirate	Rare	Variable. Consider resection if size >3 cm, main duct dilation, or other suspicious features like nodularity.
Solid pseudopapillary tumor (SPT)	"Daughter lesion" • Age ~ 25 • Almost all women	• Encapsulated cystic and solid mass • Nodular enhancing components • May be hemorrhagic • Main differential diagnoses include mucinous cystic neoplasm and neuroendocrine tumor	30% marginal or central	Low-grade malignancy. Resect.

*The differential diagnosis of a cystic pancreatic lesion also includes collections related to pancreatitis (pseudocysts and walled-off necrosis) as well as cystic neuroendocrine tumors.
CEA, carcinoembryonic antigen.

References: Cooper JA. Solid pseudopapillary tumor of the pancreas. *Radiographics* 2006;26(4):1210.

Dewhurst CE, Mortele KJ. Cystic tumors of the pancreas: imaging and management. *Radiol Clin North Am* 2012;50(3):467–486.

Low G, Panu A, Millo N, et al. Multimodality imaging of neoplastic and nonneoplastic solid lesions of the pancreas. *Radiographics* 2011;31(4):993–1015.

16   **Answer A.** Annular pancreas is an uncommon congenital anomaly. **This annular pancreas is radiologically complete**, with circumferential pancreatic tissue (arrows) surrounding the duodenum.

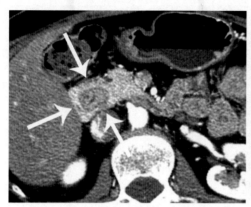 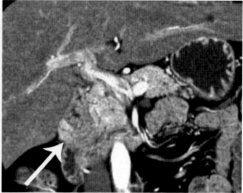

If a portion of parenchyma is thinned and not visible on CT, the annular pancreas is radiologically incomplete and may be more difficult to diagnose. However, **ERCP and MRCP could confirm an encircling duct**. The normal duodenum surrounded by pancreatic tissue may be mistaken for a pancreatic head neoplasm, but tracing the course of the duodenum should reveal duodenal continuity. In childhood, annular pancreas most frequently presents with **duodenal obstruction**. In adults, annular pancreas **can be incidental**, but if symptomatic, adults most commonly present with **pancreatitis**. In normal development, the ventral anlage passes from right to left behind the descending duodenum to fuse with the dorsal anlage, forming the uncinate process and inferior pancreatic head. Abnormal migration can result in annular pancreas. Treatment of symptomatic patients is surgical.

References: Borghei P, Sokhandon F, Shirkhoda A, et al. Anomalies, anatomic variants, and sources of diagnostic pitfalls in pancreatic imaging. *Radiology* 2013;266(1):28–36.

Sandrasegaran K, Patel A, Fogel EL, et al. Annular pancreas in adults. *AJR Am J Roentgenol* 2009;193(2):455–460.

17a   **Answer D.** There is a **hypoenhancing mass** in the pancreatic body causing upstream **pancreatic ductal dilation**, most consistent with **pancreatic ductal adenocarcinoma** (PDA). This is not a typical finding for the other answer choices (lung carcinoma, sarcoidosis, or septic emboli). In the chest, there are multiple bilateral pulmonary emboli. **The high incidence of thromboembolic disease** in patients with advanced pancreatic carcinoma is well known and is a life-threatening complication that may be incidentally noted on abdominal CT.

Regarding the other answer choices, septic emboli themselves are microscopic but manifest as multifocal infarcts in organs such as kidney and spleen, with or without abscesses. In the lungs, septic emboli manifest as peripheral pulmonary nodules that may cavitate, not as macroscopic emboli in the visible pulmonary arteries. In sarcoidosis, findings include adenopathy, nodular interstitial lung disease, and hepatosplenic nodules, but it does not usually involve the pancreas.

17b   **Answer A.** The underlying disease is **pancreatic ductal carcinoma with distant metastases** (stage IV), which is unresectable and treated with **chemotherapy**. The arrows on the images below indicate the multiple findings. Anticoagulation was initiated emergently for the bilateral pulmonary emboli. The hypovascular **liver metastases** are denser than expected for simple fluid. The omental soft tissue nodules are consistent with **peritoneal carcinomatosis**, which is not associated with ascites in this case.

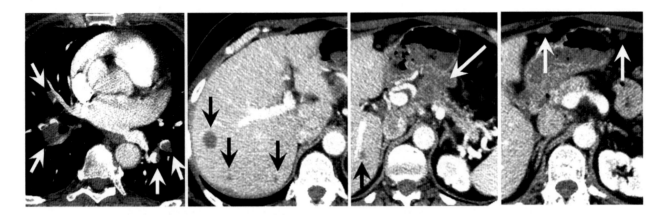

In patients without distant metastases, CT assessment of local vascular involvement is critical in determining resectability. Fewer than a quarter of patients present with resectable disease. Vascular occlusion or "encasement" (tumor contact >180 degrees of vessel circumference) of the SMA is usually considered unresectable. **A description of the vessels involved and extent of involvement is generally more appropriate than reporting the tumor as resectable or unresectable.** Abutment (tumor contact ≤180 degrees of vessel circumference) or even encasement/occlusion of arteries and veins may be considered resectable (e.g., splenic vessels) or borderline resectable with newer surgical techniques. Borderline resectable tumors may be downsized with neoadjuvant chemoradiation, followed by curative resection, potentially with vascular reconstruction. Short segments of the hepatic artery, celiac artery, portal vein, and superior mesenteric vein may be grafted or bypassed. **The criteria for resectability vary among institutions and depend on surgical expertise.** Resectability is also affected by **vascular anatomy** including normal variants and presence of adequate collateral flow.

References: Schawkat K, Manning MA, Glickman JN, Mortele KJ. Pancreatic ductal adenocarcinoma and its variants: pearls and perils. *Radiographics* 2020;40(5):1–20.

Tamm EP, Balachandran A, Bhosale PR, et al. Imaging of pancreatic adenocarcinoma: update on staging/resectability. *Radiol Clin North Am* 2012;50(3):407–428.

18 **Answer B.** MRCP shows a dark, well-defined filling defect (white arrow) within the main duct in the pancreatic body. There is **upstream dilation of the main duct and side branches** with abrupt transition at the level of filling defect. Parenchyma is atrophic. Findings are consistent with an **obstructing ductal stone in the setting of chronic pancreatitis** (CP). The stone is visible as a calcification on the fluoroscopic scout image obtained at the time of ERCP (black arrow).

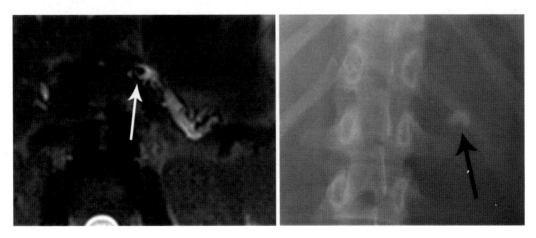

The most common finding in CP is dilation of the main duct and/or side branches, which is seen in two-thirds of patients. **Ductal dilation is caused by strictures and stone formation** in CP. Intraductal stones are demonstrated on MRCP due to the brightness of the surrounding ductal fluid on T2W images. Otherwise, calcifications scattered in the pancreas may not be visible on MRI. Other features of CP include gland atrophy, pseudocysts, pseudoaneurysm, and splenic vein thrombosis. CP in the head may cause biliary as well as pancreatic ductal dilation, resulting in the double-duct sign. Amylase-rich ascites or pleural fluid may be the sequela of pseudocyst rupture or fistulization.

Treatment of obstructing ductal strictures and stones may improve chronic pain. Endoscopic techniques include stenting and lithotripsy. Surgery with pancreaticojejunostomy or partial resection may be indicated in refractory cases. **CP is associated with an increased risk of developing pancreatic ductal adenocarcinoma.** Tumor can be difficult to distinguish from CP, and biopsy should be performed if there is concern for a coexisting malignancy.

Aside from strictures and stones in CP, **differential diagnosis of main duct dilation includes neoplasms,** such as pancreatic ductal adenocarcinoma (PDA) and intrapapillary mucinous cystic neoplasm (IPMN), but also other primary or metastatic lesions. Filling defects representing mucinous debris or nodular tumor can be present in the duct in patients with IPMN. However, these are typically not as dark as the signal voids associated with calculi.

References: Perez-Johnston R, Sainani NI, Sahani DV. Imaging of chronic pancreatitis (including groove and autoimmune pancreatitis). *Radiol Clin North Am* 2012;50(3):447–466.

Wolske KM, Ponnatapura J, Kolokythas O, et al. Chronic pancreatitis or pancreatic tumor? A problem-solving approach. *Radiographics* 2019;39(7):1965–1982.

19a **Answer B.**

19b **Answer D.** This patient was suspected to have a pancreatic head neoplasm, but findings on MRI are diagnostic for microscopic lipid due to **focal fatty infiltration, a benign incidental finding**. Shown are a contrast-enhanced CT and noncontrast MRI with gradient-echo T1W in-phase and out-of-phase images. There is mild hypoattenuation of the anterior part of the pancreatic head on CT. On the MRI, there is **signal loss on the out-of-phase** image (long arrows) compared to the in-phase image. Comparison with muscle (short arrows) as an **internal reference may be helpful when signal loss is more subtle**. The pancreatic head is brighter than muscle on in-phase image and slightly darker than muscle on out-of-phase image.

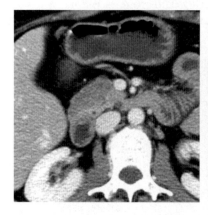 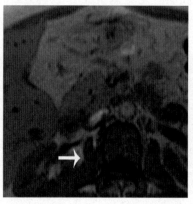 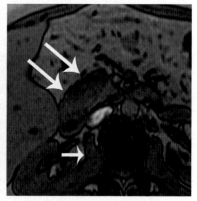

Fatty infiltration can **differentially involve the anterior and posterior portions of the pancreatic head as seen in this case**, attributed to histologic differences between the embryologic dorsal and ventral pancreas. On CT, the hypoenhancing area of fatty infiltration can be mistaken for a pancreatic head neoplasm, but the upstream pancreas (not shown) should be normal without ductal dilation nor parenchymal atrophy. This area of fatty infiltration **will enhance because it is parenchyma, so the key to diagnosis is comparing in-and-out-of-phase images**, not pre- and postcontrast images. Regarding the other answer choices, **a lipoma is composed of macroscopic fat, which would lose signal on fat-saturated images, not on out-of-phase images.** Neither pancreatic ductal adenocarcinoma nor neuroendocrine tumor have fat.

Fat- and water-bound protons precess at slightly different frequencies, and their phase shifts can be manipulated to detect microscopic lipid on the T1W GRE in-phase and out-of-phase sequences. A pixel that contains a combination of fat- and water-bound protons within an area containing microscopic lipid would lose signal during the out-of-phase images (acquired at a TE of about 2.4 msec in a 1.5 tesla magnet) compared to the in-phase images (acquired at a TE of about 4.8 msec). Pixels at fat–water interfaces also contain a combination of these protons, producing the **characteristic dark lines of the "India ink," or "etching," artifact around organs surrounded by fat on the out-of-phase images.** No fat saturation has been applied, so macroscopic fat as seen in the mesentery and retroperitoneum remains bright on both sequences.

These MR images have been performed without contrast, yet **artifactual high signal intensity can be seen in the aorta and IVC on some images due to the "entry phenomenon" on gradient-echo sequences.** Flowing blood moving into the imaging volume is inherently bright on gradient-echo sequences and **should not be mistaken for enhancement**. Signal in the IVC will be brightest on the inferior slices of the abdomen as shown here with unsaturated protons coming from below. The signal in the aorta will be brightest on the superior slices of the abdomen with the unsaturated protons coming from above.

References: Befera NT, Bashir MR, Amrhein TJ. Chapter 7: Type 2 chemical shift artifact. In: Mangrum WI (ed). *Duke review of MRI physics*, 2nd ed. Philadelphia, PA: Elsevier, Inc., 2019:65–76.

Kim HJ, Byun JH, Park SH, et al. Focal fatty replacement of the pancreas: usefulness of chemical shift MRI. *AJR Am J Roentgenol* 2007;188(2):429–432.

Pokharel SS, Macura KJ, Kamel IR, et al. Current MR imaging lipid detection techniques for diagnosis of lesions in the abdomen and pelvis. *Radiographics* 2013;33(3):681–702.

20 **Answer A. Most pancreatic neuroendocrine neoplasms (PNENs) are sporadic, but about 10% are associated with genetic syndromes.** PNENs are found in patients with **multiple endocrine neoplasia type 1 (MEN-1)** and are the **major cause of mortality.** Most of these are nonfunctioning, but the most common subtype of functioning tumors in MEN-1 is gastrinoma. Patients with MEN-1 are predisposed to developing parathyroid adenomas or hyperplasia, PNEN, and pituitary adenoma ("pa, pa, pi"). Complete surgical resection may not be possible due to **tumor multicentricity and high risk of recurrence in patients with MEN-1** compared with sporadic cases.

Von Hippel-Lindau (VHL) disease is a rare hereditary syndrome with a broad spectrum of clinical features, and pancreatic findings in VHL include simple cysts, PNEN, serous microcystic cystadenomas, and rarely ductal adenocarcinomas. Two other syndromes, **neurofibromatosis type 1** and **tuberous sclerosis**, have also been linked with PNENs. Pancreatic lesions are not a feature of MEN-2a or MEN-2b. MEN-2a is associated with medullary thyroid cancer, pheochromocytoma, and parathyroid adenomas ("me, phe, pt"). MEN-2b is associated with medullary thyroid cancer, pheochromocytoma, and neuromas ("me, phe, ne").

References: Davila A, Menias CO, Alhalabi K, et al. Multiple endocrine neoplasia: spectrum of abdominal manifestations. *AJR Am J Roentgenol* 2020:1–11.

Khanna L, Prasad SR, Sunnapwar A, et al. Pancreatic neuroendocrine neoplasms: 2020 update on pathologic and imaging findings and classification. *Radiographics* 2020;40(5):1240–1262.

21 **Answer C.** Findings are suspicious for **lymphoma** with homogeneous mass-like expansion of the pancreatic head. **The pancreatic and biliary ducts pass through the enlarged pancreatic head virtually undisturbed with no obstruction.** The pancreatic body and tail appear normal. Secondary involvement of the pancreas in non-Hodgkin lymphoma can occur in up to 30% of patients, while primary pancreatic lymphoma is very rare. Lymphoma can present as localized or diffuse infiltration. Lesions are typically homogeneous iso-to-hypoenhancing with little or no mass effect.

The main differential diagnosis is autoimmune pancreatitis (not an answer choice), which can also have a mass-like infiltrative appearance. Acute and chronic pancreatitis (not answer choices) should evolve with other findings such as surrounding inflammatory fat stranding, fluid collections, necrosis, calcification, irregular ductal dilation, or atrophy. Regarding the other answer choices, neuroendocrine tumor and leiomyosarcoma are discrete rather than infiltrative masses. Neuroendocrine tumors are typically hypervascular, not a feature in this case. The **pancreas is normally the most T1 hyperintense organ in the abdomen** due to high protein content, and this should not be mistaken for enhancement on arterial phase. Pancreatic ductal adenocarcinoma is hypovascular and can have infiltrative margins but tends to obstruct the duct even when small because of its desmoplastic nature. Pancreatic leiomyosarcoma is rare and presents as a discrete heterogeneously enhancing mass.

References: Low G, Panu A, Millo N, et al. Multimodality imaging of neoplastic and nonneoplastic solid lesions of the pancreas. *Radiographics* 2011;31(4):993–1015.

Manning MA, Paal EE, Srivastava A, et al. Nonepithelial neoplasms of the pancreas, Part 2: Malignant tumors and tumors of uncertain malignant potential from the radiologic pathology archives. *Radiographics* 2018;38(4):1047–1072.

22 **Answer B.** The two coronal and one axial image from MRCP show **pancreas divisum**. The dorsal duct continues as the accessory duct of Santorini (arrows) toward the minor papilla, **crossing anterior to the common bile duct** (black arrow on the third image) rather than converging with the CBD at the major papilla.

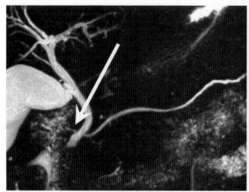 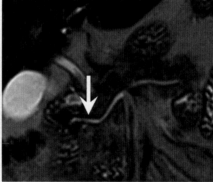 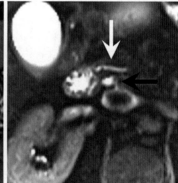

At ERCP in another patient, contrast injection of the major papilla reveals the characteristic **short branching duct within the uncinate process** (arrows) that does not communicate with the main duct.

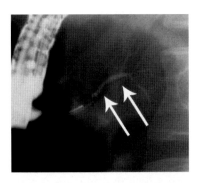

Pancreas divisum is the most common congenital pancreatic anomaly, found in about 10% of the population. There is a failure of fusion of dorsal and ventral pancreatic tissue and ducts. Divisum exposes the accessory duct to an abnormally **increased volume of pancreatic secretions, which may not be adequately drained by the minor papilla**. While pancreas divisum may be asymptomatic, some patients suffer **recurrent pancreatitis**. A focal cystic ductal dilation at the minor papilla called a **Santorinicele may develop due to obstructive physiology**. Treatment with endoscopic sphincterotomy has been found to improve flow through the minor papilla and decrease clinical symptoms.

The other answer choices are also variations of ductal anatomy in the pancreatic head. Ansa pancreatica (also known as an ansa loop) is a ductal variant in which a duct arises from the main (dorsal) duct of Wirsung in the pancreatic head and swings up to exit the minor papilla. This may be a predisposing factor for pancreatitis as well. A long common channel is an abnormal pancreaticobiliary union associated with some types of choledochal cysts, but the ducts in this case do not join. In annular pancreas, the pancreatic duct would encircle the descending duodenum.

References: Borghei P, Sokhandon F, Shirkhoda A, et al. Anomalies, anatomic variants, and sources of diagnostic pitfalls in pancreatic imaging. *Radiology* 2013;266(1):28–36.

Manfredi R, Costamagna G, Brizi MG, et al. Pancreas divisum and "santorinicele": diagnosis with dynamic MR cholangiopancreatography with secretin stimulation. *Radiology* 2000;217(2):403–408.

23 **Answer A.** The patient is status post a **Whipple procedure**. The arrows point to a **normal-appearing afferent (biliopancreatic) limb** at the level of the pancreaticojejunostomy. After resection of the pancreatic head and duodenum, the jejunum is pulled up to the region of the porta hepatis, and anastomoses are performed with the biliary and pancreatic ducts. The blind end of this limb may be demarcated by a staple line, as seen in this case adjacent the stomach. Tubular morphology with thin jejunal folds identifies this as a normal segment of the bowel. Occasionally, the afferent limb may resemble a mass or an abscess in the porta hepatis. The gallbladder has been resected as part of the Whipple procedure.

Common complications after Whipple procedure are delayed gastric emptying, wound infection, abscess, hemorrhage, anastomotic leak, peritonitis, and pancreatitis. **Dilation of the limb may indicate afferent loop syndrome.** The cause of afferent loop syndrome may be benign or malignant and may or may not be visible on CT.

References: Morgan DE. Imaging after pancreatic surgery. *Radiol Clin North Am* 2012;50(3):529–545.

Yamauchi FI, Ortega CD, Blasbalg R, et al. Multidetector CT evaluation of the postoperative pancreas. *Radiographics* 2012;32(3):743–764.

24 **Answer B.** Synthetic secretin may be administered intravenously during MRCP or ERCP to improve distention of the pancreatic ducts. Secretin is a hormone normally produced by the duodenum in response to acid, stimulating the pancreas to produce bicarbonate-rich fluid and increasing the tonicity of the sphincter of Oddi. A dynamic series of T2W images are obtained over time after secretin injection. **Structural abnormalities of the duct including strictures, stones, normal variants, and leaks may be better visualized with the improved duct distention after secretin injection.** Secretin injection also allows semiquantitative assessment of exocrine function, for example, in patients with chronic pancreatitis. A greater increase in duodenal fluid volume after secretin injection indicates better preservation of exocrine function. After a small test dose, secretin is administered slowly over 1 minute. Side effects are uncommon but up to 5% may experience nausea, flushing, and pain. Acute pancreatitis is a contraindication.

Sincalide is the pharmacologic form of **cholecystokinin** (CCK), which may be infused during Tc-99m IDA hepatobiliary studies. CCK is produced by the duodenum and primarily **causes gallbladder contraction facilitating the transit of bile into the duodenum** after a fatty meal. Sincalide is used after 1 hour if bowel activity is not seen. Subsequent bowel activity would indicate normal variation in bile transit rather than true ductal obstruction. Sincalide administration also allows for calculation of gallbladder ejection fraction when chronic cholecystitis is suspected.

Glucagon has a hypotonic effect on bowel and may be administered subcutaneously intramuscularly, or intravenously. It **decreases bowel spasm, improving distention and patient comfort** during double-contrast upper GI, barium enema, CT enterography, and CT colonography. Glucagon also **decreases bowel motion artifacts on MR enterography**. Glucagon and insulin are produced by the islet cells of the pancreas to regulate blood glucose levels. Glucagon increases and insulin decreases blood glucose.

References: Sanyal R, Stevens T, Novak E, et al. Secretin-enhanced MRCP: review of technique and application with proposal for quantification of exocrine function. *AJR Am J Roentgenol* 2012;198(1):124–132.

Tirkes T, Sandrasegaran K, Sanyal R, et al. Secretin-enhanced MR cholangiopancreatography: spectrum of findings. *Radiographics* 2013;33(7):1889–1906.

25 **Answer D.** This cystic neoplasm was **resected, revealing a mucinous cystic neoplasm (MCN)**, in this case a cystadenocarcinoma. This lesion demonstrates enhancing soft tissue nodularity, as well as a few foci of rim calcification. **The increased conspicuity of the nodular tissue against the fluid background compared to noncontrast image reflects tumor enhancement.** Chronic fluid collections such as pseudocysts and walled-off necrosis from prior pancreatitis may have features overlapping those of cystic neoplasms on imaging. Pancreatitis fluid collections can demonstrate capsular enhancement, internal debris, and rim calcification but should not exhibit enhancing soft tissue nodularity. Neoplasms sometimes present with pancreatitis secondary to duct obstruction, confounding assessment.

Some cystic neoplasms have little or no perceptible internal complexity. **Growth of a chronic cystic lesion increases suspicion for neoplasm** and should prompt further investigation or closer follow-up. Fluid collections in pancreatitis may be drained if symptomatic or infected, but not all collections require drainage. **Percutaneous or endoscopic drainage of tumors should be avoided.**

References: Kim YH, Saini S, Sahani D, et al. Imaging diagnosis of cystic pancreatic lesions: pseudocyst versus nonpseudocyst. *Radiographics* 2005;25(3):671–685.

Megibow AJ, Baker ME, Morgan DE, et al. Management of incidental pancreatic cysts: a white paper of the ACR Incidental Findings Committee. *J Am Coll Radiol* 2017;14(7):911–923.

26a **Answer D.** This is **autoimmune pancreatitis** (AIP) with the **classic peripheral halo** surrounding the gland. AIP is an immune-mediated chronic pancreatitis with lymphoplasmacytic infiltration. The three patterns of involvement on imaging are described as **diffuse, focal, or multifocal.** The diffuse pattern is associated with the classic features of AIP, including a peripheral halo or gland enlargement with effacement of the fatty interstices for a **"sausage"** appearance as shown in a different patient below.

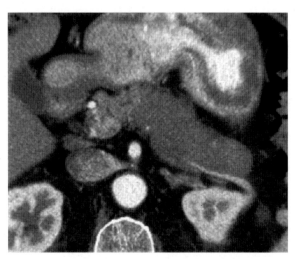

Image courtesy of Dr. Priya Bhosale, Department of Diagnostic Radiology, The University of Texas, MD Anderson Cancer Center, Houston, Texas.

The focal and multifocal patterns of involvement may have **mass-like appearance mimicking neoplasm**. If fibrosis is prominent, delayed enhancement and ductal obstruction can be seen, making distinction from pancreatic ductal adenocarcinoma difficult. The halo, if fibrotic, may also demonstrate delayed enhancement. Findings are potentially reversible with **steroid treatment**.

The other answer choices do not present with the well-circumscribed halo. The pancreas in this case enhances without evidence of necrosis. Lymphoma may present as hypovascular masses or diffuse involvement of the gland with little or no ductal dilation. Associated lymphadenopathy may be identified. Lymphoma diffusely infiltrating the gland effaces the normal fatty interstices of the gland and may mimic the sausage appearance of AIP. However, in the case shown for this question, the parenchymal architecture is preserved with no evidence of an infiltrating neoplasm.

References: Khandelwal A, Shanbhogue AK, Takahashi N, et al. Recent advances in the diagnosis and management of autoimmune pancreatitis. *AJR Am J Roentgenol* 2014;202(5):1007–1021.

Perez-Johnston R, Sainani NI, Sahani DV. Imaging of chronic pancreatitis (including groove and autoimmune pancreatitis). *Radiol Clin North Am* 2012;50(3):447–466.

26b **Answer A.** Autoimmune pancreatitis (AIP) is characterized by lymphoplasmacytic infiltration that can be (but not always) associated with elevated levels of IgG4 in serum and in tissue at FNA/biopsy. **Two types of AIP** have been described. **Type 1 AIP is far more common and accounts for >80% of cases in the United States**, with the typical patient **>50 years old** and male. Type 1 AIP is one of the manifestations of **multisystemic IgG4-related fibroinflammatory disease**. More than half of these patients exhibit extrapancreatic signs at presentation, such as retroperitoneal fibrosis, sclerosing cholangitis, sclerosing mesenteritis, orbital pseudotumor, or Riedel thyroiditis. Relapse of type 1 AIP occurs often after steroid treatment.

Type 2 AIP is seen in younger patients with a lower prevalence of IgG4 elevation. The pancreas is typically the only organ involved, although there is an association with inflammatory bowel disease in 30%. After steroid treatment, type 2 AIP rarely relapses. **The three imaging patterns of involvement (focal, multifocal, and diffuse) can be seen in both types of AIP.**

Regarding the other answer choices, CRP (C-reactive protein) is a general indicator of infection or inflammation without specificity for AIP. CA19-9 may be elevated in patients with pancreatic and biliary ductal adenocarcinoma, in which case levels can be used to track the disease. However, sensitivity and specificity of CA19-9 for malignancy are limited. Chromogranin A is a marker associated with neuroendocrine tumors.

References: Khandelwal A, Shanbhogue AK, Takahashi N, et al. Recent advances in the diagnosis and management of autoimmune pancreatitis. *AJR Am J Roentgenol* 2014;202(5):1007–1021.

Perez-Johnston R, Sainani NI, Sahani DV. Imaging of chronic pancreatitis (including groove and autoimmune pancreatitis). *Radiol Clin North Am* 2012;50(3):447–466.

27 **Answer C.** The mass in the pancreatic body enhances on arterial phase greater than venous phase, consistent with a hypervascular neoplasm. The left kidney has been resected with surgical clips visible. (The pancreatic tail extends into the nephrectomy site.) **Renal cell carcinoma (RCC) is the most common metastasis to the pancreas and often appears as a hypervascular mass.** RCC accounts for 30% of metastases to the pancreas, followed by lung cancer. Breast, colorectal, and melanoma metastases are also seen. **Metastases to the pancreas are uncommon**, representing 2% to 5% of pancreatic malignancies, with **variable appearance**. They can present as a solitary mass, multiple masses, or diffuse infiltration. The duct may be normal or obstructed, whereas pancreatic ductal adenocarcinoma being desmoplastic tends to cause duct obstruction even if the tumor is small. Patients can be asymptomatic or exhibit nonspecific symptoms such as pain or weight loss. While most other metastases develop within 3 years of primary tumor diagnosis, **RCC metastases to the pancreas can be a late manifestation occurring a decade or more after initial presentation**. The main differential diagnosis for this solitary hypervascular mass is a pancreatic neuroendocrine tumor. Melanoma metastasis and small cell lung cancer (considered a neuroendocrine neoplasm) may be hypervascular but are less common in the pancreas than RCC. Lymphoma and most other metastases are hypovascular. Secondary involvement of the pancreas in lymphoma is seen in up to 30% of patients with extensive non-Hodgkin lymphoma and is more common than primary pancreatic lymphoma.

References: Diaz de Leon A, Pirasteh A, Costa DN, et al. Current challenges in diagnosis and assessment of the response of locally advanced and metastatic renal cell carcinoma. *Radiographics* 2019;39(4):998–1016.

Low G, Panu A, Millo N, et al. Multimodality imaging of neoplastic and nonneoplastic solid lesions of the pancreas. *Radiographics* 2011;31(4):993–1015.

28a **Answer D.** There is small round outpouching (arrows on images below) from the splenic artery consistent with a **pseudoaneurysm** (PSA). It is at the margin of the pancreatic fluid collection that represents walled-off necrosis. The enhancement of the PSA **follows the density of the aorta** on both the arterial and venous phase. **Multiphase imaging can differentiate pseudoaneurysm (which maintains the same shape) and active hemorrhage (which grows and disperses).**

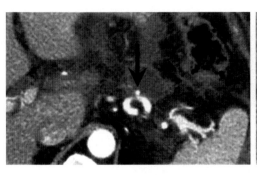 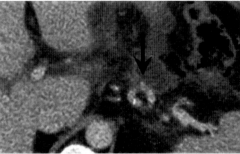

Severe pancreatitis can be complicated by vascular abnormalities secondary to enzymatic digestion or infection of the vascular wall. PSAs are a late complication and most commonly arise from the **splenic artery**, but gastroduodenal, hepatic, superior mesenteric, and left gastric arteries may also be affected. Thrombosis of the splenic or other veins can also occur. Regarding the other answer choices, a calcified ductal stone would have the same unchanging high density on all phases. Patients with chronic pancreatitis do have an increased risk of pancreatic ductal adenocarcinoma, but development of tumor is not expected within the time course of acute pancreatitis. Findings are not consistent with solid tumor on this study.

References: O'Conner O, Buckley JM, Maher MM. Imaging of the complications of acute pancreatitis. *AJR Am J Roentgenol* 2011;197:w375–w381.

Shyu JY, Sainani NI, Sahni VA, et al. Necrotizing pancreatitis: diagnosis, imaging, and intervention. *Radiographics* 2014;34(5):1218–1239.

28b **Answer A.** The splenic artery PSA has significantly enlarged, and the enhancing component is surrounded by a large heterogeneous blood clot. **Angiography** (shown below) and treatment with **embolization** is the most appropriate next step in this hemodynamically stable patient.

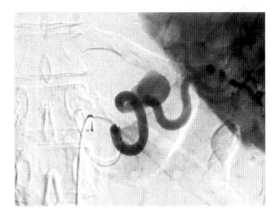

Even small PSAs can be symptomatic with life-threatening hemorrhage and require urgent treatment. Detection can be challenging, and meticulous analysis of arterial CT images in multiple planes is crucial. In patients with negative CT angiography but continued hemorrhage, repeat CTA or angiography may be considered for further evaluation. **Spontaneous hemorrhage in necrotizing pancreatitis** can occur from erosion of arteries or veins or from rupture of a pseudoaneurysm or varices. The slow rate of venous hemorrhage is usually undetectable on imaging. **High mortality of hemorrhagic pancreatitis** up to 52% has been reported.

References: O'Conner O, Buckley JM, Maher MM. Imaging of the complications of acute pancreatitis. *AJR Am J Roentgenol* 2011;197:w375–w381.

Shyu JY, Sainani NI, Sahni VA, et al. Necrotizing pancreatitis: diagnosis, imaging, and intervention. *Radiographics* 2014;34(5):1218–1239.

QUESTIONS

For patients in questions 1 to 6, select the most likely diagnosis (A to G) for the hepatic masses. Each option may be used once, more than once, or not at all.

A. Cavernous hemangioma
B. Focal nodular hyperplasia (FNH)
C. Hepatocellular adenoma (HCA)
D. Hepatocellular carcinoma (HCC)
E. Metastatic colon carcinoma
F. Cholangiocarcinoma (CCA)
G. Angiomyolipoma (AML)

1 A 63-year-old woman. Images are from an MRI using conventional extracellular gadolinium contrast.

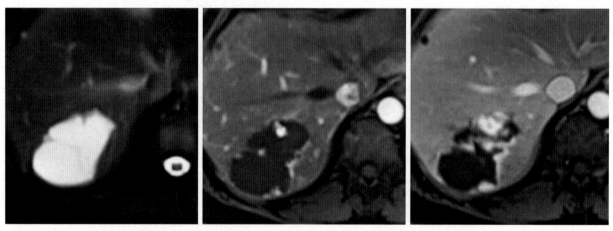

FS T2W, arterial phase T1W+gad, and delayed-phase T1W+gad.

2a A 60-year-old man.

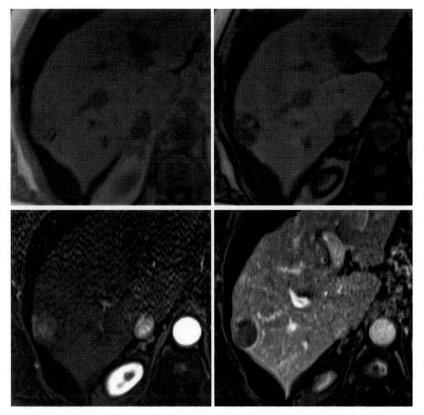

Top row: In-phase and out-of-phase T1W. **Bottom row:** Arterial and venous phase FS T1W+gad.

2b On the in-phase and out-of-phase gradient echo T1W images, this lesion
contains

    A. Macroscopic fat
    B. Microscopic fat
    C. Acute hemorrhage
    D. Old hemorrhage with hemosiderin

3 A 68-year-old man.

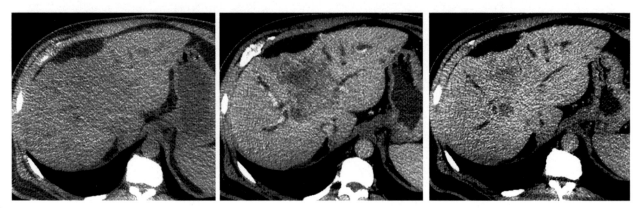

4 A 21-year-old woman was found to have an incidental liver lesion on pelvic ultrasound. Images from an MRI using hepatobiliary gadolinium contrast agent gadoxetate disodium (Eovist—Bayer HealthCare) are shown.

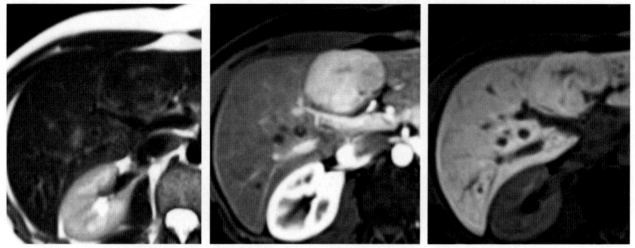

T2W, arterial phase FS T1W+hepatobiliary gad, and 20-minute FS T1W+hepatobiliary gad.

5 A 55-year-old man.

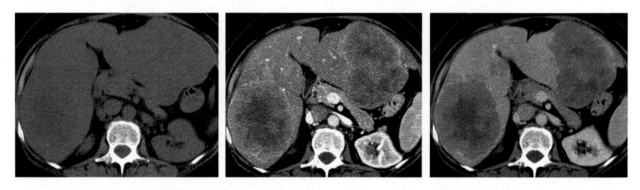

6 A 51-year-old man with hepatitis B and cirrhosis. Images from an MRI performed with hepatobiliary contrast agent are shown.

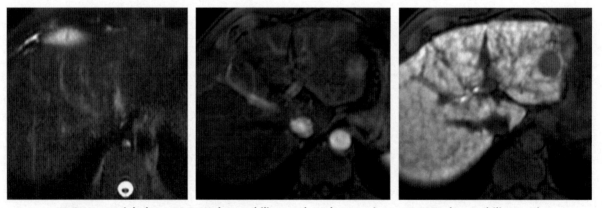

FS T2W, arterial phase FS T1W+hepatobiliary gad, and a 20-minute FS T1W+hepatobiliary gad.

7 Which of the following would be considered an ancillary feature favoring malignancy rather than a major feature according to the Liver Imaging Reporting and Data System (LI-RADS)?

A. Washout appearance
B. Capsule appearance
C. Arterial enhancement
D. Hepatobiliary phase hypointensity

8 Images from a CT on a 55-year-old man with hepatitis C and cirrhosis are shown. Arterial phase images are shown on the left, and delayed images are shown on the right. Which LI-RADS category best fits the findings?

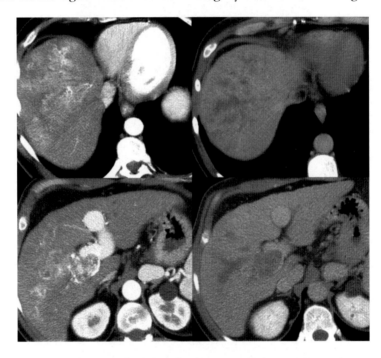

A. LR-3 (intermediate probability for hepatocellular carcinoma)
B. LR-4 (probably hepatocellular carcinoma)
C. LR-5 (definitely hepatocellular carcinoma)
D. LR-TIV (definitely tumor in vein)

9 A 71-year-old man undergoes a CT scan. What is the most likely diagnosis?

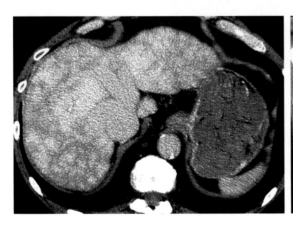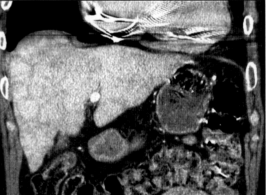

A. Metastatic disease
B. Budd-Chiari syndrome
C. Congestive hepatopathy
D. Schistosomiasis

10a A 24-year-old man with no known history of liver disease presents with epigastric pain and vomiting. A transverse image from an abdominal ultrasound is shown. What is the most likely diagnosis?

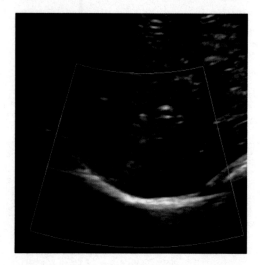

A. Hemangioma
B. Hepatocellular carcinoma
C. Angiomyolipoma
D. Metastasis

10b What finding is indicated by the arrow on this sagittal ultrasound image from the same patient?

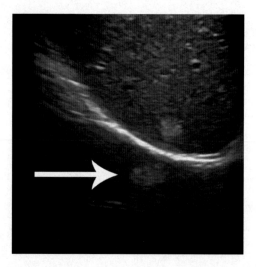

A. Lung nodule
B. Mirror artifact
C. Peritoneal nodule
D. Twinkling artifact

11 A 22-year-old patient presents with abdominal pain. A venous phase CT and hepatic venogram are shown. Which of the following is the most common known etiology of this disease process?

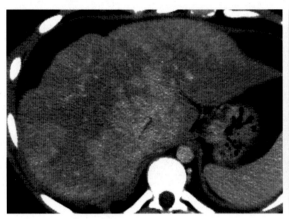 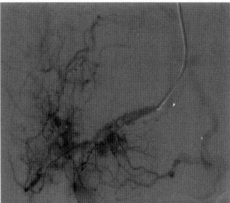

A. Thrombophilia
B. Viral hepatitis
C. Alcohol abuse
D. Congenital defect

For the patients in questions 12 to 15, select the most likely diagnosis (A to F). Each option may be used once or not at all.

A. Pyogenic abscess
B. Echinococcal (hydatid) cyst
C. Polycystic liver disease in autosomal dominant polycystic kidney disease (ADPCKD)
D. Biliary hamartomas (von Meyenburg complex)
E. Biliary cystadenoma/cystadenocarcinoma (BCA/BCAC)
F. Subcapsular hematoma

12 A 63-year-old man with pancreatic cancer status post common bile duct stent placement.

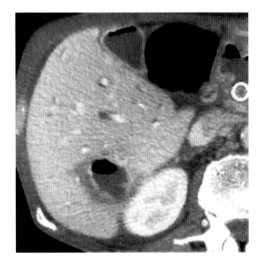

13   A 71-year-old woman status post renal transplant.

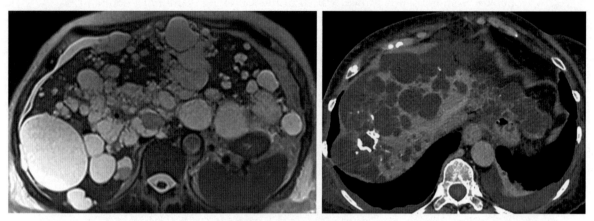

T2W MRI and venous phase CT.

14   A 46-year-old woman.

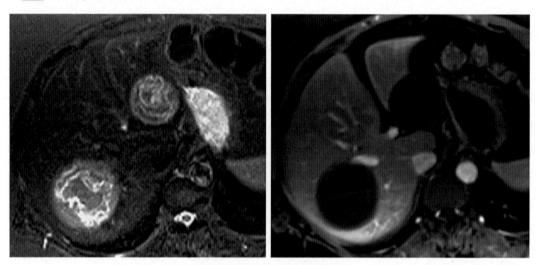

FS T2W and FS T1W+gad.

15   A 75-year-old man.

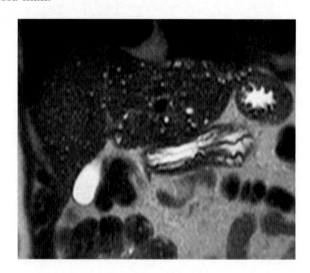

16a A 35-year-old man underwent an abdominal ultrasound as part of preoperative evaluation for renal transplant. An MRI was performed to further evaluate the liver. What is the cause of the disease process revealed on these T1W GRE in-phase and out-of-phase images?

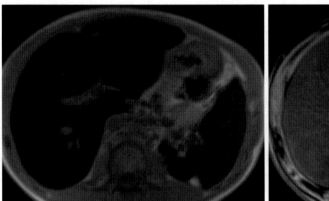 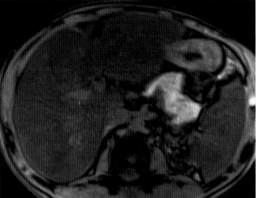

A. Viral hepatitis
B. Blood transfusions
C. Alcohol consumption
D. Hereditary depositional disease

16b Which of the following parameters would be the most effective for reducing T2* effect and susceptibility artifacts?

A. Gradient-echo sequence and shorter TE
B. Gradient-echo sequence and longer TE
C. Fast spin-echo sequence and shorter TE
D. Fast spin-echo sequence and longer TE

17 A 54-year-old man undergoes MR imaging for evaluation of a liver mass. Among the choices listed, which is the most likely diagnosis?

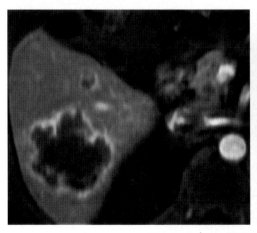 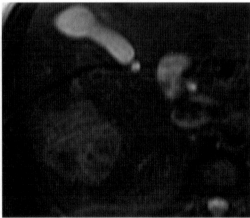

Venous phase FS T1W+gad and T2W MRI.

A. Metastasis
B. Hemangioma
C. Simple cyst
D. Focal nodular hyperplasia

18 Regarding contrast agent selection for liver MRI, which of the following indications has the best consensus for the use of a hepatobiliary contrast agent such as gadoxetate disodium (Eovist—Bayer HealthCare) over a conventional extracellular contrast agent?

A. Assessing for residual or recurrent hepatocellular carcinoma after transarterial chemoembolization

B. Differentiating between focal nodular hyperplasia and hepatocellular adenoma

C. Confirming a hemangioma

D. Screening for hepatocellular carcinoma in a patient with hemochromatosis

19 A 77-year-old woman with abdominal pain and abnormal liver function tests was imaged with CT. What is the most likely diagnosis?

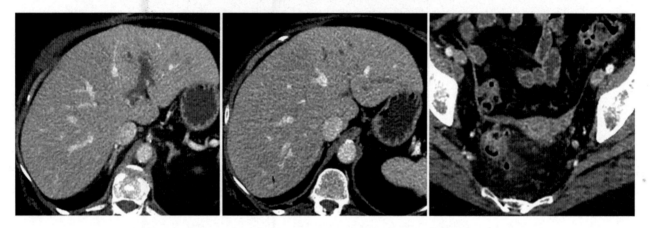

A. Portal vein thrombophlebitis

B. Biliary obstruction with cholangitis

C. Metastatic colon cancer

D. Liver laceration

20a A 19-year-old man was injured in a motor vehicle collision. Which statement is TRUE regarding the management of the liver findings on CT?

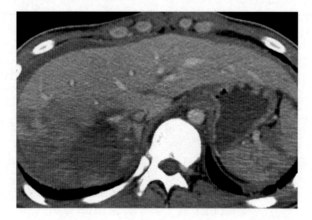

A. Partial hepatic resection is indicated for extent of laceration.

B. Angiography is indicated for embolization of a pseudoaneurysm.

C. No intervention is needed if patient is hemodynamically stable.

D. Percutaneous catheter placement is indicated for subcapsular hematoma.

20b The patient was hemodynamically stable and managed conservatively. Within 24 hours, the patient developed jaundice, which prompted an HIDA scan. What is the diagnosis?

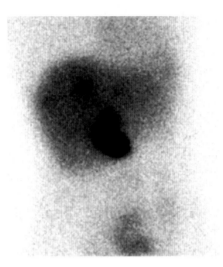

A. Intrahepatic bilomas
B. Intraperitoneal bile leak
C. Common bile duct obstruction
D. Gallbladder laceration

21 A 49-year-old woman has the following liver finding on MRI performed with conventional extracellular contrast agent. What is the diagnosis?

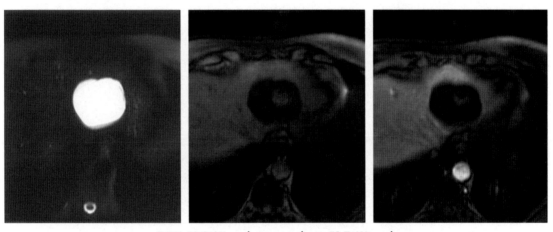

T2W, FS T1W, and venous phase FS T1W+gad.

A. Simple hepatic cyst
B. Biliary cystadenocarcinoma with enhancing nodule
C. Liquefying hematoma with residual blood clot
D. Echinococcal cyst with daughter cyst

22 A 52-year-old woman undergoes a CT scan with images shown below. Findings are consistent with which diagnosis?

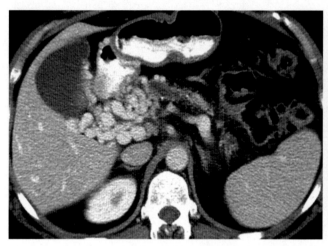 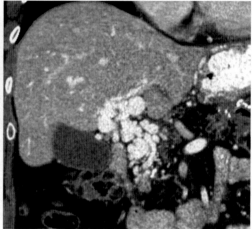

A. Cholangiocarcinoma
B. Hemangioma
C. Lymphadenopathy
D. Portal vein occlusion

23a A 46-year-old woman with breast ductal carcinoma in situ (DCIS) was found to have a liver lesion on breast MRI. Dedicated liver MRI was performed with a conventional extracellular contrast agent for further evaluation. What is the most likely diagnosis?

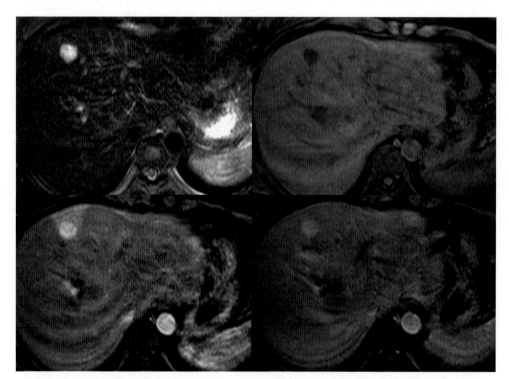

Top row: FS T2W and FS T1W. **Bottom row:** Arterial and delayed-phase FS T1W+gad.

A. Hemangioma
B. Metastatic breast cancer
C. Abscess
D. Hepatocellular carcinoma

23b This is the arterial phase postcontrast T1W image from the same case. What finding is indicated by the arrows?

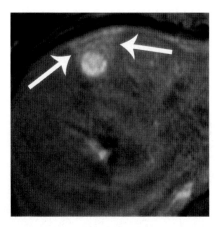

    A. Poor fat saturation
    B. Focal fatty sparing
    C. Transient hepatic intensity difference (THID)
    D. Hemorrhage

24a A 30-year-old woman is evaluated for a liver lesion that was incidentally noted at the time of a pelvic ultrasound. Which of the following statements is TRUE about the finding in the right lobe of the liver?

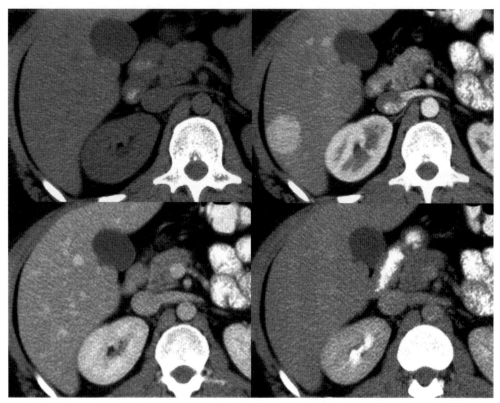

Top row: Noncontrast and arterial phase CT. **Bottom row:** Venous and delayed-phase CT.

    A. The finding demonstrates washout appearance and is most likely a malignancy.
    B. The finding is likely a mass of hepatocellular origin.
    C. The finding is likely a transient hepatic attenuation difference (THAD).
    D. The finding demonstrates a central scar.

24b Hepatocellular adenomas in which of the following groups of patients have the highest risk of malignant transformation to hepatocellular carcinomas?

   A. Women using oral contraceptives
   B. Men
   C. Patients with diabetes
   D. Patients with steatosis in the background liver

25 What is the most likely cause of the liver abnormality?

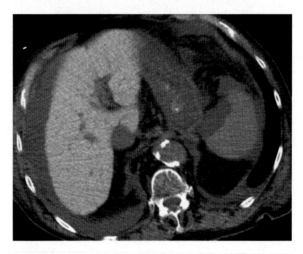

   A. Radiation therapy
   B. Total parenteral nutrition
   C. Hepatorenal syndrome
   D. Iodine deposition

26 A 77-year-old woman with unresectable pancreatic carcinoma undergoes a restaging CT. The following CT image is obtained at the level of the known right adrenal metastasis. What is the most likely etiology of the new liver finding involving the right and left lobes?

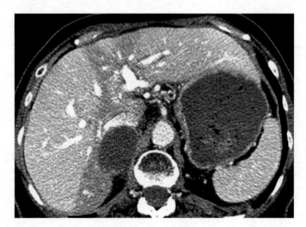

   A. Liver metastases
   B. Radiation therapy
   C. Total parenteral nutrition
   D. Portal vein thrombosis

27a A 19-year-old woman was found to have elevated liver function tests. Workup included a liver MRI with hepatobiliary contrast agent. Findings are most consistent with what diagnosis?

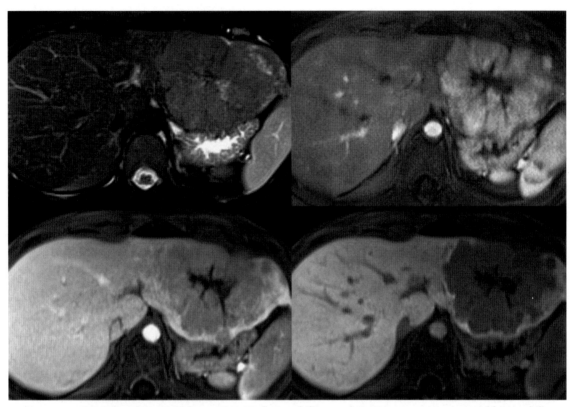

Top row: FS T2W and arterial phase FS T1W+hepatobiliary gad. **Bottom row:** Venous and hepatobiliary phase FS T1W+hepatobiliary gad.

    A. Colon carcinoma metastasis
    B. Giant cavernous hemangioma
    C. Focal nodular hyperplasia
    D. Fibrolamellar hepatocellular carcinoma

27b Which of the following statements is TRUE regarding fibrolamellar hepatocellular carcinoma (FHCC)?

    A. Five-year survival is higher compared to conventional hepatocellular carcinoma.
    B. Most patients are female.
    C. The background liver is cirrhotic in the majority of cases.
    D. There is a bimodal distribution affecting patients <40 and >60 years of age.

28 Which of the following is the most common benign liver tumor?

    A. Hepatocellular adenoma
    B. Focal nodular hyperplasia
    C. Peliosis hepatis
    D. Hemangioma

29 A 44-year-old man presents to the emergency department with fever, flank pain, and vomiting. CT and MRI were performed. What is the most likely diagnosis?

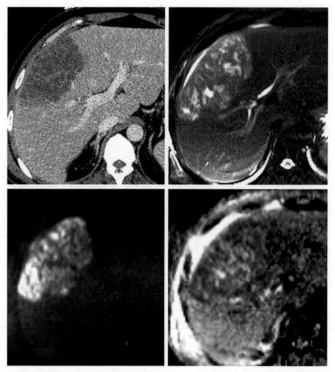

Top row: Venous phase CT and FS T2W MRI. **Bottom row:** DWI and ADC map MRI.

A. Subcapsular hematoma with T2 shine-through
B. Hepatic infarct with restricted diffusion
C. Cavernous hemangioma with T2 shine-through
D. Pyogenic abscess with restricted diffusion

30a A 29-year-old man shot in the abdomen underwent CTA after laparotomy for liver laceration. What finding is shown on the CTA images?

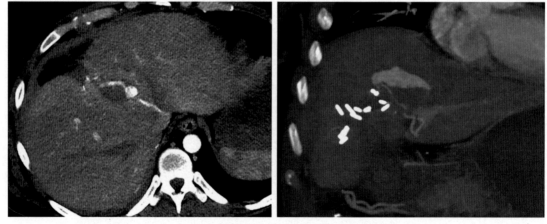

Arterial phase CT axial and coronal MIP.

A. Intrahepatic hematoma without vascular injury
B. Pseudoaneurysm with arteriovenous fistula
C. Active bleeding breaching the liver parenchyma into the peritoneum
D. Retained surgical sponge

30b What is the next best step for this patient?

    A. Consult interventional radiology for emergent angioembolization.

    B. Refer to general surgery for repeat laparotomy.

    C. Repeat CT in 1 week to assess stability/resolution.

    D. No follow-up needed.

31 A 71-year-old woman with cirrhosis undergoes an MRI using conventional extracellular contrast agent. What is the most appropriate LI-RADS category for the 2.3-cm observation in the left lobe?

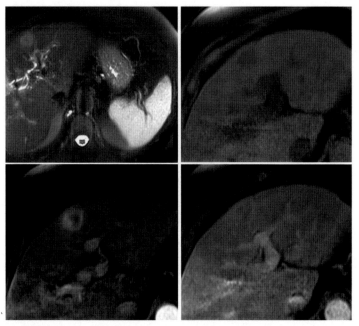

Top row: FS T2W and FS T1W. **Bottom row:** Arterial and delayed-phase FS T1W+gad.

    A. LR-2 (probably benign)

    B. LR-3 (intermediate probability of malignancy)

    C. LR-5 (definitely HCC)

    D. LR-M (probably or definitely malignant but not HCC specific)

32a A 35-year-old woman with no history of chronic liver disease or underlying malignancy presents with abdominal pain. Based on the following MR images, what is the best description of the mass in the liver?

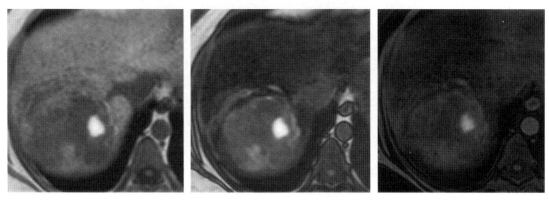

In-phase T1W, out-of-phase T1W, and FS T1W.

    A. Fat-containing mass in a background of hepatic steatosis

    B. Fat-containing mass in a background of hepatic hemochromatosis

    C. Hemorrhagic mass in a background of hepatic steatosis

    D. Hemorrhagic mass in a background of hepatic hemochromatosis

32b What is the most likely diagnosis of the mass?

    A. Focal nodular hyperplasia

    B. Hepatocellular adenoma

    C. Hepatocellular carcinoma

    D. Metastatic disease

33 A 22-year-old woman presents to the emergency department with malaise and elevated liver function tests after alcohol consumption. An ultrasound was performed. What is the most likely diagnosis?

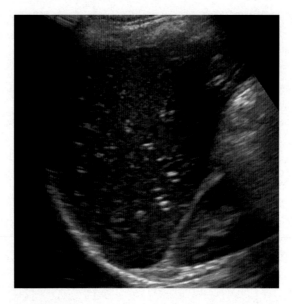

    A. Ascending cholangitis

    B. Acute hepatitis

    C. Fungal microabscesses

    D. Hemangiomas

34 A 41-year-old woman who underwent a diagnostic procedure to evaluate suspected liver disease presents with acute severe epigastric pain. What is the finding involving the lateral segment left lobe on the CT?

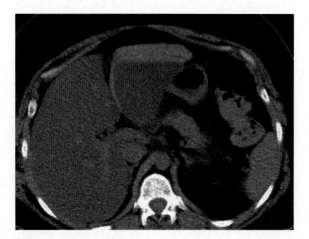

    A. Diffuse periportal edema

    B. Focal fatty sparing

    C. Subcapsular hematoma

    D. Transient hepatic attenuation difference (THAD)

35 A 60-year-old man with cirrhosis underwent MRI exams 5 months apart. Arterial phase images of the current MRI exam are shown in the top row, and arterial phase images of the prior MRI exam are shown in the bottom row with a finding (arrow) in segment VII. The patient did not receive treatment between the exams. What is the most likely explanation for the appearance of the current exam in the top row?

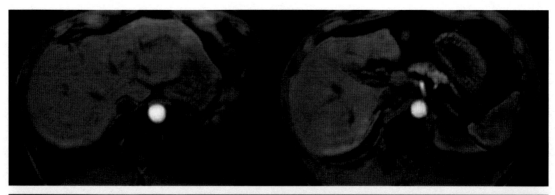

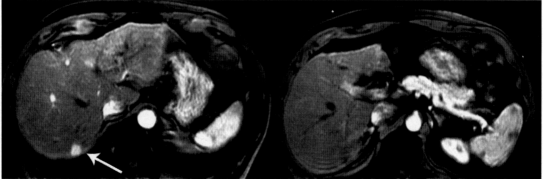

A. The arterial phase on the current exam is not optimally timed for assessment of hypervascular neoplasms.

B. There has been spontaneous resolution of a dysplastic nodule.

C. There was a hepatocellular carcinoma that responded to treatment given before both exams.

D. The finding the prior study was ghosting artifact from arterial pulsation no longer seen due to swapping of the phase- and frequency-encoding directions.

For the patients in questions 36 to 40, select the most likely underlying primary tumor (A to F) that is associated with the hepatic imaging findings. Each option may be used once or not at all.

A. Pancreatic ductal carcinoma

B. Neuroendocrine tumor

C. Non–small cell lung carcinoma

D. Breast carcinoma

E. Lymphoid tumor

F. Mucinous colorectal carcinoma

36 A 61-year-old patient with abdominal pain. Venous phase CT images are shown.

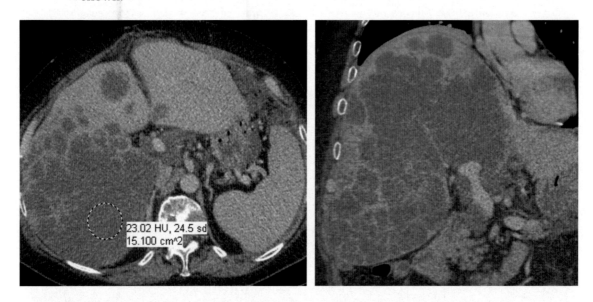

37 A 71-year-old woman.

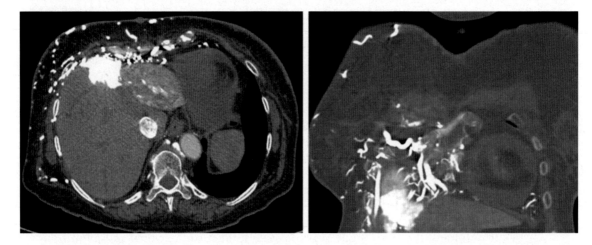

38 A 41-year-old man status post liver transplant several months ago for cirrhosis and hepatocellular carcinoma. Arterial and venous phase CT as well as ultrasound images are shown.

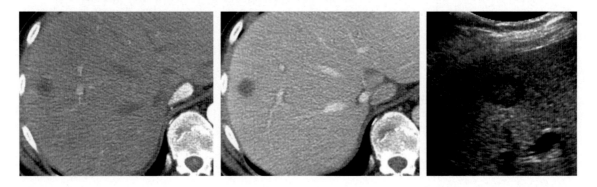

39 A 77-year-old woman. Venous phase images are shown from two CT scans performed 12 months apart.

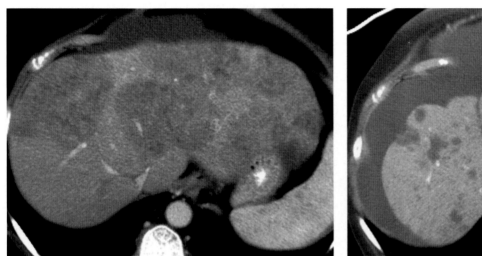
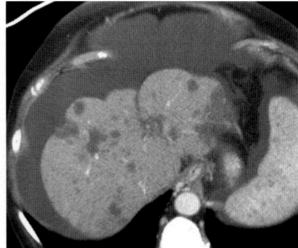

Initial CT and CT 12 months later.

40 A 39-year-old man.

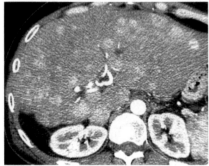
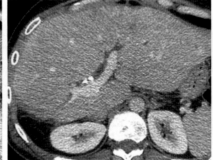
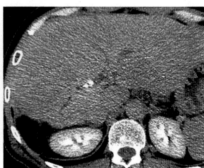

Arterial, venous, and delayed-phase CT.

41 A patient with cirrhosis and hepatocellular carcinoma is undergoing evaluation for liver transplantation. Which of the following is a contraindication to transplantation according to the Milan criteria?

A. Encephalopathy
B. Refractory variceal hemorrhage
C. Malignant portal vein thrombus
D. Solitary HCC measuring 4 cm

42 The most common etiology of graft failure after liver transplant is

A. Posttransplant lymphoproliferative disorder
B. Vascular thrombosis
C. Biliary stricture
D. Rejection

43 For the patients 1 to 3, select the most likely interpretation (A to D) of the MR elastography findings. For each patient, a T2W image, postprocessed color wave image, and color stiffness map are shown. Each option may be used once or not at all.

Patient 1.

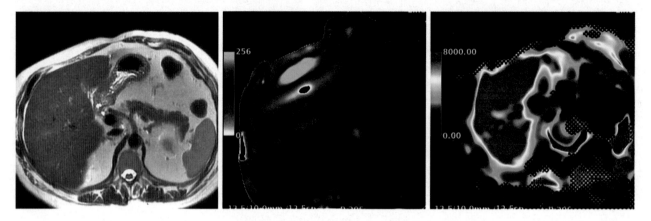

Patient 2.

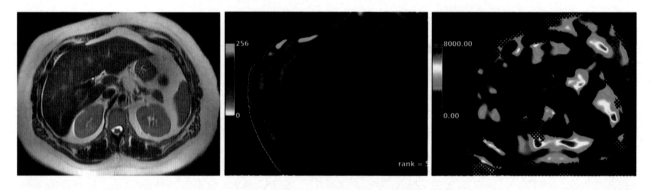

Patient 3.

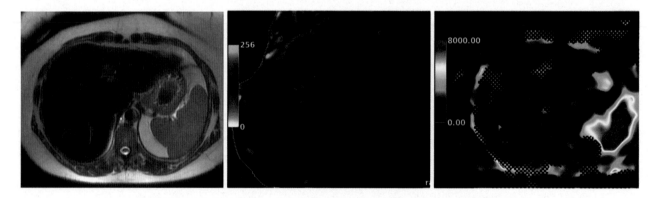

A. Nondiagnostic study due to cardiac motion artifact
B. Nondiagnostic study due to significant signal loss from hepatic iron deposition
C. Markedly elevated liver stiffness consistent with cirrhosis
D. Normal liver stiffness

44 A 63-year-old man with cirrhosis is status post-CT-guided microwave ablation of a hepatocellular carcinoma in the right hepatic lobe. Two CT scans are shown. What is the most likely diagnosis?

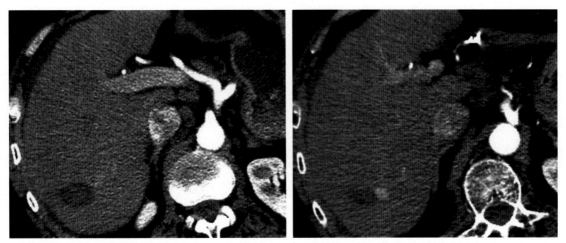

Arterial phase CT scans 6 months after ablation and 14 months after ablation.

A. Hemangioma
B. Recurrent hepatocellular carcinoma
C. Abscess
D. Dysplastic nodule

45 A patient with a liver transplant was evaluated with ultrasound followed by angiography. The arrow indicates the location of spectral Doppler interrogation. What vascular complication is demonstrated?

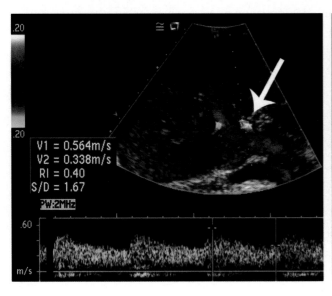
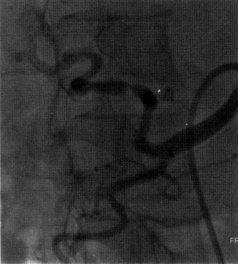

A. Hepatic artery stenosis
B. Portal vein thrombosis
C. Pseudoaneurysm
D. Arterioportal fistula

46 An MRI was performed with conventional extracellular contrast agent to evaluate a liver mass. This mass may be associated with which syndrome?

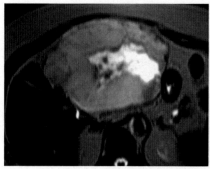 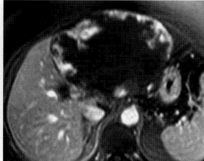 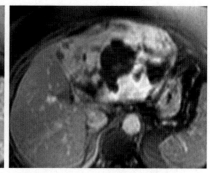

    A. Kasabach-Merritt syndrome
    B. Cushing syndrome
    C. Carcinoid syndrome
    D. Lambert-Eaton syndrome

For the patients in questions 47 to 50, select the most likely diagnosis (A to D) for the hepatic abnormalities. Each option may be used once, more than once, or not at all.

    A. Siderotic nodule
    B. Regenerative nodule, nonsiderotic
    C. Nodular steatosis
    D. Infarct

47 A 44-year-old woman with end-stage liver disease now with abdominal pain. Images from a CT scan and MRI are shown. A transjugular intrahepatic portosystemic shunt is partially imaged in the right lobe.

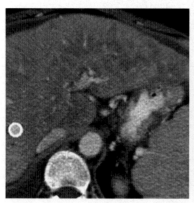 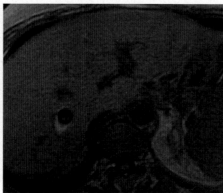 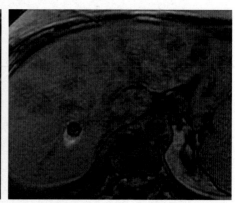

Venous phase CT, in-phase T1W MRI, and out-of-phase T1W MRI.

48 A 66-year-old man with cirrhosis. An MRI performed with hepatobiliary contrast agent is shown.

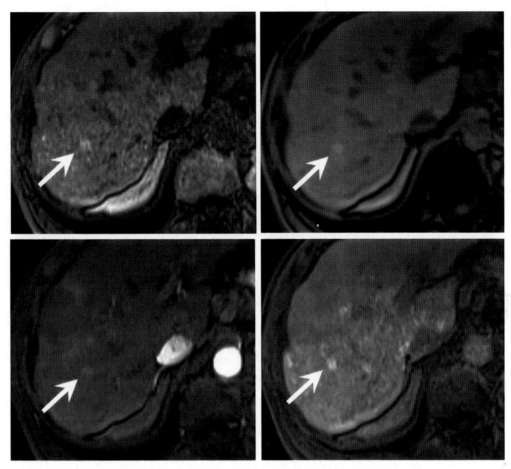

Top row: FS T1W and out-of-phase T1W. **Bottom row:** Arterial and 20-minute FS T1W+hepatobiliary gad.

49 A 39-year-old man with testicular cancer status post retroperitoneal nodal dissection. Postoperative course was complicated by large hemoperitoneum. Images from two CT scans are shown.

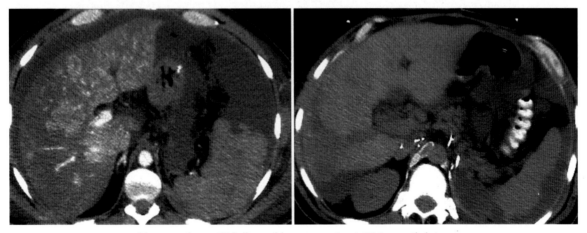

Venous phase CT followed by noncontrast CT 1 month later.

50 A 53-year-old man with chronic hepatitis B infection.

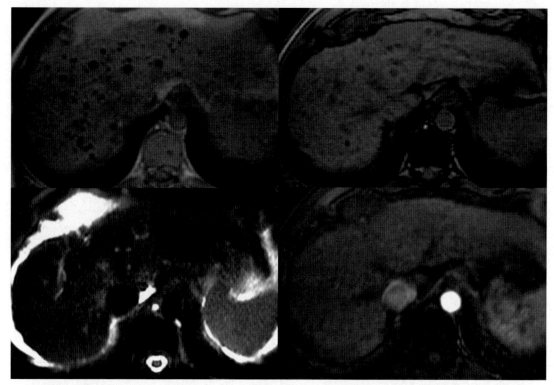

Top row: In-phase and out-of-phase T1W. **Bottom row:** FS T2W and arterial phase FS T1W+gad.

51a A 46-year-old woman underwent MRI for multiple liver lesions found on ultrasound. Arterial and delayed-phase FS T1W images from an MRI performed using conventional extracellular contrast agent are shown. This pattern of enhancement is most commonly identified with which of the following lesions?

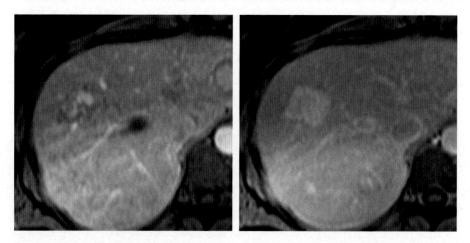

A. Cavernous hemangioma
B. Peliosis hepatis
C. Lymphoma
D. Pseudoaneurysm

51b The organisms responsible for the most common form of peliosis hepatis seen in AIDS patients are species of

A. *Bartonella*
B. *Echinococcus*
C. *Ascaris*
D. *Cryptococcus*

52 A 37-year-old woman was evaluated with abdominal US and MRI with conventional extracellular contrast agent (top row) for a liver lesion incidentally found on a lumbar MRI. She presented 1.5 years later with abdominal pain and additional imaging (bottom row) was performed. What is the most likely diagnosis?

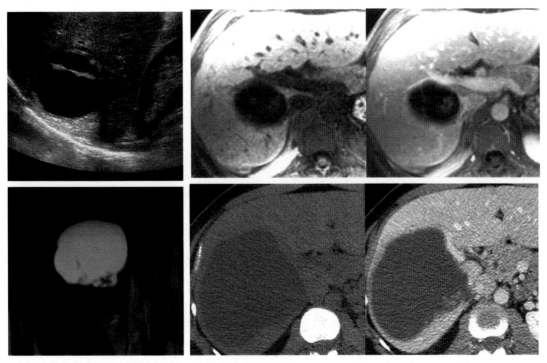

Top row: Initial imaging: sagittal US, FS T1W MRI, and venous phase FS T1W MRI+gad. **Bottom row:** Imaging 1.5 years later: Cor T2W MRI. Noncontrast and venous phase CT.

    A. Pyogenic abscess
    B. Hemorrhagic cyst
    C. Biliary cystadenoma/cystadenocarcinoma
    D. Metastatic ovarian carcinoma

53 The bright signal intensity (arrows) on the MR image below represents

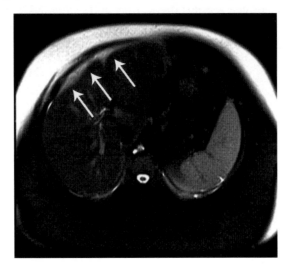

    A. Moiré fringes
    B. Focal fatty infiltration
    C. Ascites
    D. Uneven fat saturation

ANSWERS AND EXPLANATIONS

1 **Answer A.** This mass has classic imaging features of a **cavernous hemangioma**. There is a well-circumscribed lesion in hepatic segment VII, which is **"light bulb" bright on the T2W** image approaching signal intensity of cerebrospinal fluid. The mass demonstrates **peripheral, nodular, discontinuous enhancement, followed by centripetal fill-in on delayed phase**. Fill-in may be partial or complete in hemangiomas. Enhancement has been described as following blood pool. Hemangiomas are dilated venous channels with hepatic arterial supply. The great majority are asymptomatic and require no follow-up or treatment.

References: Boland GWL, Halpert RD. Chapter 6: Liver. In: Boland GWL, Halpert RD (eds). *Gastrointestinal imaging: the requisites*, 4th ed. Philadelphia, PA: Elsevier/Saunders, 2014:218–290.

Cogley JR, Miller FH. MR imaging of benign focal liver lesions. *Radiol Clin North Am* 2014;52:657–682.

2a **Answer D.** The mass shows three of the **major features of hepatocellular carcinoma** (HCC) according to the Liver Imaging Reporting and Data System (LI-RADS): (1) **non-rim arterial enhancement**, followed by (2) **washout appearance** as well as (3) **capsule appearance**. This patient is an older man with a visibly nodular cirrhotic liver at risk for HCC, eliminating entities such as focal nodular hyperplasia (FNH) and hepatocellular adenoma (HCA) from practical consideration. Signal intensity of the mass is similar to surrounding liver on in-phase T1W image, a clue that the tumor may be of hepatocellular origin.

MRI is the most sensitive and specific imaging modality for the diagnosis of HCC. Awareness of patient demographics and clinical history is critical in the evaluation of hepatic lesions. In the presence of cirrhosis, a high index of suspicion for HCC should be maintained for any enhancing liver lesion.

2b **Answer B.** This hepatocellular carcinoma (HCC) contains **microscopic intracellular fat demonstrated by signal dropout on out-of-phase** gradient echo T1W image. Macroscopic fat is unaffected on out-of-phase imaging and remains bright, as seen around the kidney and in the subcutaneous tissue. Some HCCs accumulate microscopic or macroscopic fat, and presence of fat within a focal observation is an **ancillary feature favoring HCC** in the at-risk population. HCCs can present with hemorrhage, but blood would not lose signal intensity on out-of-phase imaging. In fact, the iron in hemosiderin with old hemorrhage would create susceptibility resulting in greater signal dropout on the in-phase rather than out-of-phase images.

Hepatocellular adenomas (HCAs) and angiomyolipomas (AMLs) may contain fat, but they are not in consideration given risk for HCC. Angiomyolipoma (AML) is a benign mesenchymal tumor that is rarely found in the liver, and about half of the cases in the liver demonstrate macroscopic fat.

References: ACR Liver Imaging Reporting and Data System version 2018. American College of Radiology website. Available at https://www.acr.org/Clinical-Resources/Reporting-and-Data-Systems/LI-RADS. Accessed on August 12, 2020.

Choi JY, Lee JM, Sirlin CB. CT and MR imaging diagnosis and staging of hepatocellular carcinoma: Part II. Extracellular agents, hepatobiliary agents, and ancillary imaging features. *Radiology* 2014;273(1):30–50.

Costa AF, Thipphavong S, Arnason T, et al. Fat-containing liver lesions on imaging: detection and differential diagnosis. *AJR Am J Roentgenol* 2018;210(1):68–77.

3 **Answer F.** This is a large mass-forming intrahepatic **cholangiocarcinoma** (CCA) involving both the right and left lobes. Multiple **dilated biliary ducts** terminate in a large mass with ill-defined margins and overlying **hepatic capsular retraction**. The mass is **hypovascular with subsequent classic progressive enhancement** from venous to delayed phase, **typical of the fibrosis within this desmoplastic tumor**. This should not be mistaken for the centripetal fill-in of cavernous hemangioma, since there is no discontinuous peripheral nodular enhancement pattern following blood pool as expected of hemangioma.

CCA is a malignant tumor arising from the biliary ducts and represents the second most common primary malignancy of the liver after HCC. It can be categorized into three types based on morphology: mass-forming, periductal infiltrating, and intraductal growing types. CCA has a greater **propensity for biliary obstruction** than other liver lesions. Parenchymal atrophy can be a result of underlying biliary obstruction, fibrosis, and/or portal vein occlusion by tumor. **An atrophic area of the liver must be carefully inspected for underlying tumor, rather than assumed to be from a past benign insult** such as infarct or trauma. The differential diagnosis of this mass may include an uncommon malignancy called combined hepatocellular cholangiocarcinoma (cHCC-CCA). This is an aggressive neoplasm with a combination of imaging and pathologic features of both HCC and CCA usually found in patients with chronic liver disease.

References: Joo I, Lee JM, Yoon JH. Imaging diagnosis of intrahepatic and perihilar cholangiocarcinoma: recent advances and challenges. *Radiology* 2018;288(1):7–13.

Seo N, Kim DY, Choi JY. Cross-sectional imaging of intrahepatic cholangiocarcinoma: development, growth, spread, and prognosis. *AJR Am J Roentgenol* 2017;209(2):W64–W75.

4 **Answer B.** Findings are most consistent with **focal nodular hyperplasia** (FNH) in this premenopausal woman with an incidental liver mass. The mass demonstrates **avid arterial enhancement** and **retention of contrast at 20-minute hepatobiliary phase** on this MRI performed with Eovist contrast agent. During the portal venous phase (not shown), an FNH is usually nearly isointense to liver. A **central scar with classic T2 hyperintensity** is present. **Occasionally, a prominent feeding vessel extending toward the central scar can be identified on arterial phase** (not visible in this case). When a conventional extracellular contrast agent is used, the delayed phase may show near-isointensity of the mass as well as delayed enhancement of the central scar. **On precontrast T1W and T2W images, the lesion is usually iso- or nearly isointense to surrounding liver since it is composed of hepatocytes.** Focal nodular hyperplasia is a benign mass thought to be a hyperplastic response to a preexisting arterial malformation. It is most common in **women of reproductive age**. In 20% of cases, there are multiple lesions.

MRI with hepatobiliary contrast agent has been used to help differentiate FNH from HCA (and from the rare malignancy fibrolamellar hepatocellular carcinoma) in this young patient population. No treatment is required for FNH, while HCA may require follow-up or intervention for hemorrhage, or rarely, malignant transformation. Because FNH contains functioning hepatocytes, it accumulates hepatobiliary contrast agent and remains iso- to hyperintense to the liver on 20-minute hepatobiliary phase images. In contradistinction, HCAs and the other answer choices are usually hypointense to the liver on the hepatobiliary phase.

Unfortunately, accumulating experience is revealing that hepatobiliary phase iso- or hyperintensity is not as specific for FNH as previously believed. Although less common, other benign and malignant etiologies sometimes show hepatobiliary phase retention of contrast. These include subtypes of hepatocellular adenomas and hepatocellular carcinomas, via preservation or up-regulation of the receptor responsible for contrast uptake. Parts of fibrotic tumors, necrotic tumors, and hemangiomas may also show some hepatobiliary signal intensity via prolonged contrast retention in an expanded extracellular space. **Liver lesions must always be evaluated in the context of patient demographics, clinical scenario, and multiseries MR imaging appearance.** If there are atypical imaging features that decrease diagnostic confidence for FNH, the patient may require additional workup or follow-up.

References: Fujita N, Nishie A, Asayama Y, et al. Hyperintense liver masses at hepatobiliary phase gadoxetic acid-enhanced MRI: imaging appearances and clinical importance. *Radiographics* 2020;40(1):72–94.

Khosa F, Khan AN, Eisenberg RL. Hypervascular liver lesions on MRI. *AJR Am J Roentgenol* 2011;197(2):W204–W220.

5 **Answer E.** Large lobulated **cauliflower-like** hepatic lesions like these are commonly seen with **colon carcinoma metastases**. Colon adenocarcinoma is a common source of liver metastasis with other common primaries including lung and breast carcinoma. These metastases are usually **hypoenhancing** compared to surrounding liver on all postcontrast CT and MRI phases. There is also nonenhancing central necrosis in this case. **The continuous rim of thick, irregular soft tissue should not be mistaken for a cavernous hemangioma's peripheral nodular discontinuous enhancement.** In addition, the peripheral tumor tissue does not follow the blood pool. Biliary obstruction is uncommon even when hepatic metastases are large and widespread. In contradistinction, cholangiocarcinomas have the greatest propensity for biliary obstruction.

Even though we describe these metastases as "hypovascular" on CT and MRI, contrast-enhanced ultrasound (CEUS) has revealed that most of these metastases actually have very early arterial enhancement. This enhancement appears and disappears so rapidly that it is undetectable by the timing of CT and MRI image acquisition. "Hypervascular" lesions on CT and MRI are visible because they enhance in the late arterial phase (25 to 45 seconds from initiation of contrast injection).

References: Kim HJ, Lee SS, Byun JH, et al. Incremental value of liver MR imaging in patients with potentially curable colorectal hepatic metastasis detected at CT: a prospective comparison of diffusion-weighted imaging, gadoxetic acid-enhanced MR imaging, and a combination of both MR techniques. *Radiology* 2015;274(3):712–722.

Tirumani SH, Kim KW, Nishino M, et al. Update on the role of imaging in management of metastatic colorectal cancer. *Radiographics* 2014;34(7):1908–1928.

6 **Answer D.** This is the **typical appearance of a hepatocellular carcinoma** (HCC) on an MRI with hepatobiliary contrast agent. The mass in the left lobe of the liver shows **arterial enhancement**. It is **dark compared to surrounding liver on the hepatobiliary phase**. There is evidence of cirrhosis with bands of fibrosis, which are also hypointense on hepatobiliary phase. Other hypervascular masses such as hemangioma, hepatocellular adenoma (HCA), focal nodular hyperplasia (FNH), and metastasis are less common in the cirrhotic liver compared to the general population. The lesion is isointense to the liver on T2 images, with no evidence of "light bulb" T2 hyperintensity to suggest a hemangioma. This 51-year-old man is not in the right demographic for HCA or FNH, lesions that most commonly occur in premenopausal women.

The role of hepatobiliary contrast agents in the patients at risk for HCC continues to evolve. **In general, isointensity on hepatobiliary phase is reassuring**, and considered a benign finding such as regenerative nodule, dysplastic nodule, or arterioportal shunt with transient hepatic intensity difference (THID). **However, hyperintensity on the hepatobiliary phase occurs in about 10% to 15% of HCCs and cannot be considered a benign**

feature in this patient population. Borders of an infiltrative HCC may appear more sharply marginated on hepatobiliary phase than on other sequences, helping in the delineation of some tumors.

References: Choi JY, Lee JM, Sirlin CB. CT and MR imaging diagnosis and staging of hepatocellular carcinoma: Part II. Extracellular agents, hepatobiliary agents, and ancillary imaging features. *Radiology* 2014;273(1):30–50.

Fujita N, Nishie A, Asayama Y, et al. Hyperintense liver masses at hepatobiliary phase gadoxetic acid-enhanced MRI: imaging appearances and clinical importance. *Radiographics* 2020;40(1):72–94.

Jhaveri K, Cleary S, Audet P, et al. Consensus statements from a multidisciplinary expert panel on the utilization and application of a liver-specific MRI contrast agent (gadoxetic Acid). *AJR Am J Roentgenol* 2015;204(3):498–509.

7 **Answer D.** If a hepatobiliary agent such as gadoxetate disodium (Eovist—Bayer HealthCare) is used, **hypointensity on the 20-minute hepatobiliary phase is considered an ancillary feature that favors malignancy** in general, which may be hepatocellular carcinoma (HCC) or another malignancy, according to the Liver Imaging Reporting and Data System (LI-RADS) version 2018. Diffusion restriction and subthreshold growth are other ancillary features favoring malignancy in general. Some ancillary features that would favor HCC in particular include intralesional fat, internal blood products, and nodule-in-nodule architecture. **Ancillary features may upgrade suspicion for hepatocellular carcinoma no higher than category LI-RADS category 4 (Probably HCC).**

Hepatobiliary phase hypointensity is not "washout." On an MRI performed with a hepatobiliary contrast agent, **evaluation for "washout" is valid only as long as the portal veins appear to enhance greater than liver parenchyma (usually earlier than 2 minutes),** before the hepatobiliary phase begins to dominate. Major features for HCC in LI-RADS include "washout," "capsule," and threshold growth. Non-rim arterial enhancement and size thresholds are also included in major criteria, with masses ≥2 cm most worrisome. "Washout" and "capsule" specified in quotation marks (or washout appearance and capsule appearance) are the terms preferred by LI-RADS. This serves as a reminder that these terms are visual cues, which do not necessarily represent true loss of contrast enhancement on imaging or a true capsule at pathology.

LI-RADS is applicable only to the patient population with cirrhosis or other chronic liver disease who are at risk for (HCC). The algorithm for LI-RADS is an interactive graphic on the ACR Web site with definitions, descriptions, and examples. LI-RADS categories range from LR-1 (100% certainty that observation is benign) to LR-5 (100% certainty that observation is HCC). When an observation does not meet criteria for other categories, it is designated LR-3 indicating intermediate probability for HCC.

References: ACR Liver Imaging Reporting and Data System version 2018. American College of Radiology website. Available at https://www.acr.org/Clinical-Resources/Reporting-and-Data-Systems/LI-RADS. Accessed on August 12, 2020.

Cerny M, Chernyak V, Olivié D, et al. LI-RADS version 2018 ancillary features at MRI. *Radiographics* 2018;38(7):1973–2001.

8 **Answer D.** This **hepatocellular carcinoma (HCC) with infiltrative appearance** is an extensive heterogeneous mass with ill-defined margins. The branching thrombosis in the right portal vein demonstrates arterial **enhancement consistent with tumor thrombus.** Both the tumor and tumor thrombus show washout appearance on the delayed (equilibrium) phase. These features are consistent with **LR-TIV (definitely tumor in vein), which is a category separate from LR-5 category (definitely HCC)** in CT/MRI LI-RADS version 2018. LR-TIV should be applied when there is unequivocal tumor within the portal veins. Portal vein tumor thrombus increases the confidence level for HCC.

Portal vein thrombosis can alter the perfusion of the liver and the tumor, presenting challenges in tumor diagnosis. Tumor thrombus generally follows the imaging features of the primary HCC. Although identification of flow in the thrombus is specific for tumor thrombus, sensitivity is limited. Arterialization of the thrombus is detectable in fewer than 10% of cases. Significant expansion of the vein favors tumor over bland thrombus.

Infiltrative HCCs constitute 10% to 15% of all HCCs and have poor prognosis given their size and frequent association with tumor thrombus. Surgery decreases survival, so resection and transplantation are usually contraindicated. Response to systemic chemotherapy is poor. Intra-arterial chemo- or radioembolization may increase survival in a subset of patients with limited disease and adequate liver function.

References: ACR Liver Imaging Reporting and Data System version 2018. American College of Radiology website. Available at https://www.acr.org/Clinical-Resources/Reporting-and-Data-Systems/LI-RADS. Accessed on August 12, 2020.

Reynolds AR, Furlan A, Fetzer DT, et al. Infiltrative hepatocellular carcinoma: what radiologists need to know. *Radiographics* 2015;35(2):371–386.

9 **Answer C.** This is **congestive hepatopathy with classic "nutmeg" appearance** of the liver. The lacy reticular hypodensities are best appreciated peripherally in the venous phase and reflect heterogeneous suboptimal enhancement of the parenchyma. On delayed images, the reticular hypodensities will eventually enhance resulting in a more homogeneous appearance (not shown). The axial image shows **engorged IVC and hepatic veins**, and the coronal image also reveals cardiomegaly with a cardiac pacer lead. Reflux of contrast from the heart into the IVC might be demonstrated on early phases of enhancement (not shown). With congestive heart failure (and other causes of increased right heart pressures such as constrictive pericarditis and pericardial effusion), elevated pressures are transmitted retrograde into the IVC and hepatic veins. Impaired venous return to the heart results in hepatic congestion. Chronic passive congestion **can lead to cirrhosis.** Treatment is aimed at controlling the underlying cardiac disease.

Regarding the other answer choices, metastases would be mass-like rather than reticular. In Budd-Chiari syndrome, heterogeneity of the liver is accompanied by thrombosis or attenuation of the IVC and hepatic veins, not enlargement. Schistosomiasis is a parasitic infection that is prevalent in developing countries but uncommon in the United States. Development of calcified capsular and peripheral fibrotic bands as a reaction to ova deposition can result in the **"tortoise shell" appearance of schistosomiasis** and lead to presinusoidal portal hypertension.

References: Elsayes KM, Shaaban AM, Rothan SM, et al. A comprehensive approach to hepatic vascular disease. *Radiographics* 2017;37(3):813–836.

Wells ML, Fenstad ER, Poterucha JT, et al. Imaging findings of congestive hepatopathy. *Radiographics* 2016;36(4):1024–1037.

10a **Answer A.** The most likely diagnosis is a **hemangioma.** This incidentally discovered lesion in a young patient without significant past medical history has a **low probability for malignancy.** This lesion is in the **periphery of the liver, well defined, and hyperechoic.** Color Doppler interrogation is not sensitive or specific for malignancy, since both benign and malignant lesions may or may not have detectable color Doppler flow.

The need for follow-up or definitive characterization of a liver lesion may depend on the patient age, underlying malignancy, presence of chronic liver disease, atypical hypoechoic or heterogeneous appearance, or request by the patient or physician. Regarding imaging management:

- **Multiphase MRI is more sensitive and specific than CT**. In addition, MRI does not involve ionizing radiation. **Contrast-enhanced ultrasound (CEUS) may also be an option** for further evaluation.

- **Tc-99m red blood cell scan** could be considered if a hemangioma requires confirmation, and a low glomerular filtration rate precludes administration of MRI contrast (because of concerns about nephrogenic systemic fibrosis) or CT contrast (because of concerns about nephropathy). Lesions should be 2 cm or larger to be optimally evaluated on Tc-99m RBC scan. Increased uptake on the 1- to 2-hour blood pool images would be consistent with hemangioma.

- **Follow-up ultrasound to document stability or no further workup** may be appropriate for a lesion in young patients with low suspicion for malignancy.

References: ACR Appropriateness Criteria: liver lesion—initial characterization. American College of Radiology website. Available at https://acsearch.acr.org/docs/69472/Narrative. Published 1998. Updated 2020. Accessed on August 12, 2020.

Boland GWL, Halpert RD. Chapter 6: Liver. In: Boland GWL, Halpert RD (eds). *Gastrointestinal imaging: the requisites*, 4th ed. Philadelphia, PA: Elsevier/Saunders, 2014:218–290.

10b **Answer B.** The arrow points to a mirror artifact that mimics a mass outside the liver. **Mirror artifact is a type of reverberation artifact** as depicted below.

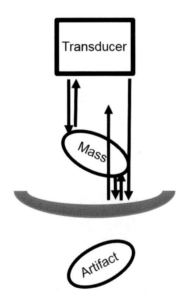

The beams that initially encounter the mass and return to the transducer are mapped correctly. However, some beams initially encounter the highly reflective surface of the diaphragm–air interface and reverberate between the diaphragm and the posterior margin of the mass before returning to the transducer. These late-returning echoes are erroneously mapped as a mirror image, **farther away but equidistant from the diaphragm on the opposite side**. The artifact can also be **in color with color Doppler imaging**. Notice that the pseudolesion shows distortion and is not precisely the same shape or size as the true lesion.

References: Feldman MK, Katyal S, Blackwood MS. Ultrasound artifacts. *Radiographics* 2009;29(4):1179–1189.

Triche BL, Nelson JT, McGill NS, et al. Recognizing and minimizing artifacts at CT, MRI, US, and molecular imaging. *Radiographics* 2019;39(4):1017–1018.

11 **Answer A.** Constellation of findings is consistent with **Budd-Chiari syndrome** (BCS), most commonly caused by **thrombophilia**. Axial contrast-enhanced image demonstrates a **heterogeneous** liver with a **macronodular** contour. There is **enlargement and increased enhancement of the caudate lobe**. The **hepatic veins are not visualized**. Hepatic venogram demonstrates **"spider-web" collateral vessels**, indicating hepatic venous obstruction consistent with Budd-Chiari syndrome (BCS).

The venous obstruction in BCS can occur from the level of the small intrahepatic veins to the IVC. **In the West, the typical patient is young and female**. Primary BCS, in which the underlying obstruction originates from intrinsic venous sources, accounts for two-thirds of cases. These patients may have risk factors for thrombophilia including myeloproliferative disorders, factor V Leiden deficiency, antiphospholipid antibody syndrome, or protein C or S deficiency. **Web-like obstruction can be congenital or acquired and is more common in Asia.** In secondary BCS, obstruction results from an extrinsic source affecting the veins, such as metastatic lesions, abscesses, or trauma. Treatment options for BCS include anticoagulation/thrombolysis, angioplasty/stenting, and management of cirrhosis including portosystemic shunting and liver transplant.

BCS can be **acute, subacute, or chronic**. Imaging findings in the acute setting include thrombosed hepatic veins/IVC, ascites, and splenomegaly. Early in a multiphase scan, there may be peripheral hypovascularity and caudate hypervascularity. On subsequent phases of enhancement, a reversal or "flip-flop" of this pattern can be seen with peripheral hypervascularity and caudate hypovascularity.

In the subacute to chronic setting, morphologic changes of cirrhosis as well as attenuation of the involved vessels can be seen. **Patients can develop nodular regenerative hyperplasia (NRH), which represents growth of otherwise normal tissue that compensates for atrophy in other parts of the liver.** NRH can lead to noncirrhotic portal hypertension. Venous and delayed-phase MR images below in a different patient with BCS demonstrate NRH, with large nodular areas of enhancement that can persist into the venous phase. There is no delayed washout appearance of these enhancing areas on delayed phase to suggest HCC, and these areas should not be mistaken for neoplasm.

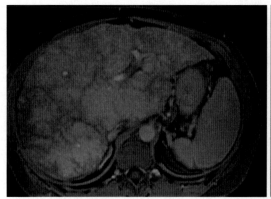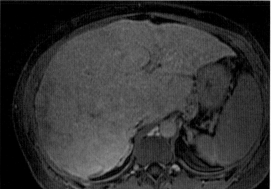

Venous and delayed-phase FS T1W MR images showing nodular regenerative hyperplasia (NRH) in patient with BCS.

References: Elsayes KM, Shaaban AM, Rothan SM, et al. A comprehensive approach to hepatic vascular disease. *Radiographics* 2017;37(3):813–836.

Ferral H, Behrens G, Lopera J. Budd-Chiari syndrome. *AJR Am J Roentgenol* 2012;199(4):737–745.

12 **Answer A.** This case demonstrates the **"double-target" sign of pyogenic (bacterial) hepatic abscess** on CT. There is a hypodense center representing necrosis, a hyperdense inner rim of enhancing granulation tissue, and a hypodense outer rim of inflammatory edema. **Occasionally, internal gas may be present.** Another CT finding is **transient surrounding geographic enhancement** that could represent inflammatory parenchymal reaction (arrows below in a different patient). Abscesses may be unilocular or multilocular. On ultrasound, they have complex cystic appearance with internal debris and posterior acoustic enhancement.

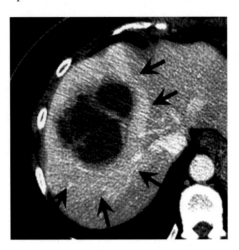

Pyogenic abscesses are the most common hepatic abscess in the United States, followed by fungal and amebic abscesses. This cancer patient with a history of biliary stenting and obstruction is at risk for development of cholangitis and hepatic abscess. Patients with history of surgery, trauma, and bacteremia are also at risk. Diverticulitis and appendicitis can cause pyogenic abscesses due to seeding via the portal venous system, but seeding is less common now due to rapid diagnosis and treatment of these diseases. Amebic abscesses tend to be unilocular and may appear similar to pyogenic abscess with thickened wall. Hepatic abscesses are associated with significant morbidity and mortality, and early intervention antibiotics and percutaneous drainage are indicated.

References: Bächler P, Baladron MJ, Menias C, et al. Multimodality imaging of liver infections: differential diagnosis and potential pitfalls. *Radiographics* 2016;36(4):1001–1023.

Borhani AA, Wiant A, Heller MT. Cystic hepatic lesions: a review and an algorithmic approach. *AJR Am J Roentgenol* 2014;203(6):1192–1204.

13 **Answer C.** The multiple renal cysts are not shown on these images, but among the choices, the most likely diagnosis is **polycystic liver disease (PLD) in the setting of autosomal dominant polycystic kidney disease (ADPCKD)** in this patient with a renal transplant. Cysts **vary in size** and have thin walls without enhancement. Cysts may have rim calcifications as in this case, typically well demonstrated on CT but not on MRI. **Cysts may develop heterogeneity or wall thickening due to infection or hemorrhage and become symptomatic.** Of note, autosomal dominant polycystic liver disease (ADPLD) is a separate disease with a different genetic mutation that can have the same appearance without renal cysts.

When more than 10 hepatic cysts are identified, a **fibropolycystic liver disease** such as PLD could be present. These cysts represent dilated abnormal bile ducts related to embryologic malformation of the ductal plate and no longer communicate with the biliary tree. Management is generally supportive, although in some cases, large cysts may be targeted for aspiration for symptomatic relief.

References: Brancatelli G, Federle MP, Vilgrain V, et al. Fibropolycystic liver disease: CT and MR imaging findings. *Radiographics* 2005;25(3):659–670.

Patel A, Chapman AB, Mikolajczyk AE. A practical approach to polycystic liver disease. *Clin Liver Dis (Hoboken)* 2019;14(5):176–179.

14 **Answer B.** This cyst demonstrates the **"water lily" sign, which is highly specific for echinococcal (hydatid) cyst** and first described in ultrasound. There is sloughing and collapse of the internal membrane resulting in a wrinkled curvilinear structure. This architecture is visible on the T2W image but not the postcontrast T1W images, where there is no enhancement that would suggest an active abscess or neoplasm. **Another pathognomonic appearance for hydatid cysts is a "mother cyst" with multiple peripheral "daughter cysts" arranged in a spoke-wheel, or rosette, pattern.**

Echinococcal cysts have **variable appearance, ranging from simple cysts to complex cystic masses** with calcification. **There may be wall enhancement** (not present in this case). Presence of fat density suggests communication with the biliary system, attributed to the lipid content in bile. When imaging features are less specific, the differential diagnosis may include biliary cystadenoma/cystadenocarcinoma or cystic/necrotic metastases. Amebic abscesses are usually unilocular and thick walled, with appearance more similar to pyogenic (bacterial) abscesses.

Hydatid disease is a parasitic infection caused by tapeworms endemic in underdeveloped parts of the world, particularly where sheep are raised. The **liver is the most common site** of involvement, seen in 75% to 80% of cases. Echinococcal cysts may be complicated by **peritoneal rupture, portal obstruction, biliary obstruction, and superinfection**. Treatment options include surgery, percutaneous aspiration, and antiparasitic agents such as albendazole.

References: Pakala T, Molina M, Wu GY. Hepatic echinococcal cysts: a review. *J Clin Transl Hepatol* 2016;4(1):39–46.

Zalaquett E, Menias C, Garrido F, et al. Imaging of hydatid disease with a focus on extrahepatic involvement. *Radiographics* 2017;37(3):901–923.

15 **Answer D.** Findings are most consistent with **biliary hamartomas, also known as von Meyenburg complex**. There are numerous subcentimeter T2 hyperintense lesions scattered throughout the liver, many of which are punctate. Biliary hamartomas are typically of **fairly uniform small size** <15 mm, while simple hepatic cysts and polycystic liver disease are more variable in size as shown in a previous question. Margins of biliary hamartomas may be angular, and **enhancement is uncommon**.

Biliary hamartomas are considered a **fibropolycystic liver disease** resulting from abnormal embryologic development of the biliary ductal plate. These lesions no longer communicate with the biliary ducts. Biliary hamartomas are **benign, asymptomatic, and do not require intervention**. The differential diagnosis for widespread, small, cystic liver lesions includes simple hepatic cysts, microabscesses (typically fungal infection), and Caroli disease.

References: Anderson SW, Kruskal JB, Kane RA. Benign hepatic tumors and iatrogenic pseudotumors. *Radiographics* 2009;29(1):211–229.

Brancatelli G, Federle MP, Vilgrain V, et al. Fibropolycystic liver disease: CT and MR imaging findings. *Radiographics* 2005;25(3):659–670.

16a **Answer D.** There is marked diffuse **loss of signal intensity in both the liver as well as the spleen on the in-phase** relative to the out-of-phase images. This is due to marked T2* effects from iron. Findings are consistent with **hemosiderosis, a form of secondary hemochromatosis**. Patients with end-stage renal disease have multifactorial iron deficiency anemia requiring repeated blood transfusions and/or intravenous iron infusion, which predispose to iron overload. Iron is deposited in the form of hemosiderin in the **reticuloendothelial system** including the liver and spleen.

In contradistinction, iron deposition in primary (hereditary) hemochromatosis involves the liver but spares the spleen. Other major organs that may be involved in primary hemochromatosis but not hemosiderosis include the **pancreas and heart**. It is an autosomal recessive hereditary disorder associated with elevated intestinal absorption of iron. **Iron deposition is toxic and leads to organ dysfunction and malignancy,** including cirrhosis, hepatocellular carcinoma, diabetes, and cardiac dysfunction. "Bronze diabetes" refers to pancreatic dysfunction and skin hyperpigmentation in these patients. Other conditions such as cirrhosis can also lead to increased iron absorption. Hemochromatosis is one of the causes of a hyperdense liver on noncontrast CT.

Techniques have been developed to quantify the degree of iron deposition with MRI sequences performed with progressively longer TE. Region-of-interest (ROI) values in the liver from each of the sequences can be used to estimate the iron concentration. Quantification can provide information on the severity of the disease and effectiveness of treatment sparing repeated biopsies.

Treatment of primary hemochromatosis is repeated phlebotomy. Since patients with hemosiderosis have underlying anemia, phlebotomy is not advised. Iron chelation using drugs like deferoxamine is an option if treatment is felt to be necessary. Liver transplant can be considered in cases of primary hemochromatosis that progress to cirrhosis.

References: Labranche R, Gilbert G, Cerny M, et al. Liver iron quantification with MR imaging: a primer for radiologists. *Radiographics* 2018;38(2):392–412.

Merkle EM, Nelson RC. Dual gradient-echo in-phase and opposed-phase hepatic MR imaging: a useful tool for evaluating more than fatty infiltration or fatty sparing. *Radiographics* 2006;26(5):1409–1418.

Queiroz-Andrade M, Blasbalg R, Ortega CD, et al. MR imaging findings of iron overload. *Radiographics* 2009;29(6):1575–1589.

16b **Answer C. T2* susceptibility effects would be diminished on spin-echo and short TE sequences** compared to gradient-echo (GRE) and longer TE sequences. **A longer TE results in greater susceptibility because it allows more time for the T2* effect of iron to degrade the transverse magnetization vector** needed to produce a signal. Therefore, signal loss on T2W (longer TE) is greater than on T1W (shorter TE) images. By convention on T1W GRE dual-echo series, the in-phase images are performed with a longer TE so the **signal loss with iron is greater on in-phase images**. (At 1.5 Tesla, TE is 4.6 msec in-phase compared to 2.3 msec out-of-phase.) **The appearance is the opposite of steatosis**, in which signal loss is greater on the out-of-phase images due to the intravoxel cancellation of the water- and fat-bound protons (chemical shift type II effect).

In the case of iron deposition as shown in the previous question, T2* effects can be helpful in diagnosis. However, these effects may produce **susceptibility artifacts** that degrade image quality. The heterogeneity of the magnetic field induced by susceptibility can result in **image distortion** and **poor fat saturation** in the area of interest. These effects are particularly noticeable with metals or at interfaces between two substances of significantly different susceptibilities. An interface that is prone to susceptibility effects is air with soft tissue (e.g., where lung bases meet the upper abdomen). Other than using fast spin-echo (FSE) and short TE sequences, **techniques to reduce susceptibility include increasing receiver bandwidth, increasing echo train length, and applying corrective reconstruction algorithms to restore spatial fidelity.**

References: Shetty AS, Sipe AL, Zulfiqar M, et al. In-phase and opposed-phase imaging: applications of chemical shift and magnetic susceptibility in the chest and abdomen. *Radiographics* 2019;39(1):115–135.

Viradia NK, Merkle EM, Song AW, et al. Chapter 8: Susceptibility artifact. In: Mangrum WI (ed). *Duke review of MRI physics*, 2nd ed. Philadelphia, PA: Elsevier, Inc. 2019:77–90.

17 **Answer A.** These MRI findings are compatible with **metastatic disease** in this patient with colon cancer. The T1W postcontrast MRI shows a mass with lobulated margins and **continuous rim enhancement,** rather than the discontinuous nodularity with cavernous hemangioma. The mass is only mildly T2 hyperintense, less than expected in a hemangioma or a fluid collection such as an abscess (not an answer choice). A smaller lesion is present anteriorly. A simple cyst would have an imperceptible wall without enhancement and marked T2 hyperintensity. Focal nodular hyperplasia does not show rim enhancement and is most often found in premenopausal women.

Metastases are the most common malignant liver lesion and have **varied appearances.** Central necrosis or a cystic/mucinous component can show increased signal on T2W images. **Most metastases are T1 hypointense and somewhat T2 hyperintense, with T2 signal intensity similar to spleen.** Most metastases are hypovascular and appear **hypointense to liver on venous phase**.

When metastatectomy or other targeted therapies are being considered, detection of every liver metastasis is important for complete treatment. Multimodality imaging with PET/CT and/or MRI increase the sensitivity for detection of metastases compared to CT alone. **On MRI, restricted diffusion and hepatobiliary phase hypointensity** when using a hepatobiliary contrast agent such as Eovist can confirm liver metastases that are more subtle, as shown below.

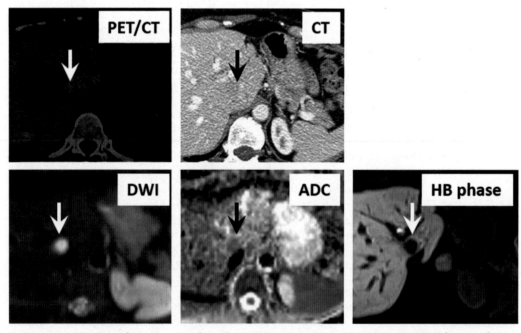

Breast cancer metastasis more conspicuous on MRI. **Top row:** A CT ¹⁸F-FDG PET/CT shows a focus of radiotracer uptake in the caudate lobe with maximum SUV of 4.3, corresponding to a subtle hypodensity on the venous phase CT performed same day. **Bottom row:** MRI performed with hepatobiliary contrast agent (Eovist). There is a hyperintense focus of restricted diffusion on high *b*-value DWI (appearing dark on ADC map) corresponding to a well-circumscribed hypointense lesion on 20-minute hepatobiliary phase. There were no other lesions identified on the MRI, and the patient was considered a candidate for metastatectomy.

References: Namasivayam S, Martin DR, Saini S. Imaging of liver metastases: MRI. *Cancer Imaging* 2007;7:2–9.

Tirumani SH, Kim KW, Nishino M, et al. Update on the role of imaging in management of metastatic colorectal cancer. *Radiographics* 2014;34(7):1908–1928.

18 **Answer B.** One of the most widely accepted indications for performing an MRI with a hepatobiliary contrast agent is **differentiating between focal nodular hyperplasia (FNH) and hepatocellular adenoma (HCA).** Accuracy remains high, although lower than previously believed. Conventional extracellular contrast agents used in CT and MRI are excreted mostly by the kidneys. While hepatobiliary agents have some extracellular activity, allowing for some degree of dynamic assessment on arterial and portal venous phases, these agents are also taken up by hepatocytes with subsequent biliary excretion. Gadoxetate disodium (Eovist—Bayer HealthCare) is an agent that has moderate (50%) uptake by hepatocytes. **Lesions without functioning hepatocytes appear hypointense on the 20-minute T1W hepatocyte phase images.** There is biliary excretion, and contrast can be seen in the ducts in the hepatobiliary phase. The following two tables list clinical scenarios and rationales for selecting a hepatobiliary contrast agent versus a conventional extracellular contrast agent.

Potential Applications of Hepatobiliary Gadolinium-Based Contrast Agents	
Scenario	**Rationale**
Distinguishing FNH vs. adenoma	FNH shows uptake and appears iso- to hyperintense on hepatobiliary phase, although specificity not as high as previously believed.
Prehepatectomy planning to assess number and distribution of colorectal metastases for curative intent	Detects more lesions, including lesions <1 cm than CT, conventional MRI, or PET/CT
Assessment of biliary anatomy in conjunction with MRCP, for example, in living-related liver donors	Improved depiction of second- and third-order biliary ducts on hepatobiliary phase
Detection of bile leaks in conjunction with MRCP	Improved detection and localization of leaks on hepatobiliary phase
Screening for new nodules in patients with cirrhosis or chronic hepatitis (evolving role)	Improved detection of HCCs, especially small lesions <1 cm

Scenarios in Which MRI or CT Using Conventional Contrast May Be Preferred	
Scenario	**Why Hepatobiliary Agents Are Suboptimal**
Confirming hemangioma	Diagnosis may be difficult due to "pseudo washout": hemangiomas become hypointense on delayed and hepatobiliary phases like most other lesions.
Assessment for treatment response after locoregional therapies (e.g., post-TACE, RFA)	Pseudolesions with arterial enhancement and hepatobiliary phase hypointensity mimic residual or recurrent HCC or hypervascular tumor. Worst within 1 month posttreatment and believed to be related to adjacent hepatocyte inflammation and injury.

(Continued)

Scenarios in Which MRI or CT Using Conventional Contrast May Be Preferred (*Continued*)	
Scenario	Why Hepatobiliary Agents Are Suboptimal
Bilirubin > 3	Reduced hepatocyte uptake of hepatobiliary contrast due to markedly decreased liver function, as indicated by elevated bilirubin.
Assessment of vasculature needed	Smaller contrast bolus of hepatobiliary agent may be suboptimal for evaluation of vessels.
Hemochromatosis	Generalized hypointensity of the liver due to iron deposition limits the utility of the hepatobiliary phase to detect lesions.

References: Jhaveri K, Cleary S, Audet P, et al. Consensus statements from a multidisciplinary expert panel on the utilization and application of a liver-specific MRI contrast agent (gadoxetic acid). *AJR Am J Roentgenol* 2015;204(3):498–509.

Seale MK, Catalano OA, Saini S, et al. Hepatobiliary-specific MR contrast agents: role in imaging the liver and biliary tree. *Radiographics* 2009;29(6):1725–1748.

19 **Answer A.** Findings are consistent with **portal vein thrombophlebitis** associated with acute diverticulitis of the sigmoid colon. Linear hypodensities in the left lobe match the expected portal vein branches. There is a subtle wedge-shaped area of altered perfusion matching the vascular distribution, which is better demonstrated with narrower window settings, as shown below. In the pelvis, there is inflammatory fat stranding adjacent to a sigmoid diverticulum. An infection from diverticulitis or appendicitis can spread via the mesenteric veins into the portal venous system resulting in thrombophlebitis.

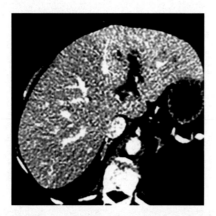

The dynamics of the **liver's dual blood supply** account for the altered perfusion seen with portal vein thrombosis. **The affected region receives increased hepatic arterial inflow to compensate for the decreased portal venous inflow**, accounting for the increased regional density in the early phases of enhancement. **The perfusion differences are transient or become less evident** on later phases as the unaffected liver progressively enhances. These areas of altered perfusion called transient hepatic attenuation or intensity differences (THADs on CT and THIDs on MRI). **An area of altered perfusion may be more noticeable than the underlying cause, and any THAD/THID should be closely evaluated** for portal vein thrombosis, mass, arterioportal shunts, or inflammation.

Bland thrombosis may be associated with cirrhosis, inflammation, hypercoagulable states, and percutaneous hepatobiliary procedures. **Tumor thrombus is most commonly due to hepatocellular carcinoma in cases of intrahepatic thrombus,** and pancreatic or gastric carcinoma if extrahepatic. Half of patients with PVT have no identifiable cause. Thrombus enhancement would be consistent with tumor thrombus but may be difficult to detect reliably with any imaging modality. Significant vein expansion tends to favor tumor over bland thrombus. Patients with acute PVT may be treated with anticoagulation and correction of underlying cause.

Regarding the other answer choices, **dilated bile ducts should run in parallel with normal enhancing portal veins.** Cholangitis remains a clinical diagnosis, but imaging may identify an underlying obstructing lesion or a complication such as abscess. There is no hepatic mass to indicate metastasis. Liver laceration extending to the vessels may be a cause of portal venous thrombus, but the overlying parenchyma is intact.

References: Colagrande S, Centi N, Galdiero R, et al. Transient hepatic intensity differences. Part 2. Those not associated with focal lesions. *AJR Am J Roentgenol* 2007;188(1):160–166.

Elsayes KM, Shaaban AM, Rothan SM, et al. A comprehensive approach to hepatic vascular disease. *Radiographics* 2017;37(3):813–836.

20a **Answer C.** The contrast-enhanced CT in this patient with blunt trauma reveals linear and patchy areas of hypodensity representing **hepatic and splenic lacerations. No intervention is needed if patient is hemodynamically stable.** The liver laceration extends centrally toward the right hepatic vein and approaches the intrahepatic IVC without frank vascular disruption. Findings are most consistent with a grade IV laceration (involving 25% to 75% of a hepatic lobe) according to the most widely used liver injury grading scale, the American Association for the Surgery of Trauma (AAST) classification.

Analogous to management for splenic injury, the trend is toward nonsurgical management. About 70% to 90% of cases are now managed nonoperatively with 90% success rate. The AAST scale ranges from grade I to grade V. The 2018 update incorporates the CT diagnosis of **"vascular injury" (defined as pseudoaneurysm and arteriovenous fistula) and active bleeding,** which **upgrade any injury to Grade III or IV. The higher the grade, the more likely the patient will fail nonsurgical management.** Stable patients with vascular injuries or active bleeding may be considered for angioembolization as part of nonsurgical management. Patients who are hemodynamically unstable proceed to surgery.

Regarding the other answer choices, there is no evidence of active arterial hemorrhage or pseudoaneurysm to embolize. No subcapsular hematoma is seen and, even if present, would not require percutaneous drainage in uncomplicated cases.

References: Brillantino A, Iacobellis F, Festa P, et al. Non-operative management of blunt liver trauma: safety, efficacy and complications of a standardized treatment protocol. *Bull Emerg Trauma* 2019;7:49–54.

Kozar RA, Crandall M, Shanmuganathan K, et al. Organ injury scaling 2018 update: spleen, liver, and kidney. *J Trauma Acute Care Surg* 2018;85(6):1119–1122.

Yoon W, Jeong YY, Kim JK, et al. CT in blunt liver trauma. *Radiographics* 2005;25:87–104.

20b **Answer A.** The HIDA scan shows contrast uptake by the liver and excretion into the bile ducts, gallbladder, and small bowel. Two foci of intrahepatic bile accumulation superior and lateral to the gallbladder are compatible with **bilomas** (arrows), which were confirmed at ERCP.

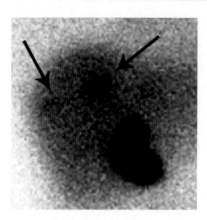

With hepatic injury being managed nonoperatively, the development of bilomas is common, seen in up to 20% of patients. Patients may complain of increased abdominal pain or have jaundice, fever, and leukocytosis. **CT may show low-density fluid collections or ascites.** Bile leaks are generally managed nonoperatively with ERCP and stenting, but percutaneous drainage or laparotomy may be indicated for superinfection of a biloma or for bile peritonitis.

References: Gupta A, Stuhlfaut JW, Fleming KW, et al. Blunt trauma of the pancreas and biliary tract: a multimodality imaging approach to diagnosis. *Radiographics* 2004;24:1381–1395.

Mettler FA, Guiberteau MJ. Chapter 7: Gastrointestinal tract. In: Mettler FA, Guiberteau MJ (eds). *Essentials of nuclear medicine imaging*, 6th ed. Philadelphia, PA: Elsevier/Saunders, 2012:237–270.

21 **Answer C.** This is a simple cyst in the left hepatic lobe. There is a **pulsatile aortic flow artifact with ghosting** on the pre- and postcontrast fat saturated T1W images that maps into the cyst, mimicking internal nodularity. The ghost is the same size and shape as the aorta. **Ghosting occurs at constant intervals in the phase-encoding direction and is also visible outside the patient (arrows)** in this case. In the abdomen, phase encoding is usually applied in the shorter anterior–posterior dimension to minimize scan time. As a result, the ghosting from the aorta often projects over the left hepatic lobe.

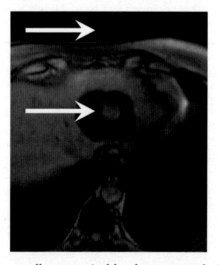

While this artifact is usually recognizable, there are techniques than can manage this artifact if necessary. The **phase- and frequency-encoding directions can be swapped** to project the ghost out of the area of interest. **Presaturation pulses ("sat bands")** can be placed above the imaged area to eliminate the signal from the incoming aortic flow (or placed below the imaged area to eliminate the signal from the incoming IVC flow). **Gradient moment nulling** involves the application of additional pulses to correct for phase shifts within moving protons. These various techniques usually lengthen the scan time.

References: Huang SY, Seethamraju RT, Patel P, et al. Body MR imaging: artifacts, k-space, and solutions. *Radiographics* 2015;35(5):1439–1460.

Morelli JN, Runge VM, Ai F, et al. An image-based approach to understanding the physics of MR artifacts. *Radiographics* 2011;31(3):849–866.

22 **Answer D.** The main portal vein is not seen. In its place, numerous tortuous periportal collateral vessels are consistent with **"cavernous transformation of the portal vein" in the setting of chronic portal vein occlusion**, in this case, from prior pancreatitis. On ultrasound, tortuous anechoic veins can demonstrate low-level hepatopedal venous waveform consistent with portal-type flow. In addition to varices, **other findings of portal hypertension that may be seen include splenomegaly and ascites**.

Varices represent portosystemic collateral pathways in the setting of portal hypertension. These may drain into the superior or inferior vena cava. The following images are from a patient with cirrhosis and portal hypertension showing extensive varices.

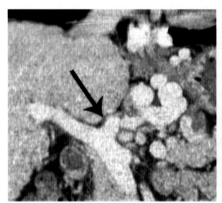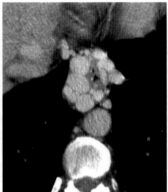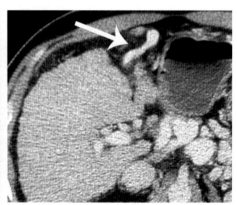

Varices in portal hypertension, including the coronary vein (*black arrow on coronal image*) arising from portal vein, esophageal varices, and "recanalized" umbilical vein (*white arrow*) in the fissure for the falciform ligament.

Portal hypertension may be classified as presinusoidal, sinusoidal (intrahepatic), or postsinusoidal. Common causes are listed in the table below.

Common Causes of Portal Hypertension	
Presinusoidal	• Portal vein thrombosis • Splenic vein thrombosis • Schistosomiasis (most common cause worldwide, with destruction of small portal branches by parasites)
Sinusoidal	• Cirrhosis (intrahepatic regenerative nodules and scarring produce resistance to portal flow)
Postsinusoidal	• Budd-Chiari syndrome (hepatic vein or IVC obstruction) • Congestive heart failure

References: Elsayes KM, Shaaban AM, Rothan SM, et al. A comprehensive approach to hepatic vascular disease. *Radiographics* 2017;37(3):813–836.

Morgan T, Qayyum A. Chapter 89: Diffuse liver disease. In: Gore RM, Levine MS (eds). *Textbook of gastrointestinal radiology*, 4th ed. Philadelphia, PA: Elsevier/Saunders, 2015:1629–1675.

23a **Answer A.** This small lesion is a **capillary ("flash-filling") hemangioma**. It is hypervascular, with homogeneous enhancement in the arterial phase. **Enhancement persists into the delayed phase, remaining greater than surrounding liver.** There is "light bulb" T2 hyperintensity as expected of hemangioma. Flash-filling hemangiomas are small, usually <2 cm. The enhancement pattern described is demonstrated on multiphase MR using conventional extracellular contrast agent and on CT. Hepatocellular carcinoma and metastases typically do not show enhancement greater than the liver on delayed imaging, and the probability for liver metastasis in this patient is low with breast DCIS. Although focal nodular hyperplasia and hepatocellular adenoma have avid arterial enhancement, they tend to be nearly isointense to surrounding liver on precontrast T1 and T2 images as well as the postcontrast venous and delayed phases.

References: Boland GWL, Halpert RD. Chapter 6: Liver. In: Boland GWL, Halpert RD (eds). *Gastrointestinal imaging: the requisites*, 4th ed. Philadelphia, PA: Elsevier/Saunders, 2014:218–290.

Silva AC, Evans JM, McCullough AE, et al. MR imaging of hypervascular liver masses: a review of current techniques. *Radiographics* 2009;29(2):385–402.

23b **Answer C.** The finding adjacent to the hemangioma represents a transient hepatic intensity difference (THID, which is analogous to a transient hepatic attenuation difference, or THAD on CT). **A THID or THAD is a wedge-shaped or geographic area of enhancement representing altered perfusion.** It is often more apparent on one phase (usually arterial) than other phases. A THID **can be seen around a rapidly enhancing lesion** such as this capillary hemangioma or other benign or malignant lesions. THIDs may also be associated with portal vein thrombosis, cholangitis, or cirrhosis. This THID is seen only on arterial phase. The other answer choices (hemorrhage, poor fat saturation, and focal fatty sparing) may appear hyperintense on T1W images but would be seen on the other postcontrast series as well.

References: Colagrande S, Centi N, Galdiero R, et al. Transient hepatic intensity differences. Part 1. Those associated with focal lesions. *AJR Am J Roentgenol* 2007;188(1):154–159.

Colagrande S, Centi N, Galdiero R, et al. Transient hepatic intensity differences. Part 2. Those not associated with focal lesions. *AJR Am J Roentgenol* 2007;188(1):160–166.

24a **Answer B.** This arterial-enhancing mass is otherwise isodense on the precontrast, venous, and delayed postcontrast images, so closely matching the surrounding liver parenchyma that it is imperceptible. This appearance may be a **clue that the mass is of hepatocellular origin**—either a focal nodular hyperplasia (FNH) or hepatocellular adenoma (HCA), when accounting for the patient's age, sex, and clinical scenario of incidental finding. Hepatocellular carcinoma (HCC), is also of hepatocellular origin, but in a young woman without chronic liver disease, HCC is much less likely. Many of these lesions likely remain unnoticed on routine CT scans because of isodensity on venous phase. HCA was the diagnosis at biopsy.

HCAs represent a heterogeneous group of tumors of hepatocellular origin. **HCAs occasionally have intralesional fat and do not typically exhibit a central scar.** MRI using a hepatobiliary contrast agent such as Eovist can be helpful in distinguishing HCA and FNH. Because hepatic adenomas lack functioning bile ducts, they should appear hypointense on hepatobiliary phase. FNH typically retains contrast in the hepatobiliary phase appearing iso- or hyperintense to surrounding liver. However, **HCAs that retain contrast on hepatobiliary phase mimicking FNH are now recognized.** Therefore, identification of atypical features that decrease diagnostic confidence for FNH such as heterogeneity and capsule appearance may prompt follow-up or further investigation for the possibility of HCA. Other imaging options that may help distinguish FNH from HCA include contrast-enhanced ultrasound (CEUS) and nuclear medicine sulfur colloid scan.

Regarding the other answer choices, washout appearance in patients without HCC risk factors is not specific, neither for HCC nor malignancy. LI-RADS criteria such as "washout" should not be applied because this patient is not at risk for HCC. Furthermore, **isodensity on the venous or delayed phases as shown in this case is not "washout."** To meet criteria for "washout," an enhancing mass should subsequently appear hypodense to the surrounding liver. **On CT and MRI, the term "washout" is often a misnomer** and should be **assessed qualitatively by visual inspection**. This appearance is mainly due to normal progression of enhancement of the surrounding liver rather than decrease in lesion enhancement. The two CT images below of an HCC in a patient with cirrhosis represent washout appearance, but there is no significant decrease in density of the neoplasm from the arterial to venous phase. **Measuring lesion density in the following manner is not appropriate in assessing for "washout"**.

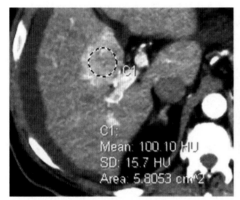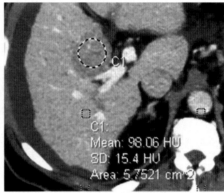

Washout appearance in this hepatocellular carcinoma is not due to decrease in lesion enhancement, but rather postarterial enhancement of surrounding parenchyma.

THADs are areas of altered perfusion in otherwise normal parenchyma that can be arterial enhancing and imperceptible on other pre- and postcontrast series. A THAD of this size should appear more geographic, not round and mass-like. This mass is homogeneous with no central scar. A central scar is also nonspecific but more common in FNH than HCA. Hypervascular metastases may have a similar enhancement pattern to HCA in which small subtle metastases are only detectable on arterial phase images. However, **hypervascular metastases of this size usually tend to be distinct from surrounding liver on pre- and postcontrast CT and MR images**. Hypervascular metastases would be much less likely than FNH or HCA in a young patient without known history of malignancy.

References: Agarwal S, Fuentes-Orrego JM, Arnason T, et al. Inflammatory hepatocellular adenomas can mimic focal nodular hyperplasia on gadoxetic acid-enhanced MRI. *AJR Am J Roentgenol* 2014;203(4):W408–W414.

Grazioli L, Bondioni MP, Haradome H, et al. Hepatocellular adenoma and focal nodular hyperplasia: value of gadoxetic acid-enhanced MR imaging in differential diagnosis. *Radiology* 2012;262(2):520–529.

Katabathina VS, Menias CO, Shanbhogue AK, et al. Genetics and imaging of hepatocellular adenomas: 2011 update. *Radiographics* 2011;31(6):1529–1543.

24b **Answer B.** Among the answer choices, **men are at greater risk** for malignant transformation of hepatocellular adenomas (HCAs). Three major subtypes of HCA had been described with different genetics and thought to represent separate entities, including inflammatory, steatotic HNF-1α–mutated, and β-catenin–mutated subtypes. As of 2017, the classification has expanded to include seven subtypes, the details of which are beyond the scope of this discussion, with an eighth group of tumors remaining unclassified. Overall, risk of **hemorrhage and rupture** is 20% to 25%, and risk of **malignant transformation to HCC** is 5% to 10%. Imaging has an important role in monitoring for growth and guiding biopsy. There may be some imaging features suggestive of a subtype, but **imaging currently does not reliably distinguish among the subtypes**. Of particular concern is the β-catenin–mutated type, which is associated with the highest risk of malignant transformation to HCC, and is not associated with a specific imaging pattern. This type occurs more commonly in men. **Biopsy may be performed** for confirmation, risk stratification, and exclusion of HCC. Initial management of HCAs involves **withdrawal of oral contraceptives or steroids and follow-up imaging.** Closer monitoring or intervention (**embolization or surgical resection**) may be considered for larger tumors (e.g., >5 cm), men, patients with glycogen storage disease, and β-catenin–mutated type as these are risk factors for complications. **Patients who have >10 tumors in number are designated as having hepatic adenomatosis,** which can apply to any subtype.

References: Grazioli L, Bondioni MP, Haradome H, et al. Hepatocellular adenoma and focal nodular hyperplasia: value of gadoxetic acid-enhanced MR imaging in differential diagnosis. *Radiology* 2012;262(2):520–529.

Katabathina VS, Menias CO, Shanbhogue AK, et al. Genetics and imaging of hepatocellular adenomas: 2011 update. *Radiographics* 2011;31(6):1529–1543.

25 **Answer D. Diffuse hepatic hyperdensity (>70 HU)** can be caused by iodine deposition in patients treated with the **cardiac antiarrhythmic drug amiodarone,** which is 37% iodine by weight. Normal density is usually 45 to 65 HU on a noncontrast CT scan obtained with conventional kVp of 120. At visual inspection, it should appear similar to the spleen, which is about 35 to 55 HU. This hyperdensity does not always indicate toxicity, and patients may be asymptomatic. However, if injury is severe, the patient may develop steatosis and cirrhosis. If there is pulmonary involvement with amiodarone toxicity, **interstitial fibrosis and high-density pulmonary opacities** may be seen.

Other less common causes of diffuse hepatic hyperdensity include hemochromatosis (iron deposition), Wilson disease (copper deposition), gold therapy, and glycogen storage disease. Thorotrast was associated with deposition of high density in a characteristic reticular pattern within the liver and spleen. The use of Thorotrast, a radioactive contrast agent, was discontinued in the 1950s when it was discovered to be carcinogenic. Total parenteral nutrition and radiation therapy are more commonly causes of steatosis and decreased liver density. Hepatorenal syndrome is unrelated to liver hyperdensity. It refers to renal failure caused by cirrhosis or fulminant hepatitis, leading to portal hypertension and ascites.

References: Coy DL, Kolokythas O. Chapter 9: Liver and biliary. In: Lin E, Coy DL, Kanne JP (eds). *Body CT: the essentials*. New York, NY: McGraw-Hill, 2015.

Morgan T, Qayyum A, Gore RM. Chapter 89: Diffuse liver disease. In: Gore RM, Levine MS (eds). *Textbook of gastrointestinal radiology*, 4th ed. Philadelphia, PA: Elsevier/Saunders, 2015:1629–1675.

26 **Answer B.** This patient completed **radiation therapy** several weeks ago to her right adrenal metastasis located behind the IVC. The metastasis is hypodense reflecting posttreatment necrosis. The liver demonstrates band-like hypodensity with the **"straight border" sign** corresponding to the radiation portal, and not matching a vascular distribution. Radiation therapy can result in hypodensity due to edema followed by steatohepatitis. If there is microscopic veno-occlusion impairing hepatic venous outflow, there can be increased enhancement compared to surrounding in the venous and delayed phase. Imaging findings of radiation therapy **may resolve or progress to fibrosis and atrophy** after 3 to 6 months.

The following CT images from a different patient show **chronic radiation effects (arrows)** in a typical distribution for pancreatic cancer treatment field at 6 months. There is atrophy with capsular concavity of the left hepatic lobe, atrophy of the medial upper poles of both kidneys, and fatty marrow replacement of the vertebrae in the radiation field.

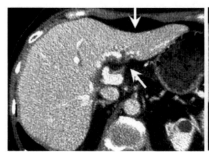 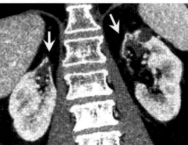 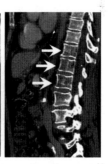

Regarding the other answer choices, in cases of portal vein thrombosis, areas of altered perfusion are typically wedge-shaped following portal vascular distribution. Sharp linear margins are not consistent with liver metastases nor hepatic steatosis from systemic treatment (such as total parenteral nutrition and chemotherapy).

References: Maturen KE, Feng MU, Wasnik AP, et al. Imaging effects of radiation therapy in the abdomen and pelvis: evaluating "innocent bystander" tissues. *Radiographics* 2013;33(2):599–619.

Viswanathan C, Truong MT, Sagebiel TL, et al. Abdominal and pelvic complications of nonoperative oncologic therapy. *Radiographics* 2014;34(4):941–961.

27a **Answer D.** Among the choices listed, **fibrolamellar hepatocellular carcinoma** (FHCC) best fits the imaging pattern. The large mass shows a **central scar**, which is found in the majority of FHCCs. There is **heterogeneous arterial enhancement**. The lesion is **hypointense on the 20-minute hepatobiliary phase**. Small satellite nodules are noted in the left lobe. About **half of the patients show regional nodal spread at presentation**.

Top differential diagnoses in a young woman with a hypervascular mass are focal nodular hyperplasia (FNH) and hepatocellular adenoma (HCA).

The mass in this case has morphology resembling FNH with lobulated margins, arterial enhancement, and central scar, but nearly all FNHs retain contrast on hepatobiliary phase, while FHCCs appear hypointense as shown here. Appearance of FHCC on CT or MRI performed with a conventional extracellular contrast agent is more variable in the venous and delayed phases, ranging from hypo- to hyperintense.

Regarding the other answer choices, colon carcinoma metastases are typically hypovascular without significant arterial enhancement. Although giant cavernous hemangiomas can be hypointense on hepatobiliary phase and contain a central scar, there is no peripheral nodular discontinuous enhancement or areas of "light bulb" T2 hyperintensity to indicate hemangioma. HCAs and hypervascular metastases are not listed among the answer choices, but they can also show arterial enhancement with hypointensity on hepatobiliary phase. However, they do not typically show a central scar.

References: Boland GWL, Halpert RD. Chapter 6: Liver. In: Boland GWL, Halpert RD (eds). *Gastrointestinal imaging: the requisites*, 4th ed. Philadelphia, PA: Elsevier/Saunders, 2014:218–290.

Ganeshan D, Szklaruk J, Kundra V, et al. Imaging features of fibrolamellar hepatocellular carcinoma. *AJR Am J Roentgenol* 2014;202(3):544–552.

27b **Answer A.** Fibrolamellar hepatocellular carcinoma (FHCC) is a rare malignancy that accounts for **fewer than 1% of HCC** and has a **higher 5-year survival rate** of about 40% compared to about 7% for conventional HCC. There is unimodal distribution with about 85% of patients **younger than 40 years of age**, whereas fewer than 5% of patients with conventional hepatocellular carcinoma (HCC) are younger than 40 years. Focal nodular hyperplasia (FNH) and hepatocellular adenoma (HCA) are more common in women, but there is **no sex predilection** in FHCC. FNH, HCA, and FHCC occur in **noncirrhotic livers**, whereas conventional HCC most often develops in the setting of cirrhosis. FHCC tumorigenesis is thought to be distinct from that of HCC. Serum α-**fetoprotein levels are normal**. Tumors are frequently **large at discovery** with nonspecific symptoms due to size.

References: Boland GWL, Halpert RD. Chapter 6: Liver. In: Boland GWL, Halpert RD (eds). *Gastrointestinal imaging: the requisites*, 4th ed. Philadelphia, PA: Elsevier/Saunders, 2014:218–290.

Ganeshan D, Szklaruk J, Kundra V, et al. Imaging features of fibrolamellar hepatocellular carcinoma. *AJR Am J Roentgenol* 2014;202(3):544–552.

28 **Answer D.** The most common benign tumor found in the liver is **hemangioma**. It is thought to have a prevalence of up to 20% of the population based on autopsy series. It is a hamartomatous proliferation of endothelium. Hemangiomas are usually asymptomatic and incidentally noted. Focal nodular **hyperplasia (FNH) is the second most common** and **hepatocellular adenoma (HCA) the third** most common benign liver tumor. Overall, **metastases are the most common malignancy** found in the liver. **Hepatocellular carcinoma (HCC) is the most common primary** liver malignancy.

Hemangioma, FNH, HCA, HCC, and some metastases are hypervascular (i.e., arterial enhancing). **When evaluating a hypervascular tumor, the first step is to determine if it is a benign hemangioma that requires no further follow-up or intervention.**

Patient demographics, clinical information, and background liver appearance are crucial in the assessment of hypervascular liver tumors. Pointers for incorporating this information into the interpretation of imaging findings are summarized in the following table.

Important Considerations in the Assessment of Hypervascular Liver Tumors	
Factor	Comment
Background Liver Appearance • Normal	• Is it a hemangioma? • HCC is rare.
• Cirrhotic	• High risk for HCC. Apply LI-RADS. • FNH, HCA, hemangioma, and metastasis are less commonly found in cirrhotic compared to normal livers.
• Fatty	• Marked hypodensity in the setting of severe steatosis may complicate assessment of dynamic enhancement pattern. • HCA is often associated with surrounding hepatic steatosis.
Demographics • Young woman	• FNH > HCA >> fibrolamellar HCC
Clinical Information • Oral contraceptive use, anabolic steroid use, glycogen storage disease, familial adenomatous polyposis	• HCA
• Known primary malignancy	• Is the primary neoplasm hypovascular or hypervascular? • Treated metastases may have atypical enhancement and appearance.
• Chronic liver disease, especially hepatitis B and C	• Increased risk for HCC. Apply LI-RADS.
• Primary sclerosing cholangitis	• Risk for cholangiocarcinoma • Risk for HCC if cirrhotic

References: Grand DJ, Mayo-Smith WW, Woodfield CA. *Practical body MRI: protocols, applications, and image interpretation.* Cambridge, UK: Cambridge University Press, 2012.

Khosa F, Khan AN, Eisenberg RL. Hypervascular liver lesions on MRI. *AJR Am J Roentgenol* 2011;197(2):W204–W220.

Silva AC, Evans JM, McCullough AE, et al. MR imaging of hypervascular liver masses: a review of current techniques. *Radiographics* 2009;29(2):385–402.

29 **Answer D.** This **pyogenic (bacterial) abscess** is heterogeneously T2 hyperintense to surrounding liver. Morphology on CT and MRI is the **"cluster-of-grapes"** appearance of liver abscess, **representing a region with multifocal areas of liquefying parenchyma rather than a collection with mass effect.** It shows **restricted diffusion**, appearing bright on diffusion series and predominantly dark on ADC map compared to surrounding liver. The movement of water molecules within thick pyogenic material is restricted. Patients with neoplasms that have necrosis or cystic changes tend not to have restricted diffusion in the liquid portions.

There is substantial overlap in the appearance of benign and malignant lesions on diffusion-weighted imaging in abdominal imaging, so images must be interpreted in conjunction with other imaging features and the clinical scenario. Neoplasms may have restricted diffusion due to hypercellularity. The appearance of restricted diffusion in the liver has been reported in metastases, hepatocellular carcinoma, adenoma, focal nodular hyperplasia, hemangioma, abscess, and hematoma. Diffusion series **may improve detection of overall number of lesions**. The spleen and lymphoid tissue are normally among the brightest structures at high *b*-value imaging, so diffusion series **can be useful to identify lymph nodes. Diffusion series should be reviewed for incidental bright foci** and correlation made with other series to determine if the foci may represent significant lesions. **Subtle neoplasms may be incidentally detected** and most conspicuous on diffusion series, including neuroendocrine tumors, gastrointestinal stromal tumor, pancreatic carcinoma, renal cell carcinoma, and peritoneal carcinomatosis. **Hemangiomas and other markedly T2 hyperintense lesions may show T2 shine-through** correlating with brightness on ADC map.

Regarding the other answer choices, while an acute infarct can show restricted diffusion, liver infarcts are rare and occur in the setting of a major event compromising both the hepatic arterial and portal venous dual blood supply. An infarct, hemangioma, or hematoma would not have "cluster of grapes" architecture. **Blood products alter the diffusion series and ADC map in various ways** and can appear to have restricted diffusion, T2 shine-through, or signal loss from hemosiderin susceptibility effects on both diffusion and ADC map. **Diffusion imaging in any part of the body should be interpreted with caution and may be nondiagnostic when blood is present.**

References: Kanematsu M, Goshima S, Watanabe H, et al. Detection and characterization of focal hepatic lesions with diffusion-weighted MR imaging: a pictorial review. *Abdom Imaging* 2013;38(2):297–308.

Lee NK, Kim S, Kim DU, et al. Diffusion-weighted magnetic resonance imaging for non-neoplastic conditions in the hepatobiliary and pancreatic regions: pearls and potential pitfalls in imaging interpretation. *Abdom Imaging* 2015;40(3):643–662.

30a **Answer B.** There is a **traumatic pseudoaneurysm (PSA) with hepatic artery to hepatic venous fistula.** These arterial images show the segment IV branch of the hepatic artery coursing superiorly to a large irregular ovoid contrast collection matching aortic blood pool, consistent with a hepatic arterial pseudoaneurysm (white arrows). Axial image also shows an adjacent ovoid hypodense area, which may be parenchymal hematoma/laceration or a thrombosed portion of the pseudoaneurysm. The axial image also shows a line of contrast extending posteriorly from the pseudoaneurysm to the IVC (black arrows), compatible with early filling of the middle hepatic vein and indicating a hepatic artery–hepatic vein fistula. No contrast extravasation is shown into the peritoneal cavity. Surgical sponge would not be expected to look like this.

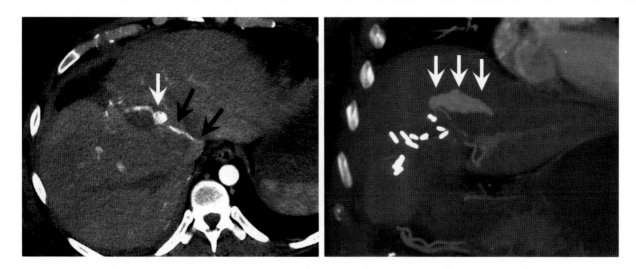

30b **Answer A.** Interventional radiology should be consulted for emergent angioembolization. Hepatic artery pseudoaneurysm, with or without arteriovenous fistula, is detected during follow-up of approximately 6% of hepatic injuries. Most are found incidentally on follow-up CT, but **all of these vascular injuries should be treated as soon as possible because of the high risk of rupture**. Arteriovenous fistulas (to hepatic or portal veins) are amenable to percutaneous angioembolization. The digital subtraction angiography image shown from selective injection of the common hepatic artery (CHA) shows the segment IV HA (HA seg IV) leading to the pseudoaneurysm (PSA), which in turn results in early filling of the middle hepatic vein (MHV) and inferior vena cava (IVC), confirming pseudoaneurysm with arteriohepatic venous fistula. The injury was successfully embolized.

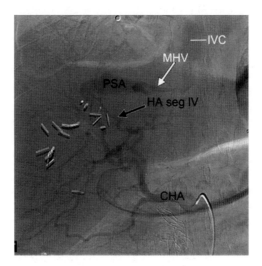

References: Brillantino A, Iacobellis F, Festa P, et al. Non-operative management of blunt liver trauma: safety, efficacy and complications of a standardized treatment protocol. *Bull Emerg Trauma* 2019;7:49–54.

Iacobellis F, Scaglione M, Brillantino A, et al. The additional value of the arterial phase in the CT assessment of liver vascular injuries after high-energy blunt trauma. *Emerg Radiol* 2019;26:647.

Yoon W, Jeong YY, Kim JK, et al. CT in blunt liver trauma. *Radiographics* 2005;25:87–104.

31 **Answer D.** The appropriate LI-RADS classification because of **targetoid (rim) arterial enhancement is LR-M (probably or definitely malignant but not HCC specific)**. Although this observation could still represent an HCC, raising the possibility of a non-HCC malignancy can change patient management and prognosis. LR-M classification **can prompt additional investigation for other malignancies and subsequent biopsy, in this particular patient revealing intrahepatic cholangiocarcinoma (CCA)**. Biopsy is often not needed prior to treatment when there is high suspicion for HCC such as with observations categorized as LR-5 (definitely HCC) or LR-4 (probably HCC).

Targetoid (rim) arterial enhancement is the main feature of LR-M. This rim arterial enhancement **should not be mistaken for the capsule appearance**, which is a major feature for HCC and **refers to rim enhancement on venous or delayed phase that is not present on arterial phase**. LR-M may also be applied when there are other features that in the radiologist's judgment suggest non-HCC malignancy. Another LR-M feature demonstrated in this particular case is the **persistent enhancement that appears greater than liver on the delayed phase. This is a feature of CCA** due to presence of fibrosis rather than of HCC. This delayed enhancement **should not be mistaken for hemangioma**. This mass has continuous peripheral rim enhancement rather than the discontinuous peripheral nodular enhancement expected of hemangioma. **In addition, the degree of T2 hyperintensity of this mass is closer to the spleen on long TE sequences, rather than the "light bulb" T2 hyperintensity that is expected of hemangioma.**

This CCA also had restricted diffusion (not shown). In LI-RADS, this is an **ancillary feature that favors malignancy** but is nonspecific and can be associated with various benign and malignant lesions. Large CCAs may have targetoid restricted diffusion, with bright diffusion restriction in the periphery due to hypercellularity and sparing in the central portion due to fibrosis. **Associated obstruction of adjacent bile ducts (not seen in this case) would be another finding suspicious for CCA**, although not always present, especially if masses are subcapsular like this one. If a hepatobiliary contrast agent such as gadoxetate disodium (Eovist—Bayer HealthCare) is used in MRI, **CCA is typically hypointense on the 20-minute hepatobiliary phase**. However, **in some large tumors, a central hazy "cloud" of hyperintensity in hepatobiliary phase** has been described due to prolonged contrast pooling within the expanded extracellular spaces of the fibrosis, as shown in a different patient below.

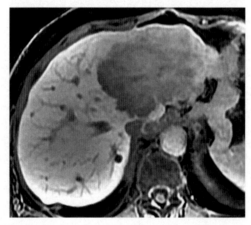

Large CCA with gadoxetate "cloud" on hepatobiliary phase MRI.

References: ACR Liver Imaging Reporting and Data System version 2018. American College of Radiology website. Available at https://www.acr.org/Clinical-Resources/Reporting-and-Data-Systems/LI-RADS. Accessed on August 12, 2020.

Joo I, Lee JM, Yoon JH. Imaging diagnosis of intrahepatic and perihilar cholangiocarcinoma: recent advances and challenges. *Radiology* 2018;288(1):7–13.

Kim YY, Kim MJ, Kim EH, et al. Hepatocellular carcinoma versus other hepatic malignancy in cirrhosis: performance of LI-RADS version 2018. *Radiology* 2019;291(1):72–80.

32a **Answer C.** There is a mass with internal hemorrhage in a background of hepatic steatosis. The first two MR images are T1W in-phase and out-of-phase images showing diffuse **loss of signal intensity on out-of-phase images of the background liver parenchyma compatible with intracellular lipid.** In hemochromatosis, the liver would lose signal intensity on the in-phase images due to increased effects of magnetic susceptibility on longer TE images. The mass contains **a small focus of T1 hyperintensity that persists on the fat-saturated T1W image, indicating hemorrhage rather than macroscopic fat.**

32b **Answer B. In a young woman with a hemorrhagic liver mass in a background of hepatic steatosis, the most likely diagnosis is hepatocellular adenoma (HCA).** While focal nodular hyperplasia (FNH) is more common than HCA, FNH does not have propensity to hemorrhage and rupture. In light of the patient's age and absence of risk factors for hepatocellular carcinoma (HCC) or primary malignancy, HCC and metastatic disease are unlikely.

HCAs are most commonly found in **women of childbearing age taking oral contraceptives,** but as discussed in a previous question, they also develop in patients with glycogen storage disease and those taking exogenous androgens. HCAs can be heterogeneous due to intralesional fat, hemorrhage, or malignant transformation. Intervention including embolization or surgical resection could be considered in lesions >5 cm or those with hemorrhage.

References: Fisher A, Siegelman ES. MR techniques and MR of the liver. In: Siegelman ES (ed). *Body MRI*. Philadelphia, PA: Elsevier Saunders, 2005:4–5.

Katabathina VS, Menias CO, Shanbhogue AK, et al. Genetics and imaging of hepatocellular adenomas: 2011 update. *Radiographics* 2011;31(6):1529–1543.

33 **Answer B.** Ultrasound of the liver shows a "starry-sky" appearance. Diffuse edema causes the appearance of decreased echogenicity of the liver parenchyma. The walls of the portal venules become more conspicuous and represent the "stars" against the night "sky" of the edematous parenchyma. **The most common cause of "starry-sky" appearance is acute hepatitis.** In this patient, acute alcoholic hepatitis was thought to be the cause. However, "starry-sky" appearance has also been described with other processes that cause liver edema or infiltration, such as toxic shock, right heart failure, leukemia, and lymphoma.

The diagnosis of acute hepatitis is usually based on clinical history, liver function tests (LFTs), and serologic tests. **Imaging such as ultrasound is useful to evaluate for alternate diagnoses such as biliary pathology that may require intervention.** Treatment of patients with acute hepatitis is supportive, with mild-to-moderate cases manageable on an outpatient basis. Severe or fulminant cases of acute hepatitis may require intensive hospital care.

References: Abu-Judeh HH. The "starry sky" liver with right-sided heart failure. *AJR Am J Roentgenol* 2002;178(1):78.

Morgan T, Qayyum A, Gore RM. Chapter 89: Vascular disorders of the liver and splanchnic circulation. In: Gore RM, Levine MS (eds). *Textbook of gastrointestinal radiology*, 4th ed. Philadelphia, PA: Elsevier/Saunders, 2015:1629–1675.

34 **Answer C.** Noncontrast image of the liver shows crescentic high attenuation conforming to the margins of the lateral segment left lobe of the liver. This is consistent with a **subcapsular hematoma** in this patient who had a percutaneous liver biopsy earlier in the day. The sudden pain is attributed to acute distention of the Glisson capsule of the liver. **CT is the study of choice for evaluation of suspected hemorrhage.** The density of an acute hematoma (1 to 3 days) decreases as the hematoma evolves, and a pseudocapsule may develop in 2 to 4 weeks. Mixed density can be seen with layering clot (hematocrit effect) or hemorrhage of different ages. Subcapsular hematomas are typically **crescentic or biconvex (lenticular)** in shape. Management of hemorrhage may include blood transfusion and transcatheter arterial embolization if clinically warranted. This patient was **hemodynamically stable and treated conservatively** without intervention.

This patient does have diffuse hepatic steatosis, accounting for diffuse low density of the liver, which makes the unenhanced vessels visible on this noncontrast exam, but the crescentic subcapsular configuration of the high-density area is not typical for fatty sparing. Transient hepatic attenuation difference (THAD) refers to altered parenchymal enhancement that tends to disappear on later phases and would not be applicable to this noncontrast exam. Periportal edema may be seen with trauma, acute hepatitis, and congestion and manifests as a halo of low density around the portal triads, not seen here.

References: Boland GWL, Halpert RD. Chapter 6: Liver. In: Boland GWL, Halpert RD (eds). *Gastrointestinal imaging: the requisites*, 4th ed. Philadelphia, PA: Elsevier/Saunders, 2014:218–290.

Casillas VJ, Amendola MA, Gascue A, et al. Imaging of nontraumatic hemorrhagic hepatic lesions. *Radiographics* 2000;20(2):367–378.

35 **Answer A.** The **arterial phase on the current study is too early, limiting evaluation for hypervascular neoplasms.** Images in a liver protocol MRI or CT **should be acquired in the late arterial phase, when there is a heterogeneous blush of contrast in the main portal vein** (long arrow) as seen on the prior MRI exam. The current exam shows no contrast in the main portal vein (short arrow).

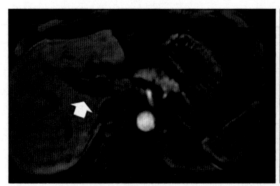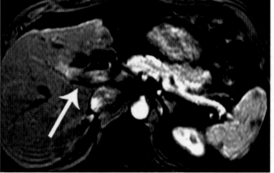

In the late arterial phase, sinusoidal enhancement of the spleen and corticomedullary phase enhancement of the kidneys are expected. However, on the current MRI in the top row, there is no contrast in the portal vein and no organ enhancement. (The pancreas has inherent T1 hyperintensity and normally appears brighter than other organs on an unenhanced T1 image.) A subsequent MRI 6 weeks later (not shown) revealed that the lesion was still present and slightly increased in size. The lesion was considered to be a hepatocellular carcinoma and treated with radiofrequency ablation. **If the arterial phase is suboptimal on MRI or CT, the other pre- or postcontrast**

series might still reveal a lesion. In particular, **other phases should be scrutinized for foci of enhancement or washout appearance.** LI-RADS category **LR-NC** (not categorizable) can be assigned when an observation cannot be categorized due to image degradation or omission.

Spontaneous regression or resolution of hypervascular true nodules in the cirrhotic liver has been reported but is rare, postulated to be due to interruption of arterial blood supply to small dysplastic nodules or even HCCs. There is no vessel in line with the liver finding in the right lobe that would account for ghosting. Small benign arterial portal shunts (not an answer choice) are typically tiny hypervascular foci commonly seen in the cirrhotic liver and may account for transient hepatic intensity differences (THIDs). These may seem to appear and disappear from study to study, perhaps due to slight differences in bolus timing.

References: Boll DT, Merkle EM. Diffuse liver disease: strategies for hepatic CT and MR imaging. *Radiographics* 2009;29(6):1591–1614.

Gandhi SN, Brown MA, Wong JG, et al. MR contrast agents for liver imaging: what, when, how. *Radiographics* 2006;26(6):1621–1636.

36 **Answer F.** This patient has **metastatic mucinous colorectal carcinoma**. The liver is enlarged by confluent hypodense masses with **density of the mucin at 23 HU slightly greater than the upper limit expected for simple fluid of 20 HU.** This **appearance can be mistaken for a group of benign cysts** such as in polycystic liver disease. In this case, there are other findings consistent with a malignant process including low-density **metastatic periportal lymphadenopathy** that encases and narrows the portal vein best seen on the coronal image, as well as peritoneal carcinomatosis. At pathology, a tumor is defined as mucinous when >50% of the tumor is composed of mucin. Mucinous hepatic metastases are **most frequently from colorectal carcinoma** (CRC), with 10% to 20% of colorectal carcinomas meeting criteria. **Calcification** is more frequently seen in mucinous compared to nonmucinous CRC. Other mucinous primaries are less common than CRC but may be from the breast, ovary, pancreas, or other sites in the gastrointestinal tract.

Metastases can also appear cystic because of necrosis before or after treatment, with variable amounts of soft tissue visible internally. The differential diagnosis of a multilocular cystic lesion may include biliary cystadenoma/cystadenocarcinoma and various infections in the appropriate clinical setting.

References: Ko EY, Ha HK, Kim AY, et al. CT differentiation of mucinous and nonmucinous colorectal carcinoma. *AJR Am J Roentgenol* 2007;188(3):785–791.

Qian LJ, Zhu J, Zhuang ZG, et al. Spectrum of multilocular cystic hepatic lesions: CT and MR imaging findings with pathologic correlation. *Radiographics* 2013;33(5):1419–1433.

37 **Answer C.** This patient has the CT equivalent of the **"hot spot" sign** (originally described in Tc-99m sulfur colloid scans), which is diagnostic for superior vena cava (SVC) obstruction. **SVC obstruction is due to lung cancer in up to 75% of cases**, usually non–small cell carcinoma. Classically, there is **intense early enhancement of the medial segment left hepatic** lobe without underlying liver mass. This is associated with an extensive network of collateral veins in the chest wall, mediastinum, and around the liver, representing caval-to-portal pathways of venous return. This could be considered a transient hepatic attenuation difference (THAD) due to altered perfusion. It usually has geographic margins and a pathognomonic appearance but could be mistaken for a hypervascular mass.

Catheter-related thrombosis is an increasing cause of SVC obstruction and may account for 15% to 40% of cases. **Lymphoma** as a cause of SVC obstruction accounts for 10% of cases. SVC obstruction may cause shortness of breath and redness and swelling of the face, neck, upper extremities, and chest wall. Management includes treating the underlying malignancy with chemotherapy and radiation, but endovascular therapy with metallic stenting may be palliative in some cases.

References: Kapur S, Paik E, Rezaei A, et al. Where there is blood, there is a way: unusual collateral vessels in superior and inferior vena cava obstruction. *Radiographics* 2010;30(1):67–78.

Sheth S, Ebert MD, Fishman EK. Superior vena cava obstruction evaluation with MDCT. *AJR Am J Roentgenol* 2010;194(4):W336–W346.

38 **Answer E.** This patient several months after a liver transplant has a lymphoid tumor consistent with **posttransplant lymphoproliferative disorder** (PTLD). Biopsy revealed lymphoma. The imaging findings in this case are nonspecific, with a hypodense lesion on the arterial and venous phase CT and a **"bull's-eye"** appearance on ultrasound. The differential diagnosis in this patient mainly includes abscess, PTLD, and recurrent hepatocellular carcinoma (HCC) with an atypical hypovascular appearance. Among the choices listed for this question, lymphoid tumor (PTLD) is the most likely diagnosis.

PTLD is a heterogeneous group of disorders **ranging from benign hyperplasia to poorly-differentiated lymphoma**, but most lesions are monoclonal. The majority of cases are B-cell proliferations thought to be induced by Epstein-Barr virus (EBV). **In the abdomen, bowel is the most commonly involved organ, while the liver is the most commonly involved solid organ**. PTLD in the liver **most often presents as solitary or multiple masses with low attenuation on CT** best seen on venous phase. Other manifestations of PTLD and lymphoid tumors are ill-defined infiltration of the parenchyma and periportal masses. Lymphoid tumors may encase periportal vessels without narrowing them, a feature that has been described as the "vessel penetration" sign. On ultrasound, lymphoid masses are typically hypoechoic, although lesions can be nearly anechoic or have a "bull's-eye" appearance with a hyperechoic center and hypoechoic rim, as seen in this patient. **Because imaging features overlap with opportunistic infections and other neoplasms in this immunosuppressed patient population, biopsy is usually required to make the diagnosis.**

In adult transplant patients, PTLD is overall the second most common tumor (after nonmelanoma skin cancer). It is most often diagnosed within 1 year of transplant but can occur at any time. Treatment includes reduction in immunosuppression, with chemotherapy and radiation for frankly malignant tumors and refractory cases.

References: Camacho JC, Moreno CC, Harri PA, et al. Posttransplantation lymphoproliferative disease: proposed imaging classification. *Radiographics* 2014;34(7):2025–2038.

Katabathina VS, Menias CO, Tammisetti VS, et al. Malignancy after solid organ transplantation: comprehensive imaging review. *Radiographics* 2016;36(5):1390–1407.

39 **Answer D.** This woman has **breast cancer with widespread liver and splenic metastases. Pseudocirrhosis** has developed after treatment with hepatic atrophy and lobulated contour. Pseudocirrhosis is a form of posttreatment sequela after chemotherapy for liver metastases. This condition has a predilection for breast cancer metastases for uncertain reasons and is **uncommonly seen with other primary tumors**. The liver contour can be finely or coarsely nodular, with areas of capsular retraction. The caudate lobe may also enlarge, as seen in some cases of cirrhosis. In some cases, nodular regenerative hyperplasia (NRH) with atrophy of intervening parenchyma without fibrosis has been found. In other cases, there is a desmoplastic response incited by an extensively infiltrating breast cancer.

Although the true histopathologic findings of cirrhosis are not found in pseudocirrhosis, some patients nevertheless develop portal hypertension with varices and ascites. Other changes that can be found after treatment of liver metastasis include altered enhancement patterns, cystic/necrotic degeneration, and calcification.

References: Faria SC, Ganesan K, Mwangi I, et al. MR imaging of liver fibrosis: current state of the art. *Radiographics* 2009;29(6):1615–1635.

Jha P, Poder L, Wang ZJ, et al. Radiologic mimics of cirrhosis. *AJR Am J Roentgenol* 2010;194(4):993–999.

40 **Answer B.** This patient has **neuroendocrine tumor** metastases. There are multiple small masses on the CT with arterial enhancement, indicating a hypervascular neoplasm. Most of the metastases are nearly isodense to liver on subsequent phases. This patient previously had a Whipple procedure to resect a pancreatic neuroendocrine tumor.

Neuroendocrine tumor metastases **can be subtle on imaging**. Most are **slow growing**, so assessment for enlargement on follow-up imaging is also a challenge. However, newer techniques have been helpful in increasing the sensitivity for detection these metastases. The **PET/CT scan using Gallium-68 dotatate** (NETSPOT) images somatostatin receptors and is **becoming the standard for whole-body evaluation** of neuroendocrine neoplasm, but can miss small liver lesions. When MRI is performed with hepatobiliary contrast agent such as Eovist, a small metastasis may be more conspicuous as a focus of **hypointensity in the hepatobiliary phase**. Careful inspection for **restricted diffusion** on diffusion-weighted images (DWI) can also improve sensitivity for detection of small metastases.

Among the choices given, a subset of breast metastases can appear hypervascular, but this patient is male, which makes the diagnosis highly unlikely. Non–small cell lung cancer, colon cancer, and lymphoid tumors are hypovascular. Note that small cell lung cancer (not an answer choice) is considered a neuroendocrine neoplasm and may show hypervascular metastases. Hypervascular neoplasms to consider are included in the mnemonic "**MR CT**" are **M**elanoma, **R**enal cell carcinoma, **C**arcinoid (i.e., neuroendocrine tumor) or **C**horiocarcinoma, and **T**hyroid carcinoma.

References: Khosa F, Khan AN, Eisenberg RL. Hypervascular liver lesions on MRI. *AJR Am J Roentgenol* 2011;197(2):W204–W220.

Silva AC, Evans JM, McCullough AE, et al. MR imaging of hypervascular liver masses: a review of current techniques. *Radiographics* 2009;29(2):385–402.

41 **Answer C.** Malignant portal vein thrombosis (PVT) is a contraindication to liver transplantation by the Milan criteria. Patients with malignant PVT have advanced hepatocellular carcinoma (HCC) and poor prognosis, with a high rate of recurrence after transplant. **Liver transplantation has found to be an effective treatment for some patients with HCC that is unresectable because of tumor location, multifocality, or severe hepatic insufficiency.** Transplantation has the potential for correcting liver dysfunction as well as removing the malignancy. Prognosis of HCC was generally poor regardless of treatment. However, patient selection for liver transplantation using the Milan criteria has been associated with positive outcomes, including 4-year overall survival of 85% and recurrence rate of 8%. Patients meeting criteria have a single tumor ≤5 cm or up to three tumors each ≤3 cm. **Vascular invasion and extrahepatic metastases are exclusion criteria.** The Milan criteria have been adopted by the United Network for Organ Sharing (UNOS) and Medicare to identify patients with HCC to determine eligibility for transplant.

Hepatic encephalopathy and refractory variceal bleeding are among the acceptable indications for liver transplant.

References: Bhargava P, Vaidya S, Dick AA, et al. Imaging of orthotopic liver transplantation: review. *AJR Am J Roentgenol* 2011;196(3 Suppl):WS15–WS25; Quiz S35–S38.

Mazzaferro V, Regalia E, Doci R, et al. Liver transplantation for the treatment of small hepatocellular carcinomas in patients with cirrhosis. *N Engl J Med* 1996;334(11):693–699.

42 **Answer D.** The most common cause of graft failure after liver transplant is rejection. Imaging evaluation when a liver transplant complication is suspected usually begins with ultrasound. Elevated resistive indices of >0.8 may be seen on ultrasound in rejection but are nonspecific. **The main role of imaging is to identify correctable structural abnormalities that clinically mimic rejection, including vascular and biliary complications.** CT, MRI, and nuclear medicine hepatobiliary scans may be helpful for subsequent problem solving. Biopsy is required for definitive diagnosis of rejection.

References: Camacho JC, Coursey-Moreno C, Telleria JC, et al. Nonvascular post-liver transplantation complications: from ultrasound screening to cross-sectional and interventional imaging. *Radiographics* 2015;35(1):87–104.

Norton PT, DeAngelis GA, Ogur T, et al. Noninvasive vascular imaging in abdominal solid organ transplantation. *AJR Am J Roentgenol* 2013;201(4):W544–W553.

43 **Answers:**

Patient 1: C. Markedly elevated liver stiffness consistent with cirrhosis.

Patient 2: D. Normal liver stiffness.

Patient 3: B. Nondiagnostic study due to significant signal loss from hepatic iron deposition.

Elastography is the analysis of the propagation of mechanical waves to evaluate the properties of tissue. One application of elastography is the **assessment of liver stiffness for identification and staging of liver fibrosis.** Although liver biopsy remains the reference standard, it is an invasive procedure with potential complications and limited by small size of biopsy specimen. MR and US elastography are among the imaging techniques in use for the staging of liver fibrosis, with **MR elastography (MRE) currently the most accurate and reproducible noninvasive study,** in addition to providing a larger map than other studies. **Fibrosis staging has implications in the diagnosis and treatment of liver disease,** since lower stages of fibrosis are potentially reversible. MR elastography is often performed in conjunction with other MR techniques to quantify fat deposition in hepatic steatosis or iron deposition in hemachromatosis.

For MRE, a device generating mechanical shear waves is strapped to patient's right upper quadrant over the liver. On the postprocessed color wave image from patient 1 shown below, the device presses on the abdominal wall (long arrows). The long arrows indicate the direction of propagation of the generated waves. **Waves propagate faster and deeper into stiffer tissue compared to softer tissue.** In this patient, the waves (small arrows) appear thick and propagate deeply, indicating abnormally elevated liver stiffness. Stiffness is expressed in units of pressure, the kiloPascal (kPa), with **red on the color stiffness map indicating the highest stiffness.** Occasionally, there is heterogeneity of fibrosis, manifesting as color heterogeneity in different areas. According to the Mayo Clinic standard protocol and classification, > 5kPa is compatible with stage 4 fibrosis (cirrhosis). In this patient, calculations revealed an average stiffness of 9.75 kPa.

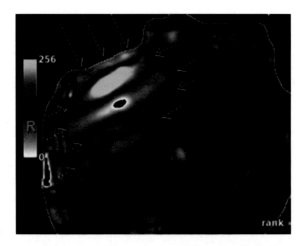

Patient 2 has **normal liver stiffness (i.e., low stiffness)**. On the color wave image, the **waves appear thin and remain superficial near the liver surface**. On the color stiffness image, the liver is blue and purple in color representing the low end of scale on the color bar. The calculated average stiffness was 2.03 kPa. According to the Mayo Clinic classification, <2.5 kPa is normal.

Patient 3 has primary **hemochromatosis**. The **amount of iron deposition in this case was large enough to result in a nondiagnostic study** from significant signal loss. MRE sequences have a relatively long TE, making them particularly **sensitive to loss of signal by susceptibility artifact**, such as from iron deposition. The color wave images are uninterpretable, showing **artifactual speckled dots of color over the liver**, which do not conform to the expected curvilinear arcs of wave propagation. The **crosshatching over the liver on the color stiffness map indicates areas that are statistically unreliable** and must be excluded from calculating stiffness. In this patient, the entire liver is crosshatched, and stiffness cannot be reliably measured anywhere. The clue to hemochromatosis is the **very dark liver on the T2W long TE series**. This series is performed as part of MRE to show anatomy.

Motion artifacts such as from respiratory or cardiac motion can degrade the exam and can manifest as disruption or distortion of the waves on the color wave map. Motion artifact is not shown in any of the cases. Cardiac motion can degrade quality particularly in the left lobe of the liver, and in those cases, the left lobe should be excluded from the region of interest (ROI) for quantification.

Sometimes, elevation in liver stiffness is not due to fibrosis. Liver stiffness can be increased by increased blood flow from recent meal, acute hepatitis, hepatic congestion, or an infiltrative process. Studies should be performed after a 4- to 6-hour fast and interpreted in light of the clinical scenario.

References: Guglielmo FF, Venkatesh SK, Mitchell DG. Liver MR elastography technique and image interpretation: pearls and pitfalls. *Radiographics* 2019;39(7):1983–2002.

Hoodeshenas S, Yin M, Venkatesh SK. Magnetic resonance elastography of liver: current update. *Top Magn Reson Imaging* 2018;27(5):319–333.

44 **Answer B.** The most recent scan shows a nodular focus of arterial enhancement at the margin of the ablation cavity where no enhancement was present several months before. Findings are consistent with **recurrent hepatocellular carcinoma**. The appropriate LI-RADS category is LR-TR viable (treated, probably or definitely viable). Notice that both arterial images were obtained with appropriate timing in the late arterial phase with a blush of contrast seen in the main portal vein. Scans performed too early or too late may miss hypervascular liver lesions. Imaging after locoregional therapy such as chemo- or radioembolization as well as radiofrequency or microwave embolization is performed to assess treatment response and evaluate for new or recurrent malignancy. Studies performed a short interval (<1 month) after ablation can demonstrate **ring-like or ill-defined perilesional altered enhancement thought to represent postprocedural injury and inflammation**. This enhancement may mimic residual or recurrent neoplasm. **For ⁹⁰Y (yttrium-90) transarterial radioembolization, changes of edema, hemorrhage, inflammation, and necrosis can persist longer than other types of locoregional therapy**, sometimes accompanied by increased size and perilesional enhancement mimicking tumor progression. As a result, radioembolization treatment response may be difficult to accurate evaluate before 3 to 6 months. Postprocedural changes should improve or resolve as the normal tissue heals around the cavity. New nodular foci that develop afterward would be suspicious for recurrent neoplasm.

References: Sainani NI, Gervais DA, Mueller PR, et al. Imaging after percutaneous radiofrequency ablation of hepatic tumors: Part 2. Abnormal findings. *AJR Am J Roentgenol* 2013;200(1):194–204.

Spina JC, Hume I, Pelaez A, et al. Expected and unexpected imaging findings after 90Y transarterial radioembolization for liver tumors. *Radiographics* 2019;39(2):578–595.

45 **Answer A.** This patient has imaging findings consistent with **hepatic artery stenosis** (HAS). Spectral Doppler waveform is being recorded in the hepatic artery (white arrow) at the porta hepatis. This is a **classic tardus et parvus waveform in the vessel downstream from a stenosis**, with delayed arterial upstroke and decreased peak velocity resulting in a **low resistive index (RI) of <0.5** (yellow arrow, RI = 0.4). The stenosis is revealed on the selective arteriogram as focal narrowing (black arrow).

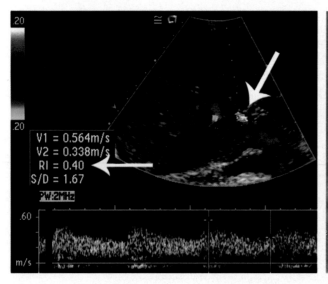
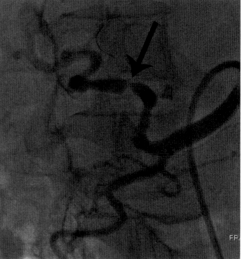

The most common vascular complications following liver transplant involve the hepatic artery. Hepatic artery stenosis and thrombosis each occur in up to 12% of transplants. HAS occurs most frequently at the anastomosis. Findings typical of HAS besides downstream parvus et tardus waveform on ultrasound include **elevated velocity of >200 cm/s and focal aliasing** immediately beyond the stenosis. Angiography can be diagnostic and therapeutic.

Because the hepatic artery is the sole source of vascular supply to the bile ducts, arterial compromise **can lead to biliary ischemia with formation of bilomas and graft dysfunction**. The small hepatic hypodensities (arrows) on the following CT image in the same patient represent developing bilomas.

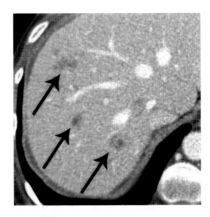

The other vascular complications (portal vein thrombosis, pseudoaneurysm, and arterioportal fistulas in the answer choices) are possible in liver transplant patients but less common and are not compatible with the imaging findings. The main portal vein is patent on the color Doppler image with appropriate direction of flow (red in this case representing hepatopedal flow toward the liver as indicated by the color reference bar on the left). A pseudoaneurysm is an enlargement, not narrowing, of the artery. An arterioportal shunt would show early venous opacification on arteriogram.

References: Crossin JD, Muradali D, Wilson SR. Ultrasound of liver transplants: normal and abnormal. *Radiographics* 2003;23(5):1093–1114.

Singh AK, Nachiappan AC, Verma HA, et al. Postoperative imaging in liver transplantation: what radiologists should know. *Radiographics* 2010;30(2):339–351.

46 **Answer A.** **Giant cavernous hemangiomas** (GCAs) can be associated with **Kasabach-Merritt syndrome**. In this syndrome, **thrombocytopenia is caused by sequestration and destruction of platelets** within a GCA. The syndrome is usually seen in infants but can also be observed in adults. Various size criteria for giant cavernous hemangiomas have been proposed ranging from >4 to >10 cm in size. GCAs usually exhibit the classic peripheral nodular discontinuous enhancement of cavernous hemangiomas as shown in this case. They may have a **T2 bright central scar that does not fill in completely** on delayed imaging, also demonstrated in this patient. The **heterogeneity and atypical appearance of some GCAs occasionally present a diagnostic challenge**. GCAs account for fewer than 10% of hemangiomas and uncommonly become symptomatic. Complications include pain, rupture, or Kasabach-Merritt syndrome.

Carcinoid syndrome is flushing and diarrhea that can be seen in some patients with metastatic neuroendocrine tumors. Cushing syndrome is related to hypercortisolism, which can manifest as weight gain, androgen excess, glucose intolerance, and bone loss, among other symptoms. Lambert-Eaton syndrome is a neuromuscular condition manifesting as muscle weakness. It may a paraneoplastic syndrome associated with small cell lung cancer.

References: Boland GWL, Halpert RD. Chapter 6: Liver. In: Boland GWL, Halpert RD (eds). *Gastrointestinal imaging: the requisites*, 4th ed. Philadelphia, PA: Elsevier/Saunders, 2014:218–290.

Coumbaras M, Wendum D, Monnier-Cholley L, et al. CT and MR imaging features of pathologically proven atypical giant hemangiomas of the liver. *AJR Am J Roentgenol* 2002;179(6):1457–1463.

47 **Answer C.** **Multifocal steatosis is seen in a patchy nodular distribution** in the liver. The CT shows areas of decreased density. These areas correspond to **loss of signal intensity on the out-of-phase images** compared to the in-phase image in keeping with microscopic fat. On imaging, steatosis may be diffuse, focal, or multifocal. Classic locations of focal steatosis include areas **periportal regions, around the gallbladder fossa, and around the falciform ligament** anteriorly. Some cases show **striking perivascular distribution** as shown in this case and on the following venous phase CT image from a different patient. Multifocal steatosis can mimic metastatic disease or infiltrative malignancy, but there is no underlying parenchymal distortion, displacement of vessels, or other mass effect. **Areas of steatosis will show enhancement since they represent hepatocytes with intracellular lipid**, although they remain hypodense relative to the surrounding liver on the different phases.

References: Cassidy FH, Yokoo T, Aganovic L, et al. Fatty liver disease: MR imaging techniques for the detection and quantification of liver steatosis. *Radiographics* 2009;29(1):231–260.

Hamer OW, Aguirre DA, Casola G, et al. Fatty liver: imaging patterns and pitfalls. *Radiographics* 2006;26(6):1637–1653.

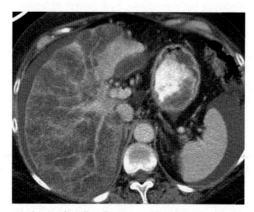

Perivascular distribution of hepatic steatosis.

48   **Answer B.** There is a heterogeneous nodular cirrhotic liver. The small nodule indicated by the arrow is slightly hyperintense on the arterial phase. However, correlation with the precontrast T1 image reveals that the **nodule is inherently T1 bright on all series including hepatobiliary phase, without arterial enhancement**. There are multiple other similar lesions scattered in the liver. This constellation of findings is reassuring for benignity and most consistent with regenerative nodules.

T1 hyperintense lesions in the diseased liver are not uncommon and often represent regenerative nodules, although on occasion, dysplastic nodules or hepatocellular carcinomas (HCCs) show T1 hyperintensity. T1 hyperintensity has been attributed to steatosis, glycogen, copper, or hemorrhage. In this case, the nodule remains **bright on the out-of-phase T1W image with no evidence of microscopic fat** and **bright on the FS T1W image with no evidence of macroscopic fat**. Regenerative and dysplastic nodules usually retain contrast on 20-minute hepatobiliary phase with iso- or hyperintensity as demonstrated in this case. The small percentage of HCCs with hepatobiliary phase hyperintensity should also demonstrate other imaging features of HCC. Nodules that are T1 hyperintense may be better evaluated on CT, if they are not bright on precontrast CT images.

References: Boland GWL, Halpert RD. Chapter 6: Liver. In: Boland GWL, Halpert RD (eds). *Gastrointestinal imaging: the requisites*, 4th ed. Philadelphia, PA: Elsevier/Saunders, 2014:218–290.

Hanna RF, Aguirre DA, Kased N, et al. Cirrhosis-associated hepatocellular nodules: correlation of histopathologic and MR imaging features. *Radiographics* 2008;28(3):747–769.

49   **Answer D.** This patient has **hepatic infarction**. The liver on the initial CT is heterogeneous with multiple areas of **hypoenhancement**, worst in the right lobe. This has a **peripheral, geographic appearance without displacement of vessels or mass effect**. Note the perisplenic high density consistent with hemoperitoneum as stated in the history. This patient suffered severe shock as a result of the large hemorrhage, leading to the infarct. On noncontrast CT a month later, there is a wedge-shaped hypodensity with atrophy and capsular retraction in the right lobe consistent with evolution of the infarct and scarring.

Hepatic infarction is uncommon because the liver has dual blood supply from the hepatic arterial and portal venous systems. Causes for hepatic infarct may include shock, anesthesia, sepsis, trauma, metastases, and percutaneous hepatic interventions such as transarterial embolization and percutaneous ablation. Hepatic infarct is difficult to diagnose early, and imaging findings may be subtle. Margins become sharper and better defined with time. Infiltrative hepatocellular carcinoma (HCC) can also be heterogeneous and ill-defined but tends to show some arterial enhancement and without atrophy. Geographic areas of hypodensity without mass effect resemble areas of steatosis, but findings were acute compared to a recent prior CT, and steatosis does not evolve into a focal scar.

References: Gore RM, Ba-Ssalamah A. Chapter 90: Vascular disorders of the liver and splanchnic circulation. In: Gore RM, Levine MS (eds). *Textbook of gastrointestinal radiology*, 4th ed. Philadelphia, PA: Elsevier/Saunders, 2015:1676–1705.

Torabi M, Hosseinzadeh K, Federle MP. CT of nonneoplastic hepatic vascular and perfusion disorders. *Radiographics* 2008;28(7):1967–1982.

50 **Answer A.** There are multiple small T1 and T2 hypointense nodules in a cirrhotic liver. These **lose signal on the in-phase** compared to out-of-phase images, most consistent with **iron-containing siderotic nodules**. There is no arterial enhancement. Although siderotic nodules may be regenerative or dysplastic, they **rarely contain malignancy**. It is hypothesized that nodules that transition to hepatocellular carcinoma lose the ability to store iron. Patients with cirrhosis and other chronic liver diseases can have abnormally increased iron absorption causing foci of hepatic iron deposition.

References: Baron RL, Peterson MS. From the RSNA refresher courses: screening the cirrhotic liver for hepatocellular carcinoma with CT and MR imaging: opportunities and pitfalls. *Radiographics* 2001;21(Spec No.):S117–S132.

Curvo-Semedo L, Brito JB, Seco MF, et al. The hypointense liver lesion on T2W MR images and what it means. *Radiographics* 2010;30(1):e38.

51a **Answer B.** This lesion has a **centrifugal inner-to-outer enhancement** pattern, which has been described as the **most common pattern associated with peliosis hepatis** (from the Greek *pelios* meaning "dusky" or "purple"). This is the **opposite of the centripetal outer-to-inner pattern of fill-in seen with hemangiomas**. Peliosis hepatis is a rare benign vascular disorder characterized by dilated sinusoids and blood-filled cavities lined by endothelium. On arterial phase in this case, there is **central globular enhancement, which progresses outward toward the periphery and remains hyperdense** to surrounding liver on the delayed phase. On late phases, peliosis may show persistent enhancement indicating blood pooling as in this case or isointensity to surrounding liver. Peliosis may exhibit other patterns of enhancement. Note that **centrifugal enhancement is not entirely specific for peliosis** and may occasionally be seen with metastases. However, in this case, the persistent enhancement greater than liver on delayed phases favors peliosis over metastases. Lymphoma secondarily involving the liver is more common than primary hepatic lymphoma and is an incorrect answer choice because it is hypoenhancing. Cholangiocarcinoma (not an answer choice) can show delayed enhancement, but the mass typically shows little arterial enhancement and may be associated with biliary ductal dilation.

Peliosis hepatis **tends to have little mass effect** on adjacent vessels compared to hemangiomas and other tumors. This is demonstrated below on the CT of a different patient with multiple hypoenhancing foci of peliosis hepatis. A branch of the right hepatic vein (black arrow) passes along the margin of the dominant lesion undisturbed. Involvement may be diffuse or focal, with lesions of variable size. Lesions may have variable internal density from blood products (white arrow showing a level between fluids of two different densities). Peliosis may involve other organs such as the spleen, lymph nodes, lungs, and skin.

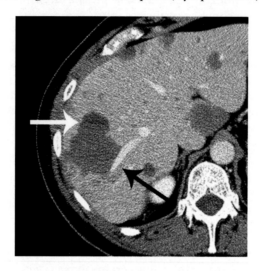

References: Iannaccone R, Federle MP, Brancatelli G, et al. Peliosis hepatis: spectrum of imaging findings. *AJR Am J Roentgenol* 2006;187(1):W43–W52.

Torabi M, Hosseinzadeh K, Federle MP. CT of nonneoplastic hepatic vascular and perfusion disorders. *Radiographics* 2008;28(7):1967–1982.

51b **Answer A. The pathogenesis of peliosis hepatis is unclear although drugs, toxins, and infections have been implicated.** Up to half of cases are idiopathic. *Bartonella henselae* and *Bartonella quintana* are the bacteria responsible for a type of peliosis called **bacillary peliosis** that is seen in **AIDS patients**. Most patients are asymptomatic and diagnosed incidentally, although there are reports of rupture and progression to cirrhosis and portal hypertension. Additional imaging modalities, follow-up imaging, and biopsy may factor into patient management because lesions may be mistaken for metastases or other primary hepatic tumors. Lymphadenopathy may be prominent in bacillary peliosis caused by *B. henselae*. Lesions can regress after treatment of the underlying cause. Bacillary peliosis caused by *Bartonella* infections is treated with antibiotics.

References: Elsayes KM, Shaaban AM, Rothan SM, et al. A comprehensive approach to hepatic vascular disease. *Radiographics* 2017;37(3):813–836.

Savastano S, San Bortolo O, Velo E, et al. Pseudotumoral appearance of peliosis hepatis. *AJR Am J Roentgenol* 2005;185(2):558–559.

52 **Answer C.** The complex cystic hepatic mass in this woman is suspicious for **biliary cystadenoma (BCA) or biliary cystadenocarcinoma (BCAC)**, which are uncommon **mucinous cystic neoplasms**. The initial US and MRI show a complex multiseptated cystic mass in the right lobe of the liver. There is **enhancement of the thickened irregular septations** at the medial part of the lesion, manifesting as increased conspicuity of this tissue on the postcontrast compared to precontrast images. On the CT 1.5 years later, the cyst has **significantly enlarged, and nodular enhancing tissue is demonstrated medially**. The enlargement and symptomatic presentation of these lesions can be secondary to hemorrhage, infection, and/or tumor enlargement.

Features of BCA and BCAC overlap. **Even if appearance favors benignity, resection should be considered since the risk of malignant transformation in BCAs is as high as 20%.** Solid enhancing components would increase suspicion for cystadenocarcinoma. Calcifications may be present. Mean patient age at presentation is 45 years for BCAs with about 90% occurring in women. For BCAC, the mean patient age is about a decade older, with more even distribution between women and men. Surgical pathology in this case revealed biliary cystadenoma with foci of high-grade dysplasia. **Ovarian-type stroma is found in a majority of these neoplasms**. These lesions can be difficult to fully resect, and **recurrence rate is as high as 90%**.

Regarding the other answer choices, there is no rim thickening or edema/hyperemia of the surrounding liver parenchyma to strongly suggest a pyogenic abscess on the initial or follow-up imaging. A hemorrhagic cyst does not have enhancing components. In ovarian carcinoma, peritoneal carcinomatosis scalloping the liver margin is much more common than hematogenous metastases. Hematogenous metastases from serous or mucinous cystic ovarian carcinoma into the liver may appear solid or cystic, with multiple lesions appearing late in disease, which does not match the clinical scenario in this patient. The differential diagnosis of a multiseptated cystic lesion in the liver would include infections such as echinococcal (hydatid) cyst (not an answer choice) if there is relevant travel history.

References: Averbukh LD, Wu DC, Cho WC, Wu GY. Biliary mucinous cystadenoma: a review of the literature. *J Clin Transl Hepatol* 2019;7(2):149–153.

Borhani AA, Wiant A, Heller MT. Cystic hepatic lesions: a review and an algorithmic approach. *AJR Am J Roentgenol* 2014;203(6):1192–1204.

53 **Answer D.** Areas of bright signal intensity are seen on this fat-saturated T2W spin-echo image in the perihepatic fat anteriorly denoted by the arrows, as well as within the subcutaneous fat peripherally. These represent areas of poor fat saturation as the result of field inhomogeneity. **Poor fat saturation should not be mistaken for pathology such as ascites or fatty infiltration.** A clue to uneven fat saturation artifact is location in areas prone to magnetic field inhomogeneity and susceptibility artifacts—at the image periphery, at interfaces with the lung, or near metallic objects. Among the choices, moiré fringes are artifacts that also occur in the periphery but have a distinctive appearance of curvilinear banding not seen in this case.

The effectiveness of frequency-selective fat saturation depends on the uniformity of the magnetic field. Factors that cause field inhomogeneity will unpredictably shift the frequency of the fat peak, preventing the fat peak from being identified and crushed (saturated) by the spoiler gradient. **To improve fat saturation and generally decrease the effects of susceptibility:**

- Move the anatomy of interest toward the **isocenter**, where the magnetic field is more homogeneous.
- Perform **shimming**, which adjusts the radiofrequency transmission elements to improve homogeneity of the magnetic field.
- Apply **sequences that are less affected** by susceptibility artifacts:
  - A short tau inversion recovery (**STIR**) sequence achieves fat suppression without relying on frequency selection of the fat peak and would produce better results at the expense of signal-to-noise ratio.
  - **Spin-echo sequences and sequences with shorter TE** are less affected by susceptibility than gradient-echo and longer TE sequences.

References: Huang SY, Seethamraju RT, Patel P, et al. Body MR imaging: artifacts, k-space, and solutions. *Radiographics* 2015;35(5):1439–1460.

Morelli JN, Runge VM, Ai F, et al. An image-based approach to understanding the physics of MR artifacts. *Radiographics* 2011;31(3):849–866.

QUESTIONS

1 A 34-year-old woman presents to the emergency department with fever and abdominal pain. What is the most likely cause of the CT findings?

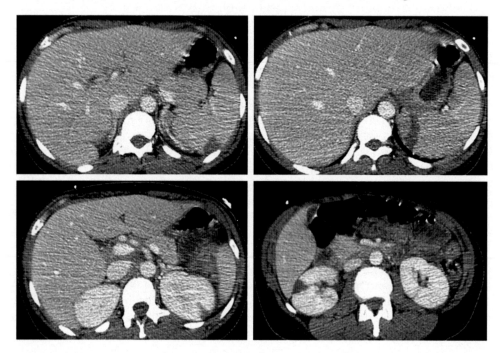

A. Emboli
B. Sarcoidosis
C. Metastases
D. Fibromuscular dysplasia

2 A CT angiogram was performed to evaluate the mesenteric vessels in a 78-year-old man with postprandial epigastric pain. Regarding the finding in the spleen, what is the most appropriate next step?

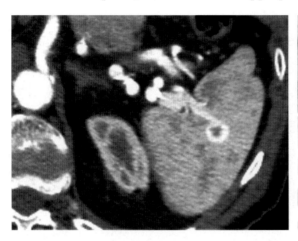 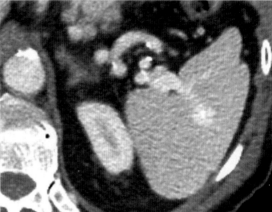

   A. PET/CT scan
   B. Percutaneous biopsy
   C. Antifungal treatment
   D. No further workup or treatment

3 A 66-year-old woman presents with a palpable mass. A CT scan was performed. What is the most likely explanation for the appearance of the spleen?

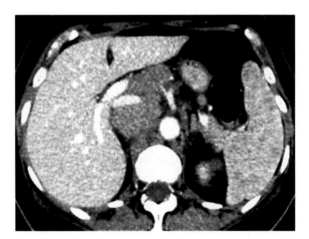

   A. Gaucher disease
   B. Normal early enhancement pattern
   C. Lymphoma
   D. Blunt trauma

4a A 38-year-old woman presents for evaluation of diffuse abdominal pain, bloating, and anorexia. The patient has a history of surgery after a fall as a child. Two images from a CT scan are shown. Which is the most appropriate test for confirmation of the suspected diagnosis?

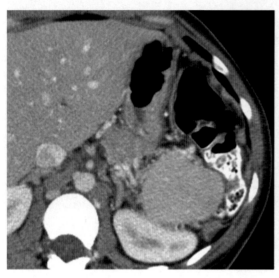
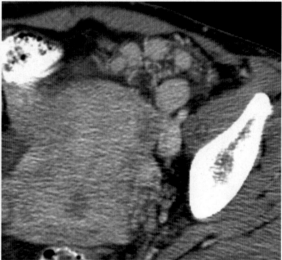

A. MRI without and with contrast
B. PET/CT
C. Sulfur colloid scan
D. Hepatobiliary iminodiacetic acid (HIDA) scan

4b A Tc-99m sulfur colloid scan was performed. Based on the following image from the scan, what is the diagnosis?

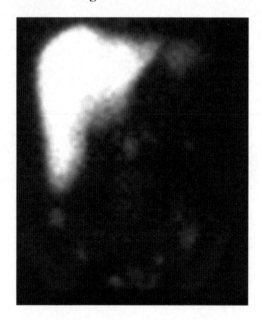

A. Peritoneal carcinomatosis
B. Splenosis
C. Tuberculosis
D. Lymphoma

5 A 38-year-old man presenting with abdominal pain underwent an MRI to further evaluate a finding in the left upper quadrant seen on ultrasound. What is the most likely diagnosis?

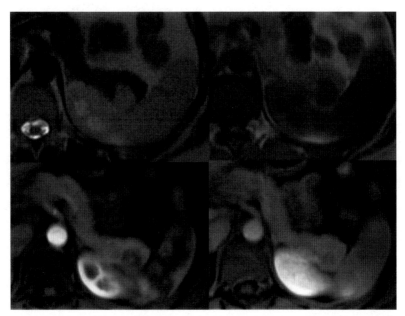

Top row: T2W and T1W. **Bottom row:** arterial and venous phase FS T1W+gad.

A. Pancreatic adenocarcinoma
B. Splenule
C. Peritoneal carcinomatosis
D. Splenic artery aneurysm

6 A 59-year-old man with a history of melanoma presents for routine surveillance imaging. A CT was performed with image shown below. What is the most likely diagnosis of the finding in the spleen?

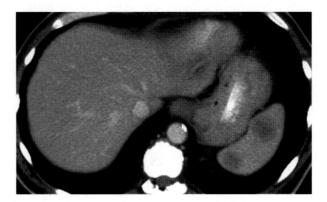

A. Littoral cell angiomas
B. Lymphangiomas
C. Pyogenic abscesses
D. Metastases

7 The following CT image is from a patient with a history of liver transplant. What is the most common organism that causes these splenic and hepatic findings?

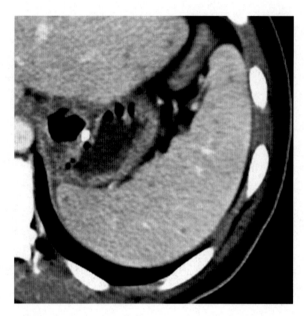

A. *Candida* species
B. *Mycobacterium avium* complex
C. *Bartonella henselae*
D. *Pneumocystis jiroveci*

8a A 59-year-old man fell off a horse one month ago. At that time, he was diagnosed with rib fractures at an outside hospital and discharged. On the day of current admission, he developed abrupt abdominal pain and presented to the hospital. A noncontrast abdominopelvic CT is shown. What is the most likely cause of the patient's symptoms?

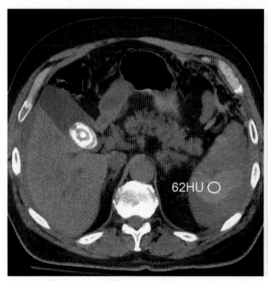
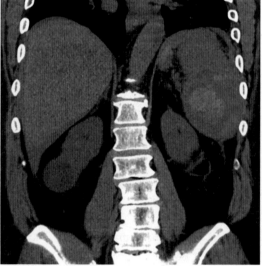

A. Acute pancreatitis
B. Acute calculous cholecystitis
C. Splenic pseudoaneurysm rupture
D. Capsular irritation from subacute subcapsular splenic hematoma

8b Which of the following types of CT examination is most sensitive and specific for diagnosing and characterizing splenic injuries following blunt trauma?

A. Noncontrast and arterial phase CT
B. Arterial phase CT only
C. Arterial phase and venous phase CT
D. Venous phase CT only

9 The following images are from a 60-year-old man. The appearance of the spleen is most consistent with

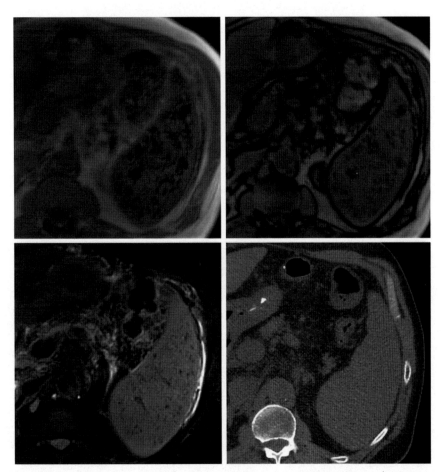

Top row: T1W in-phase and out-of-phase MRI. **Bottom row:** FS T2W MRI and noncontrast CT.

A. Microabscesses
B. Calcified granulomas
C. Gamna-Gandy bodies
D. Old infarcts

10 A 61-year-old man underwent a CT scan. What is the diagnosis?

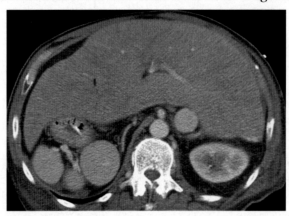

   A. Situs solitus
   B. Situs inversus
   C. Asplenia
   D. Polysplenia

11 A 55-year-old man with head and neck cancer presents for staging evaluation. An abdominal MRI examination was performed. What is the most likely diagnosis of the splenic finding?

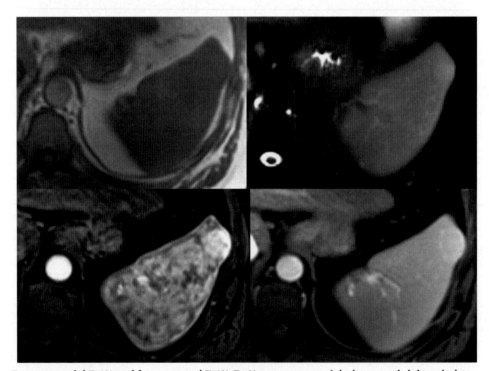

Top row: axial T1W and fat-saturated T2W. **Bottom row:** arterial phase and delayed phase.

   A. Lymphangioma
   B. Metastasis
   C. Hamartoma
   D. Angiosarcoma

12 A 49-year-old man presents with fatigue. What is the most likely diagnosis?

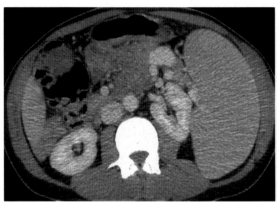
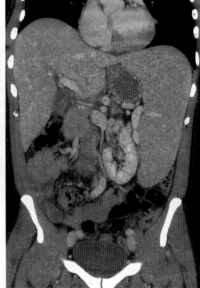
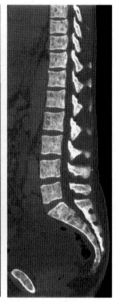

    A. Prostate carcinoma
    B. Multiple myeloma
    C. Mononucleosis
    D. Myelofibrosis

13 A patient with limb hemihypertrophy and port wine stains underwent an abdominal CT scan shown below. What do these splenic lesions represent?

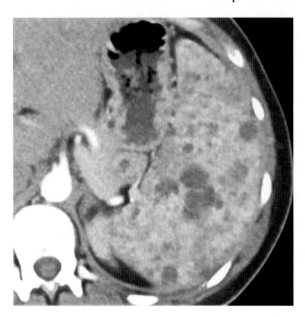

    A. Angiomas
    B. Neurofibromas
    C. Hemangioblastomas
    D. Gaucheromas

14 Match the splenic imaging findings in patients 1 to 3 with the most likely diagnosis A to C. Each option may be used only once.

Patient 1. A 74-year-old woman with CT and ultrasound images.

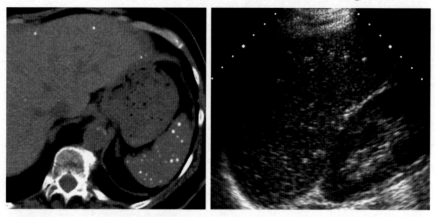

Patient 2. A 78-year-old man.   Patient 3. A 26-year-old man.

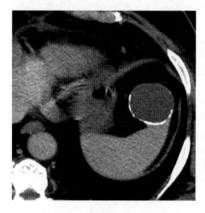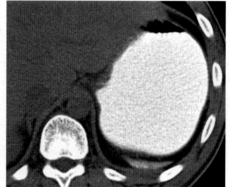

A. Sickle cell anemia
B. Posttraumatic sequela
C. Old healed granulomatous infection

15 A 43-year-old man with no significant past medical history presents with upper abdominal pain. The patient was afebrile with a normal white blood cell count. Images from a contrast-enhanced CT scan and PET/CT scan are shown. Which diagnosis is most consistent with the imaging findings and clinical scenario?

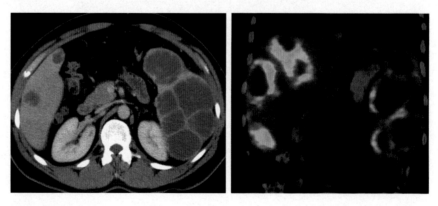

A. Angiosarcoma
B. Leukemia
C. Multiple lymphangiomas
D. Multiple hemangiomas

ANSWERS AND EXPLANATIONS

1 **Answer A.** Multiple wedge-shaped hypodensities in the periphery of the spleen and kidneys are consistent with small **infarcts**. The most common causes include emboli from atrial fibrillation and endocarditis, as well as hematologic disorders such as sickle cell disease and leukemia. Other causes of infarcts include thrombosis or aneurysm of the splenic vessels, splenomegaly, blunt trauma, and collagen vascular disease. This patient used IV drugs and presented with infarcts from septic emboli in the spleen, kidneys, and brain. **Embolic infarcts in multiple organs related to intravenous (IV) drug use and infective endocarditis are increasingly identified in younger patients**. In these patients, multiorgan manifestations of embolic disease may be identified, including in bowel (ischemia), lungs (septic emboli nodules), heart (endocarditis vegetations), spine (discitis), joints (septic arthritis), and vessels (mycotic aneurysms). The liver is less susceptible to infarcts because of dual blood supply.

Splenic infarcts may have atypical round or mottled appearance or involve the entire spleen. **Occasionally, there is a "rim" sign representing sparing of the capsule** due to separate vascular supply from capsular arteries. The margins of an infarct become better defined over time as it evolves into a residual linear scar with capsular retraction. Regarding the other answer choices, sarcoidosis and metastases in the spleen are nodular rather than wedge-shaped. Fibromuscular dysplasia (FMD) most commonly involves renal and carotid arteries rather than mesenteric arteries. FMD is usually associated with systemic hypertension rather than infarction of the kidneys.

References: Bates DDB, Gallagher K, Yu H, et al. Acute radiologic manifestations of America's Opioid Epidemic. *Radiographics* 2018;38(1):109–123.

Vos PM, Barnard SA, Cooperberg PL. Chapter 105: benign and malignant lesions of the spleen. In: Gore RM, Levine MS (eds). *Textbook of gastrointestinal radiology*, 4th ed. Philadelphia, PA: Elsevier/Saunders, 2015:1923–1964.

2 **Answer D.** This lesion has imaging characteristics of a splenic hemangioma. There is rim enhancement in the arterial phase with centripetal fill-in in the venous phase, and enhancement remains greater than surrounding splenic tissue. This was an isolated incidental finding unrelated to the symptoms. In this setting, no further workup is required.

Overall, most splenic lesions are benign. Splenic hemangioma is the most common benign primary neoplasm of the spleen. Suspicion for malignancy and active infection is low in this setting, so PET/CT, percutaneous biopsy, and antifungal treatment are not indicated. Patients with fungal microabscesses are immunocompromised and have multiple subcentimeter lesions. Microabscesses are usually identified as hypodense lesions relative to spleen on CT, although some can show early ring or targetoid central enhancement.

Splenic hemangiomas show a wide spectrum of appearances. Most splenic hemangiomas do not show the peripheral nodular discontinuous enhancement classically seen with hepatic cavernous hemangiomas. In this case, the rim enhancement appears continuous. Lesions range from solid to cystic with variable internal complexity and enhancement. Hemangiomas tend to be echogenic on ultrasound and tend to be very bright on T2W MRI sequences.

References: Thipphavong S, Duigenan S, Schindera ST, et al. Nonneoplastic, benign, and malignant splenic diseases: cross-sectional imaging findings and rare disease entities. *AJR Am J Roentgenol* 2014;203(2):315–322.

Vos PM, Barnard SA, Cooperberg PL. Chapter 105: Benign and malignant lesions of the spleen. In: Gore RM, Levine MS (eds). *Textbook of gastrointestinal radiology*, 4th ed. Philadelphia, PA: Elsevier/Saunders, 2015:1923–1964.

3 **Answer C.** This patient was diagnosed with non-Hodgkin lymphoma (NHL). The spleen is diffusely heterogeneous with ill-defined hypodensities. Bulky abdominal lymphadenopathy is also seen. Together, these findings are highly suspicious for lymphoma. The PET/CT subsequently performed on this patient is shown below and demonstrates avid FDG uptake in the spleen and the lymphadenopathy.

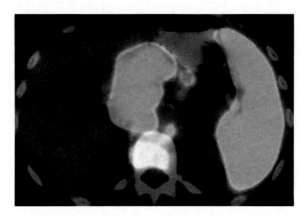

Lymphoma is the most common malignancy involving the spleen. Secondary involvement is much more common than primary splenic lymphoma. For staging, the spleen is considered a nodal site in Hodgkin disease and extranodal in NHL. Involvement may be **focal or diffuse**. Lymphoma is typically hypoenhancing to surrounding parenchyma, and the spleen may be normal in size or enlarged. **T2 hypointensity relative to surrounding spleen on MRI is occasionally seen and has been described as a feature that favors lymphoma** over metastatic disease. Untreated lymphoma is usually homogeneous in appearance, but occasionally, a large lesion or bulky lymphadenopathy shows cystic or necrotic changes. Splenic metastases would be in the differential diagnosis but much less common, usually occurring in the setting of widespread metastases to other organs.

Gaucher disease is the most common glycogen storage disease and is diagnosed in childhood or early adulthood rather than patients of this age. Patients have progressive marked hepatosplenomegaly, greater than seen in this case, due to accumulation of lipid-laden macrophages. Focal splenic lesions may represent "Gaucheromas," infarcts, or foci of extramedullary hematopoiesis. Lymphadenopathy is possible but not a salient feature of Gaucher disease.

The CT scan in this patient was obtained in the venous phase, with the hepatic and portal veins in the liver well opacified. In this phase, the spleen should demonstrate homogeneous enhancement. **The classic curvilinear sinusoidal enhancement pattern is a normal arterial phase phenomenon**, as shown on the CT below on a different patient. This enhancement has been referred to as moiré, arciform, or zebra spleen. It reflects the variable flow rates through the tortuous splenic sinusoids and should not be mistaken for pathology. Blunt trauma can result in hypoattenuating areas relative to surrounding enhancing parenchyma on a contrast-enhanced CT, representing laceration or intraparenchymal hematoma, but in this case, the clinical scenario and imaging findings do not fit with injury.

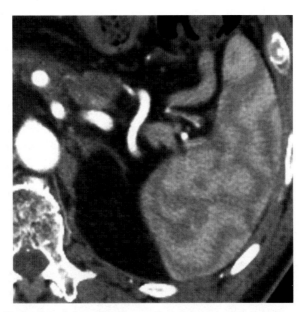

Normal moiré, arciform, or zebra spleen in arterial phase.

References: Thipphavong S, Duigenan S, Schindera ST, et al. Nonneoplastic, benign, and malignant splenic diseases: cross-sectional imaging findings and rare disease entities. *AJR Am J Roentgenol* 2014;203(2):315–322.

Thomas AG, Vaidhyanath R, Kirke R, et al. Extranodal lymphoma from head to toe: part 2, the trunk and extremities. *AJR Am J Roentgenol* 2011;197(2):357–364.

4a **Answer C.** Sulfur colloid scan.

4b **Answer B.** This patient has splenosis with multiple smooth round foci of splenic tissue (arrows) in the abdomen and pelvis that show Tc-99m sulfur colloid uptake. The patient underwent a splenectomy as a child after a fall. The largest focus of residual splenic tissue is shown in the left upper quadrant. **Splenosis is the sequela of splenic trauma, and patients often have a remote history splenectomy.** Fragments of the shattered spleen scatter in the peritoneal cavity, recruit vascular supply, and slowly grow. Intrathoracic splenosis in the mediastinum or pleural space may be found if the diaphragm was breached. These foci have the characteristics of normal splenic tissue, appearing smooth, round, and homogeneous on venous phase CT and MRI. **A Tc-99m sulfur colloid scan is usually adequate for confirmation of splenosis**, although Tc-99m heat-damaged red blood cell scan is more sensitive and specific and can also be used for diagnosis. Splenosis is a benign condition that is asymptomatic but may be mistaken for malignancy. Recognition of splenosis can prevent unnecessary biopsy. Lymphoma, tuberculosis, and carcinomatosis can present with soft tissue masses in the peritoneal cavity but do not show uptake on Tc-99m sulfur colloid or heat-damaged red blood cell scans.

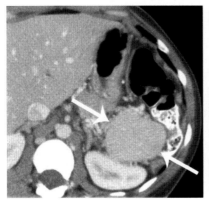
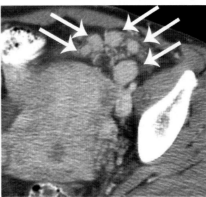
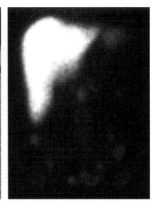

References: Lake ST, Johnson PT, Kawamoto S, et al. CT of splenosis: patterns and pitfalls. *AJR Am J Roentgenol* 2012;199(6):W686–W693.

Levy AD, Shaw JC, Sobin LH. Secondary tumors and tumorlike lesions of the peritoneal cavity: imaging features with pathologic correlation. *Radiographics* 2009;29(2):347–373.

5 **Answer B.** There is a smooth, well-circumscribed mass at the pancreatic tail that matches the signal intensity of spleen on all pre- and postcontrast series. This mass also demonstrates sinusoidal enhancement pattern matching the spleen on arterial phase. Findings are compatible with an intrapancreatic splenule (accessory spleen). Splenules are common incidental findings on CT scans. **A splenule may be difficult to distinguish from a hypervascular neuroendocrine tumor (not an answer choice) if closely associated with the pancreatic tail.** The sinusoidal enhancement typical of a splenule may not be clearly identified in small lesions, and equivocal cases may require follow-up or further evaluation such as with sulfur colloid scans.

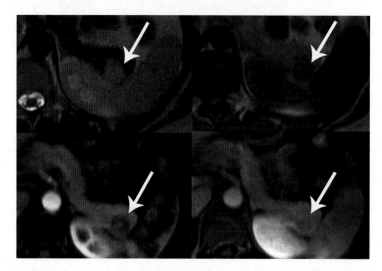

Aneurysms have signal intensity and enhancement following the aorta on all series. Pancreatic adenocarcinoma does not show arterial enhancement. Peritoneal carcinomatosis can present as a solid or cystic lesions at the periphery of the spleen, but the tumors that commonly spread by carcinomatosis (ovarian and gastrointestinal malignancies) are usually not arterial enhancing. Carcinomatosis and pancreatic adenocarcinoma are not primary considerations in this young patient.

References: Lake ST, Johnson PT, Kawamoto S, et al. CT of splenosis: patterns and pitfalls. *AJR Am J Roentgenol* 2012;199(6):W686–W693.

Levy AD, Shaw JC, Sobin LH. Secondary tumors and tumorlike lesions of the peritoneal cavity: imaging features with pathologic correlation. *Radiographics* 2009;29(2):347–373.

6 **Answer D.** The patient has melanoma metastases in the spleen. The CT image in the venous phase shows round, hypoenhancing, heterogeneous lesions with ill-defined margins. The spleen appears normal in size. **Although the imaging appearance is not specific, findings are highly suspicious for melanoma metastases given the clinical scenario.** In the setting of imaging surveillance, malignant lesions would be **new or growing** compared to prior studies.

Metastases to the spleen are uncommon. **They are usually encountered in patients with widespread metastatic disease, and isolated splenic metastasis is rare except with melanoma.** Among metastases found in the spleen, the most common pathology is lung cancer. **Among primary neoplasms, the one that has the greatest predilection for metastases to the spleen is melanoma,** with splenic metastases found in up to a third of patients at autopsy. On CT, typical imaging features of splenic metastases include solitary or multiple hypoenhancing lesions. There may be variable amounts of necrosis and cystic change. **A subset of melanoma metastases produce melanin and may appear hyperintense on T1W MRI.** Hematogenous splenic metastases are also found with lung, breast, and colon cancer. Ovarian cancer involves the spleen predominantly via spread through the peritoneal cavity. **Direct spread of cancer from adjacent organs** to the spleen can occur with gastric, pancreatic, or renal cancer.

Splenic littoral cell angioma, a primary benign vascular tumor of the spleen arising from cells in the red pulp sinuses, may present with multiple hypoenhancing splenic lesions, but it is rare and is almost always associated with splenomegaly. Splenic lymphangiomas are benign cystic tumors without enhancement. Splenic pyogenic abscesses are most commonly due to hematogenous spread of infection and can appear similar with low-attenuation lesions but do not fit with this patient's clinical scenario. Internal septations or foci of gas may be seen within a pyogenic abscess.

Incidental splenic lesions are often presumed benign. Furthermore, in the setting of widespread metastases or lymphoma, making the diagnosis of splenic involvement may not change management. However, if further characterization of an indeterminate splenic lesion is felt to be warranted, additional imaging may be helpful. An MRI may be better able to distinguish cysts and hemangiomas from solid masses. Follow-up CT scans showing stability would be reassuring. A PET/CT may confirm suspicion for metastases or lymphoma. Although traditionally percutaneous biopsy of the spleen was avoided due to concerns about the risk of hemorrhage, more recent evidence shows that it may be a safe option in certain clinical situations.

References: Gaetke-Udager K, Wasnik AP, Kaza RK, et al. Multimodality imaging of splenic lesions and the role of non-vascular, image-guided intervention. *Abdom Imaging* 2014;39(3):570–587.

Thipphavong S, Duigenan S, Schindera ST, et al. Nonneoplastic, benign, and malignant splenic diseases: cross-sectional imaging findings and rare disease entities. *AJR Am J Roentgenol* 2014;203(2):315–322.

7 **Answer A.** This immunocompromised patient has a disseminated opportunistic fungal infection with multiple tiny hypodensities representing microabscesses in the spleen and liver. **Microabscesses are usually fungal** in etiology, most commonly *Candida*, *Aspergillus*, and *Cryptococcus* species. **Microabscesses may be too small to visualize on any imaging modality, although MRI may be more sensitive than CT.** On MRI, the lesions are T2 hyperintense and can show ring or targetoid central enhancement.

Bacterial abscesses that occur in the spleen tend to be larger and are most often caused by septic emboli. Clinical history is important for suggesting the diagnosis of infection since other benign and malignant processes may present with multiple small hypoattenuating lesions in the spleen, including hemangiomas, lymphangiomas, sarcoid, lymphoma, and metastases.

The other answer choices are infectious causes of multiple splenic hypodensities but less common. *Mycobacterium avium* complex (a group of atypical mycobacteria) and *Pneumocystis jiroveci* (a fungus) can also affect immunocompromised patients. *Bartonella henselae* is the bacterium responsible for catscratch disease. Patients with catscratch disease are usually young, and hepatosplenic involvement is uncommon. In immunocompromised patients, especially those with AIDS, *Bartonella* species can cause bacillary angiomatosis, a condition with multiple vascular peliosis-type lesions in the liver as well as the spleen. Treatment of these various disseminated infections is a drug regimen targeting the underlying organism.

References: Karlo CA, Stolzmann P, Do RK, et al. Computed tomography of the spleen: how to interpret the hypodense lesion. *Insights Imaging* 2013;4(1):65–76.

Thipphavong S, Duigenan S, Schindera ST, et al. Nonneoplastic, benign, and malignant splenic diseases: cross-sectional imaging findings and rare disease entities. *AJR Am J Roentgenol* 2014;203(2):315–322.

8a **Answer C.** Delayed splenic pseudoaneurysm rupture.

8b **Answer C.** In this case, the hyperdensity of the hematoma involving the spleen suggests acute hemorrhage rather than subacute or chronic hematoma from the prior traumatic injury. This is likely due to **delayed rupture of a splenic pseudoaneurysm** (PSA). Splenic PSAs after blunt trauma may be diagnosed at initial CT or detected on follow-up. **The best imaging study includes arterial and venous phases**. PSAs are best seen on arterial phase, while the venous phase is necessary for characterization of the splenic parenchymal injury. Furthermore, the second phase (venous or delayed) is useful to assess for active bleeding. A noncontrast CT is generally not useful for evaluation of splenic lacerations or vascular injuries other than identification of perisplenic and intraperitoneal hematoma. About 20% of patients will require splenectomy after splenic injury, but **most patients can be successfully treated nonoperatively. A subset of patients would benefit from angiography and embolization of vascular injuries to avert subsequent splenectomy.** In general, patients who are hemodynamically unstable require surgery. The patient does have a calcified gallstone, but there is no inflammatory change in the fat around the gallbladder. While pancreatitis can be caused by trauma or by gallstones, there is no inflammatory change around the pancreas to suggest this diagnosis.

Analogous to management for hepatic injury, the trend is toward nonsurgical management for splenic preservation. The American Association for the Surgery of Trauma (AAST) scale for splenic injury ranges from grade I to grade V. The 2018 update incorporates the diagnosis of vascular injury by CT. **Detection of "vascular injury" (defined as pseudoaneurysm and arteriovenous fistula) or active bleeding upgrades any injury to Grade IV or V.** Multiphase CTA helps determine whether a contrast blush is active extravasation with contrast dispersal, versus a contained hemorrhage such as pseudoaneurysm or arteriovenous fistula. **The higher the grade, the more likely the patient will fail nonsurgical management.** Patients with hemodynamic instability proceed to surgery for splenectomy.

References: Furlan A, Tublin ME, Rees MA, et al. Delayed splenic vascular injury after nonoperative management of blunt splenic trauma. *J Surg Res* 2017;211:87–94.

Kozar RA, Crandall M, Shanmuganathan K, et al. Organ injury scaling 2018 update: spleen, liver, and kidney. *J Trauma Acute Care Surg* 2018;85(6):1119–1122.

Zarzaur BL, Dunn JA, Leininger B, et al. Natural history of splenic vascular abnormalities after blunt injury: a Western Trauma Association multicenter trial. *J Trauma Acute Care Surg* 2017;83:999–1005.

9 **Answer C.** This patient with cirrhosis has **Gamna-Gandy bodies** throughout the spleen. Gamna-Gandy bodies are subcentimeter foci representing the sequela of microhemorrhages and are most commonly seen in the setting of **portal hypertension**. The lesions do not enhance and contain a combination of iron, fibrosis, and sometimes calcium. They are usually not visible on CT, but MRI sequences that are sensitive to iron make these lesions conspicuous.

The MR images in this patient demonstrate the **expected features of iron-containing lesions, with hypointensity on all sequences and additional loss of signal on the gradient-echo T1W in-phase** compared to the out-of-phase images. On a 1.5-tesla magnet, the in-phase images are performed with a longer TE of about 4.8 msec compared to the out-of-phase TE of 2.4 msec, and therefore, the in-phase images are more sensitive to T2* susceptibility effects of the iron in the hemosiderin. Gamna-Gandy bodies are found in about 10% of patients with portal hypertension and also in patients with sickle cell disease.

Calcifications are not reliably detectable by MRI. Occasionally, foci of calcification produce susceptibility effects and demonstrate hypointensity on these MR sequences, typically to a lesser degree than iron. The CT, which is the most sensitive imaging modality for calcification, shows no hyperdensities that would indicate calcified granulomas. Foci of air also are not reliably detected by MRI but would appear dark on all MR sequences, as well as dark on CT. Old infarcts are wedge-shaped or linear with capsular retraction. Microabscesses are T2 hyperintense without susceptibility effects.

References: Luna A, Ribes R, Caro P, et al. MRI of focal splenic lesions without and with dynamic gadolinium enhancement. *AJR Am J Roentgenol* 2006;186(6):1533–1547.

Vos PM, Barnard SA, Cooperberg PL. Chapter 105: Benign and malignant lesions of the spleen. In: Gore RM, Levine MS (eds). *Textbook of gastrointestinal radiology*, 4th ed. Philadelphia, PA: Elsevier/Saunders, 2015:1923–1964.

10 **Answer D.** This patient has **polysplenia**, which is in the spectrum of heterotaxy syndromes. Multiple splenic nodules are seen in the right abdomen. The stomach is on the right, the liver is midline, and the IVC is on the left. Heterotaxy syndromes are congenital disorders of abnormal positioning of internal organs. Organ positioning may be referred to as situs solitus (normal), situs inversus (mirror image), or situs ambiguus (variable). In situs inversus, the liver is on the left rather than midline, and the intact spleen is on the right. **Situs ambiguus is a spectrum but generally subdivided into polysplenia and asplenia.** In polysplenia, the multiple splenic nodules may exist on the left or right sides, usually accompanying the stomach. In the chest, there may be bilateral left-sidedness with two bilobed lungs.

In asplenia, there is bilateral right-sidedness with two trilobed lungs. The liver is also midline, but the spleen is absent. **There is a higher association of congenital anomalies with asplenia compared to polysplenia, especially cardiovascular anomalies.** Asplenia is more often fatal.

References: Applegate KE, Goske MJ, Pierce G, et al. Situs revisited: imaging of the heterotaxy syndrome. *Radiographics* 1999;19(4):837–852; discussion 853–834.

Fulcher AS, Turner MA. Abdominal manifestations of situs anomalies in adults. *Radiographics* 2002;22(6):1439–1456.

11 **Answer C.** T1W and fat-saturated T2W MR images demonstrate a subtle ovoid lesion within the spleen that is nearly isointense to surrounding spleen and associated with a smooth contour bulge. Arterial phase T1W image reveals diffuse, mildly heterogeneous hyperenhancement relative to splenic parenchyma, and delayed phase image shows isointensity such that it is barely perceptible relative to splenic parenchyma. **Given its isointensity or near-isointensity to the spleen on most series, this is most likely a splenic hamartoma.** Splenic hamartoma is a benign nonneoplastic lesion that is composed of mixtures of disorganized splenic tissue—white pulp, red pulp, or both. Focal fibrosis or cystic change may be seen, particularly with larger lesions. It is typically solitary but may be multiple in patients with tuberous sclerosis or Wiskott-Aldrich syndrome (also known as eczema–thrombocytopenia–immunodeficiency syndrome).

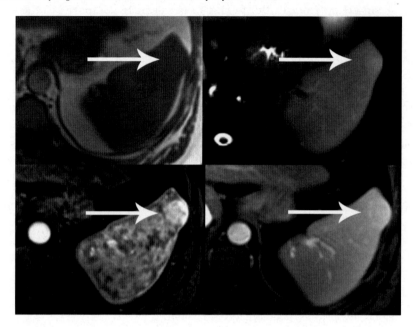

Splenic hemangioma (not an answer choice) usually shows more conspicuous T2 hyperintensity and delayed enhancement. Splenic lymphangiomas have a cystic appearance without enhancement, with some demonstrating internal complexity such as septations or proteinaceous content. Splenic metastases are uncommon and typically have some degree of T1 hypointensity and T2 hyperintensity relative to surrounding splenic parenchyma. Splenic angiosarcoma is very rare and usually appears as a heterogeneous complex solid and cystic mass.

References: Abbott RM, Levy AD, Aguilera NS, et al. From the archives of the AFIP: primary vascular neoplasms of the spleen: radiologic-pathologic correlation. *Radiographics* 2004;(4):1137–1163.

Thipphavong S, Duigenan S, Schindera ST, et al. Nonneoplastic, benign, and malignant splenic diseases: cross-sectional imaging findings and rare disease entities. *AJR Am J Roentgenol* 2014;203(2):315–322. doi: 10.2214/AJR.13.11777.

12 **Answer D.** The combination of **marked splenomegaly and osteosclerosis** is most suggestive of **myelofibrosis**. Splenomegaly represents **extramedullary hematopoiesis as a result of marrow dysfunction**. Other extramedullary hematopoiesis such as masses in the liver or paraspinal regions may also be present (not demonstrated in this case). Other myeloproliferative disorders or lymphoma are less likely with this combination of findings. Regarding the other answer choices, prostate carcinoma metastases can result in diffuse bony sclerosis but is not associated with splenomegaly. Multiple myeloma manifestations include osteopenia and lytic bone lesions with no splenomegaly. Mononucleosis is a common infectious cause of splenomegaly in young patients (usually 30 years or younger) without bony sclerosis.

Myelofibrosis is a chronic clonal stem cell abnormality considered a myeloproliferative disorder along with polycythemia vera, essential thrombocythemia, and chronic myeloid leukemia (CML). There is a risk of transformation into frank malignancy such as acute myeloid leukemia (AML). **Patients with splenomegaly from any cause are at increased risk for**

traumatic and nontraumatic ("spontaneous") splenic rupture. The enlarged spleen can extend below the protection of the ribcage and is prone to injury. Spontaneous rupture with hemoperitoneum is a rare cause of acute abdomen but may occur with minor activities such as coughing or sneezing. Patients with splenomegaly are also prone to splenic infarcts as perfusion to parts of the enlarged organ may be suboptimal. An enlarged spleen may sequester platelets resulting in thrombocytopenia.

Various methods have been proposed to define splenomegaly. The easiest methods are subjective assessment or a single maximum measurement, for example, 13 cm or greater. Normal size varies depending on individual stature. **A broad spectrum of disease can cause splenomegaly, the most common of which is congestion from portal hypertension.** Other categories of pathology causing splenomegaly besides myeloproliferative disorders include malignancy (e.g., chronic lymphocytic leukemia (CLL) and lymphoma), infection (e.g., mononucleosis with Epstein-Barr virus), storage disease (e.g., Gaucher disease), and autoimmune disease (e.g., rheumatoid arthritis).

References: Boland GWL, Halpert RD. Chapter 7: Spleen. In: Boland GWL, Halpert RD (eds). *Gastrointestinal imaging: the requisites*, 4th ed. Philadelphia, PA: Elsevier/Saunders, 2014:291–314.

Oon SF, Singh D, Tan TH, et al. Primary myelofibrosis: spectrum of imaging features and disease-related complications. *Insights Imaging* 2019;10(1):71.

13 **Answer A.** The spleen is diffusely involved with multiple lesions, which are predominantly hypoattenuating, although there is some variation. While the imaging appearance is not specific, these findings are compatible with **angiomatosis in this patient with Klippel-Trenaunay syndrome** (KTS). These vascular malformations may represent hemangiomas and/or lymphangiomas in the spleen. KTS is a syndrome of angiomatosis with a triad of limb hypertrophy, port wine stains, and varicose veins. **Visceral angiomatosis with gastrointestinal and genitourinary vascular malformations may occur and increases the risk of a life-threatening internal hemorrhage.**

Beckwith-Wiedemann syndrome and neurofibromatosis type I are associated with limb hypertrophy and hepatosplenomegaly but not port wine stains or multiple splenic lesions. Patients with von Hippel-Lindau syndrome develop multiple benign and malignant neoplasms, most importantly renal cell carcinoma and central nervous system hemangioblastomas, but the disease does not involve the spleen. Gaucher disease is the most common glycogen storage disease. Patients have progressive marked hepatosplenomegaly due to accumulation of lipid-laden macrophages. Focal splenic lesions may represent "Gaucheromas," infarcts, or foci of extramedullary hematopoiesis. The disease is not associated with limb hemihypertrophy or port wine stains.

References: Cha SH, Romeo MA, Neutze JA. Visceral manifestations of Klippel-Trénaunay syndrome. *Radiographics* 2005;25(6):1694–1697.

Louis TH, Sanders JM, Stephenson JS, et al. Splenic hemangiomatosis. *Proc (Bayl Univ Med Cent)* 2011;24(4):356–358.

14 **Answers:**
Patient 1: C. Old healed granulomatous infection.
Patient 2: B. Posttraumatic sequela.
Patient 3: A. Sickle cell anemia.

This series of cases shows calcification in the spleen. Patient 1 has multiple bright foci scattered in the spleen on noncontrast CT and ultrasound consistent with **calcified granulomas.** A few foci are demonstrated in the liver on CT as well. These foci are often identified incidentally after the lesions have healed with no clinical implications at the time of discovery. The granulomatous infections that tend to heal with calcification like these are histoplasmosis, which is endemic in the central United States, and tuberculosis. In AIDS patients, disseminated infection with *Pneumocystis jiroveci* (a yeast-like fungus initially misclassified as a protozoa and formerly known as *Pneumocystis carinii*) can produce this appearance. Occasionally, treated healed vasculitis or lymphoma will show multiple small calcifications.

Patient 2 has a cyst with a thin partial rim of calcification. Central density was measured to be 16 HU consistent with simple fluid. Among the choices, this is most likely a pseudocyst (false cyst lined by fibrosis) as the result of a prior splenic insult such as trauma or infarct. **Pseudocysts are thought to be more common than congenital epithelial cysts** (true cysts lined by epithelium). Both types can exhibit thickened walls, septations, and calcifications. Areas of internal density may represent proteinaceous fluid or hemorrhage but should not enhance. Lymphangiomas, which are slow-growing benign congenital neoplasms, may manifest as single or multiple cystic nonenhancing lesions of variable sizes with some internal complexity. Worldwide, parasitic cysts (usually echinococcal) are the most common cause of splenic cysts and can calcify. The appearance of echinococcal (hydatid) infection can range from simple cysts to complex solid and cystic masses.

Patient 3 has experienced an **autosplenectomy** and now has an end-stage nonfunctioning spleen. The spleen is very atrophic and diffusely calcified, seen as a small curved density posterior to the contrast-filled stomach on the CT image. This appearance is **classic for sickle cell disease**. It can be visible on radiographs as demonstrated on the following image from a different patient also with sickle cell disease (arrows).

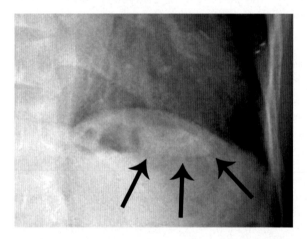

Autosplenectomy is one of the most common complications involving the spleen in sickle cell disease and is the result of repeated splenic infarction. Before autosplenectomy, patients with sickle cell disease are at risk for splenic sequestration crisis and abscess formation. **A small, scarred, high-density spleen can be seen with other processes that cause repetitive splenic infarction or fibrosis such as radiation therapy and Thorotrast exposure.** Thorotrast was a radioactive contrast agent containing an α-particle–emitting radionuclide of thorium that was used until the 1950s when it was found to be carcinogenic.

References: Consul N, Javed-Tayyab S, Lall C, et al. Calcified Splenic Lesions: Pattern Recognition Approach on CT With Pathologic Correlation. *AJR Am J Roentgenol* 2020;214(5):1083–1091.

Vos PM, Barnard SA, Cooperberg PL. Chapter 105: Benign and malignant lesions of the spleen. In: Gore RM, Levine MS (eds). *Textbook of gastrointestinal radiology*, 4th ed. Philadelphia, PA: Elsevier/Saunders, 2015:1923–1964.

15 **Answer A.** This patient has angiosarcoma, a rare and aggressive malignancy that may originate in the spleen or liver. Angiosarcomas typically have a complex cystic appearance with central necrosis and irregular foci of internal nodularity, as seen in this case in lesions throughout the spleen and liver. Lesions may be hypervascular with arterial enhancement, but degree of enhancement can be variable. They may be mistaken for hemangiomas. There is a propensity for spontaneous hemorrhage as well as early metastasis to the liver, bone, and lung.

Because angiosarcoma is very rare, the initial considerations in the differential diagnosis of complex cystic masses within the spleen that have PET/CT uptake should include metastatic disease and infection (not among the answer choices). Splenic and hepatic angiosarcomas are associated with Thorotrast exposure. Hepatic angiosarcoma has been linked to vinyl chloride and arsenic exposure, but these exposures have not been linked with splenic angiosarcoma.

Patients with leukemia have elevated white blood cell counts and diffuse splenomegaly. The white blood cell count in this patient was normal. (Focal chloromas in the setting of leukemia are possible but uncommon and usually solid.) While lymphoma is the most common malignancy to involve the spleen, the appearance of lymphoma (not an answer choice) on CT and PET/CT is typically more uniform. Complex appearance is occasionally seen with treated lymphoma or larger lesions. Lymphangiomas and hemangiomas are benign entities that do not demonstrate uptake on PET/CT.

References: Abbott RM, Levy AD, Aguilera NS, et al. From the archives of the AFIP: primary vascular neoplasms of the spleen: radiologic-pathologic correlation. *Radiographics* 2004;24(4):1137–1163.

Thompson WM, Levy AD, Aguilera NS, et al. Angiosarcoma of the spleen: imaging characteristics in 12 patients. *Radiology* 2005;235(1):106–115.

1 What is the most likely diagnosis on this ultrasound image of the gallbladder?

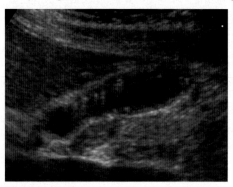

    A. Emphysematous cholecystitis
    B. Adenomyomatosis
    C. Gallstones
    D. Gallbladder carcinoma

2 A 55-year-old woman with right upper quadrant pain undergoes an MRCP. What is the diagnosis?

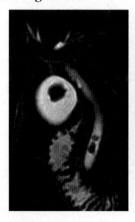 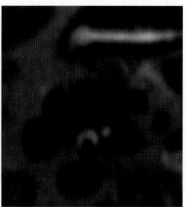

    A. Pneumobilia
    B. Cholangiocarcinoma
    C. Choledocholithiasis
    D. Ascariasis

3 A 78-year-old man presents with right upper quadrant pain. What is the most likely diagnosis?

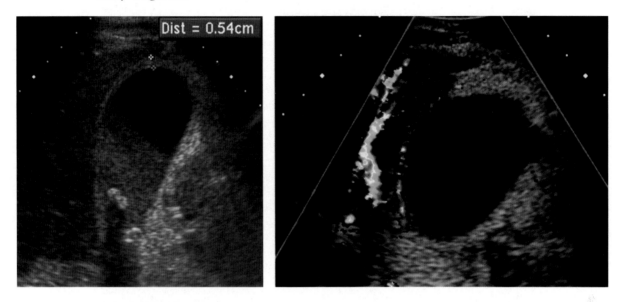

A. Acute cholecystitis
B. Acute hepatitis
C. Hepatic abscess
D. Adenomyomatosis

4 For patients 1 to 4, match the gallbladder intraluminal finding with the most likely diagnosis. Each option may be used only once.

Patient 1:

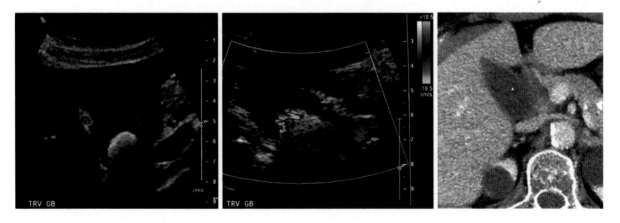

Patient 2:

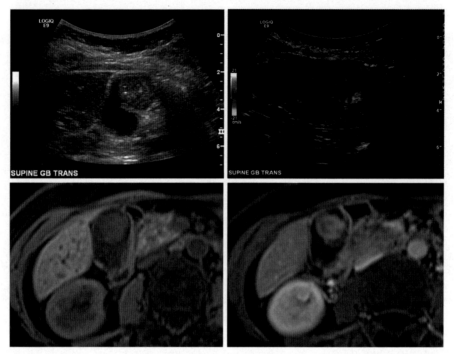

Top row: Gray scale and color Doppler ultrasound. **Bottom row:** FS T1W and FS T1W+gad MRI.

Patient 3:

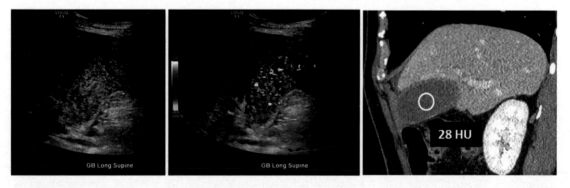

Patient 4:

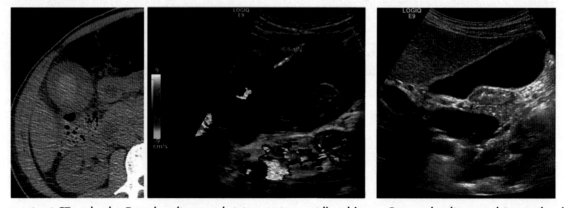

Noncontrast CT and color Doppler ultrasound status post recent liver biopsy. Gray scale ultrasound 1 month prior.

    A. Hematoma
    B. Sludge
    C. Gallstone
    D. Gallbladder carcinoma

5 What is the most common cause of a benign biliary stricture?

    A. Prior hepatobiliary surgery
    B. Primary sclerosing cholangitis
    C. Recurrent pyogenic cholangitis
    D. Pancreatitis

6a An 18-year-old woman status post recent cholecystectomy presents with signs and symptoms of peritonitis. Based on the CT and MRCP shown below, what is the most likely diagnosis?

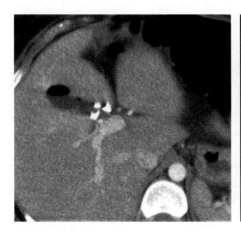 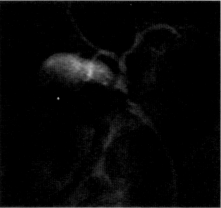

    A. Bile leak
    B. Pseudoaneurysm with active hemorrhage
    C. Gallbladder remnant
    D. Duplicated gallbladder

6b The patient in Question 6a underwent treatment including exploratory laparotomy to evacuate peritoneal fluid collections, drain placement, and antibiotics. Two months later, the patient presents with jaundice and the following MRCP. What is the diagnosis?

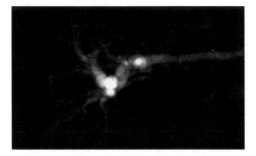

    A. Recurrent bile leak
    B. Cholangiocarcinoma
    C. Sclerosing cholangitis
    D. Posttraumatic stricture

7 Three patients presented with right upper quadrant pain and underwent ultrasound and CT scan. Match the ultrasound image for each patient (1 to 3) with that patient's corresponding CT image (A to C). Each option may be used only once.

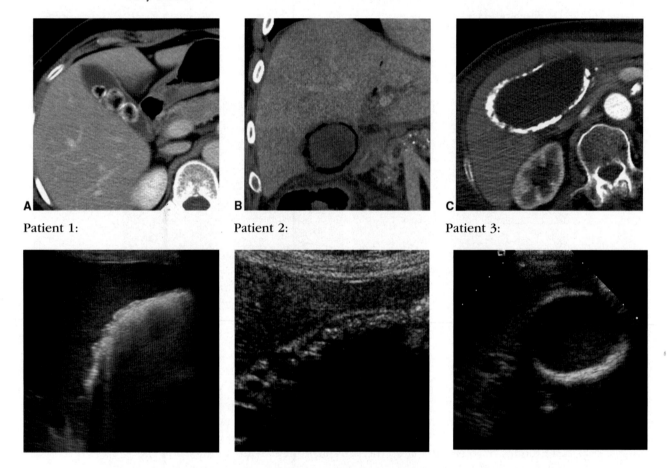

Patient 1:   Patient 2:   Patient 3:

8 The majority of patients with the disease process revealed on the following ERCP also have which of the following diseases?

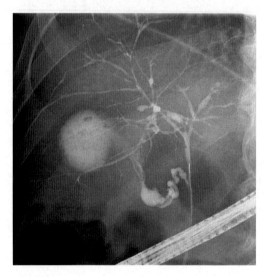

A. Cholangiocarcinoma
B. AIDS
C. Inflammatory bowel disease
D. Parasitic infection

9a A 49-year-old woman has a history of multiple episodes of right upper quadrant pain. What is the finding?

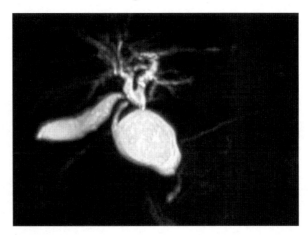

A. Duodenal duplication cyst
B. Choledochal cyst
C. Duodenal diverticulum
D. Pancreatic mucinous cystic neoplasm

9b Additional US, MR, and CT images in the same patient are shown. What is associated with the lesion?

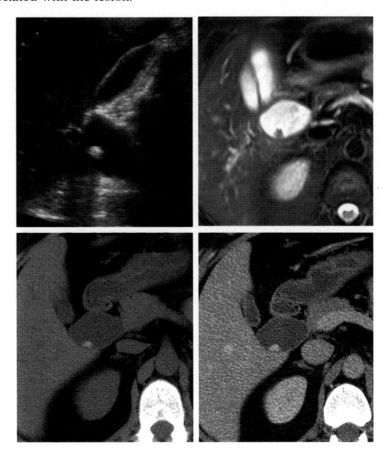

A. Hematoma
B. Stone
C. Cholangiocarcinoma
D. Cholesterol polyp

10 A 39-year-old-woman presented with acute abdominal pain. What is the most likely diagnosis?

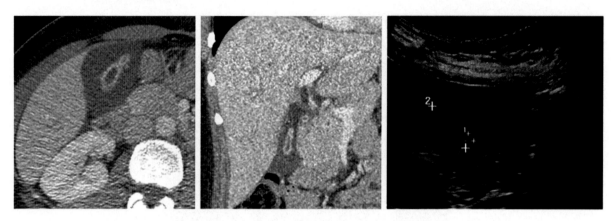

A. Acute hepatitis
B. Acute cholecystitis
C. Adenomyomatosis
D. Gallbladder carcinoma

11 Images from MRCP and CT are shown. What is the diagnosis?

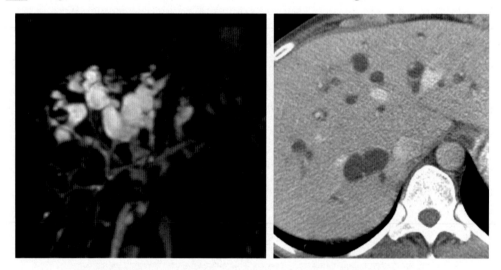

A. Caroli disease
B. Biliary cystadenocarcinoma
C. Pyogenic abscesses
D. Biliary hamartomas

12 Three contrast-enhanced CT images of the right upper quadrant are shown. What is the most likely diagnosis?

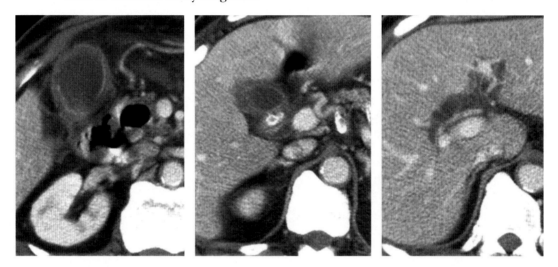

A. Mirizzi syndrome
B. Gallbladder carcinoma
C. Metastatic periportal adenopathy
D. Klatskin tumor

13a A 71-year-old man with jaundice is evaluated with CT and MRI (top row). After further investigation and treatment, an MRI was obtained 6 months later (bottom row). What is the diagnosis?

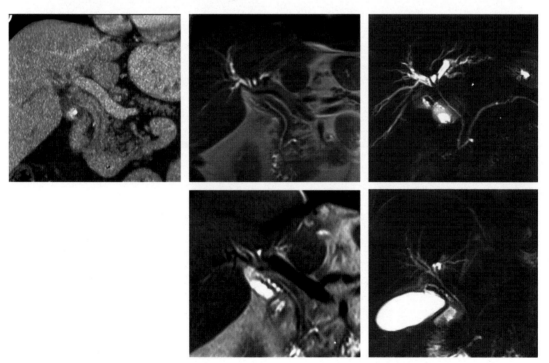

Top row: CT and MRCP at presentation. **Bottom row:** MRCP 6 months later.

A. Cholangiocarcinoma
B. Autoimmune cholangitis
C. Primary sclerosing cholangitis
D. Periportal metastatic adenopathy

13b What treatment did the patient receive?

    A. Surgical resection
    B. Chemotherapy
    C. Liver transplant
    D. Steroids

For each patient in Questions 14 to 19, select the most likely diagnosis (A to I). Each option may be used once, more than once, or not at all.

    A. Gangrenous cholecystitis
    B. Adenomyomatosis
    C. Phrygian cap
    D. Gallbladder laceration
    E. Duodenal duplication cyst
    F. Choledochal cyst
    G. Dropped gallstone with abscess
    H. Bouveret syndrome
    I. Remnant gallbladder infundibulum

14 An 87-year-old woman. Coronal and sagittal CT images are shown.

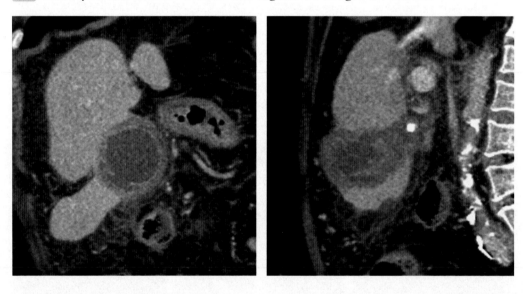

15 A 92-year-old woman.

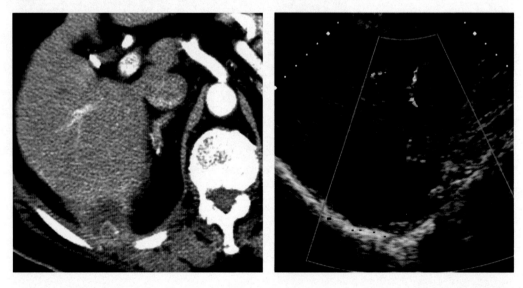

16 A 70-year-old woman. Two images from an MRCP are shown. Identify the structure indicated by the arrow.

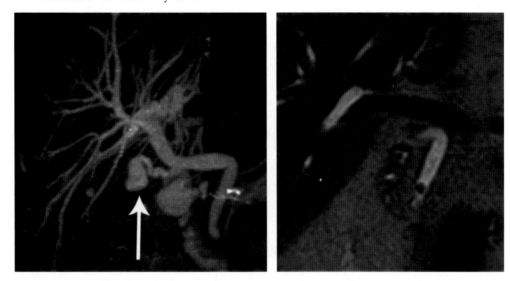

17 A 61-year-old woman. Identify the structure indicated by the arrow.

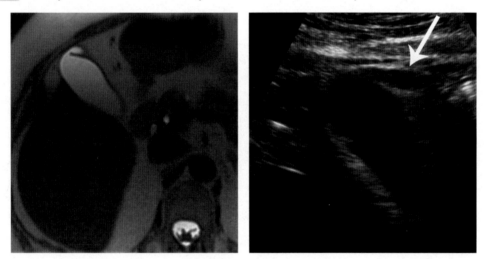

18 A 72-year-old man with vomiting.

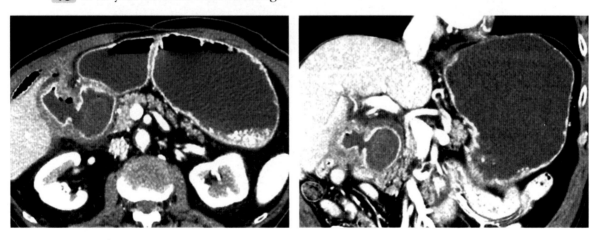

19 A 57-year-old woman for evaluation of incidentally discovered gallbladder lesion. Axial and coronal MR images are shown.

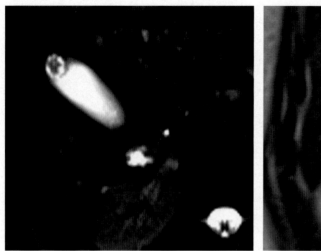 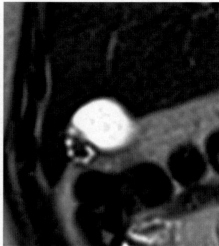

20 Match the CT images of patients 1 to 5 with the best diagnosis or description of the finding (A to E). Each option may be used once, more than once, or not at all.

Patient 1:   Patient 2:   Patient 3:

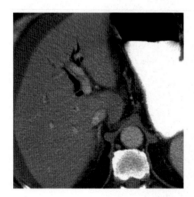 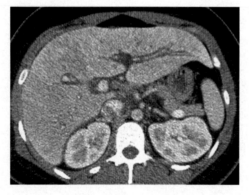 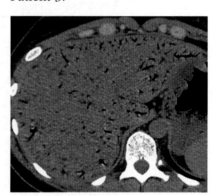

Patient 4:   Patient 5:

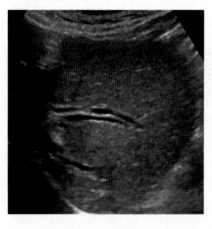 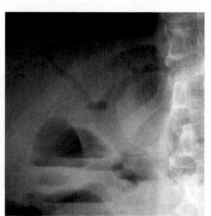

A. Pneumobilia
B. Portal venous gas
C. Periportal edema
D. Portal venous thrombosis
E. Biliary obstruction

21 Match the images from the ^{99m}Tc hepatobiliary iminodiacetic acid (HIDA) scan images of patients 1 to 5 with the most likely diagnosis (A to E) among the options listed. Each option may be used once, more than once, or not at all.

Patient 1: Images at 57 to 60 minutes and 5 hours.

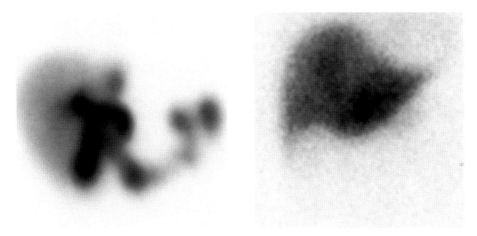

Patient 2: Image at 25 to 27 minutes.   Patient 3: Image at 57 to 60 minutes.

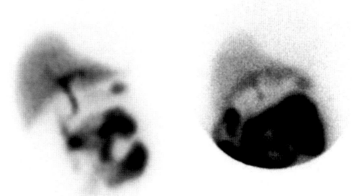

Patient 4: Anterior images with patient in right lateral decubitus position at 26 minutes and supine position at 30 minutes.

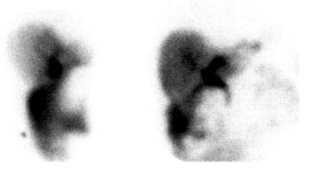

Patient 5: Images at 57 to 60 minutes and then 28 to 30 minutes after IV morphine injection.

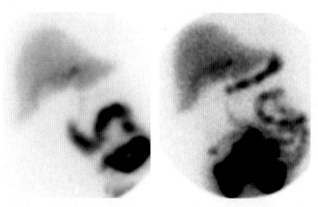

   A. Within normal limits
   B. Acute high-grade bile duct obstruction
   C. Bile leak
   D. Acute cholecystitis
   E. Chronic cholecystitis

22 A 64-year-old man presented with right upper quadrant pain. Images from his CT scan are shown. Which of the following feature if present would be most suggestive of gallbladder adenocarcinoma over perforated cholecystitis?

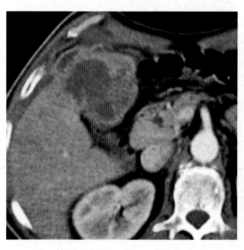 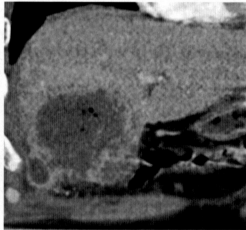

   A. Abnormal enhancement of adjacent hepatic parenchyma
   B. Gallbladder wall thickness >10 mm
   C. A 4-cm heterogeneous porta hepatis lymph node
   D. Intrahepatic biliary dilatation

23a A 52-year-old man who immigrated from the Philippines presents with worsening right upper quadrant pain. An ultrasound and CT scan were performed. Images are shown of the right hepatic lobe, but similar findings were also seen in the left lobe. What is the finding?

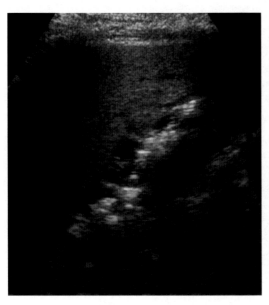
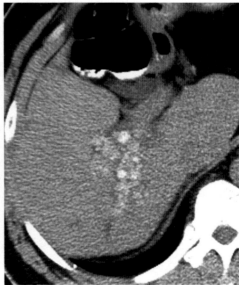

A. Calcification in a branching pattern
B. Enhancing mass in a branching pattern
C. Multifocal fat in a branching pattern
D. Air in a branching pattern

23b An MRI was performed in the same patient with images shown below. What is the most likely diagnosis?

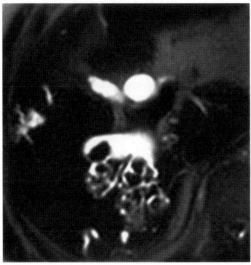
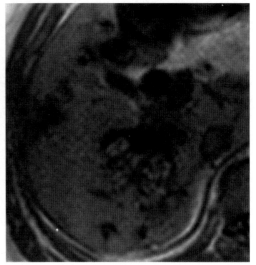

T2W and T1W

A. Ischemic bowel with portal venous gas
B. Hepatocellular carcinoma with portal venous thrombus
C. Ascariasis
D. Recurrent pyogenic cholangitis

24a A 34-year-old patient presents with a CD4 count of 46/mm³. What is the most common infectious agent associated with these ERCP findings?

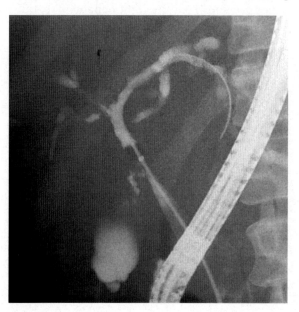

A. Kaposi sarcoma herpesvirus (human herpesvirus 8)
B. *Cryptosporidium*
C. Epstein-Barr virus (human herpesvirus 4)
D. *Microsporidia*

24b Which is the most common feature in the majority of patients with AIDS cholangiopathy?

A. Papillary stenosis
B. Long extrahepatic bile duct stricture
C. Intrahepatic biliary stones
D. Biliary diverticula

25 A 67-year-old man with cirrhosis and portal hypertension undergoes CT and MRI. What is the diagnosis?

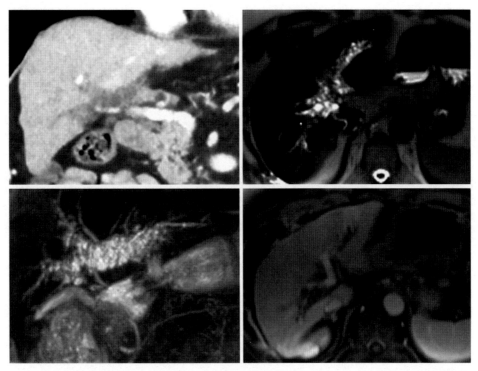

Top row: Coronal venous phase CT and axial MRCP. **Bottom row:** 3D MIP coronal MRCP and venous phase FS T1W+gad.

    A. Acute hepatitis with periportal edema
    B. Cholangiocarcinoma with biliary obstruction
    C. Primary sclerosing cholangitis with beading of the ducts
    D. Peribiliary cysts associated with severe liver disease

For patients presenting with jaundice in Questions 26 to 30, match the imaging findings with the most likely diagnosis (A to E). Each option may be used once, more than once, or not at all.

    A. Ascariasis
    B. Cholangiocarcinoma
    C. Pancreatic ductal adenocarcinoma
    D. Ampullary carcinoma
    E. Choledocholithiasis

26 A 92-year-old woman.

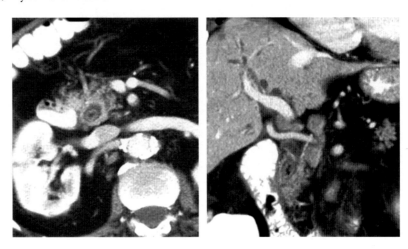

27 A 66-year-old woman.

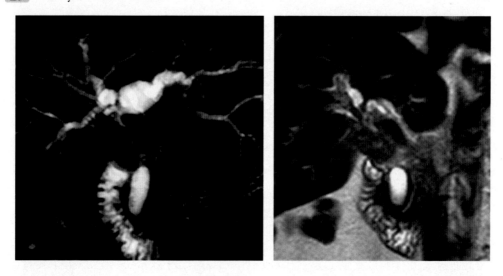

28 A 58-year-old woman.

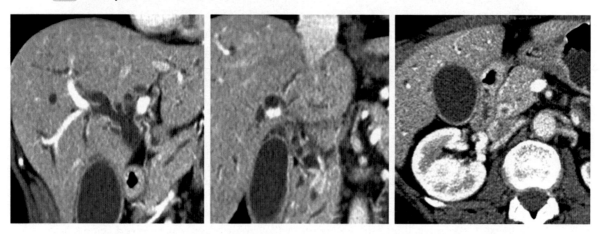

29 A 78-year-old woman.

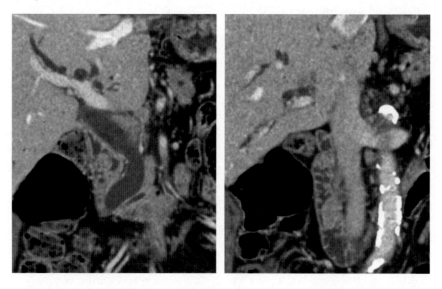

30 A 65-year-old woman.

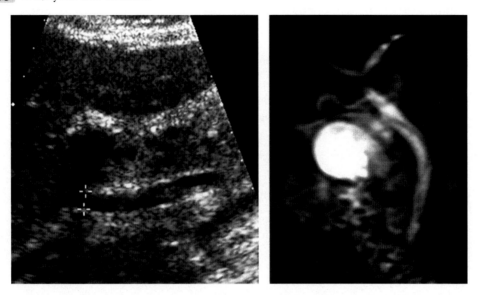

31 What is the gallbladder finding in this 70-year-old woman with shortness of breath who was evaluated with a CT pulmonary angiogram? For comparison, a contrast-enhanced CT performed 13 hours earlier is shown on the right.

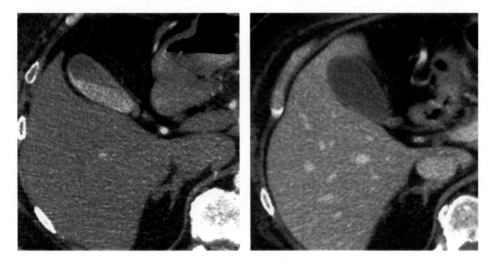

A. Acute cholecystitis
B. Milk of calcium
C. Vicarious excretion of contrast
D. Hydrops

32 Match the MRCP images for patients 1 to 4 below with the correct description of biliary ductal anatomy (A to E). Each option may be used once or not at all.

Patient 1:

Patient 2:

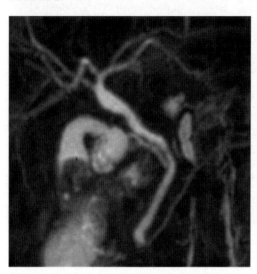

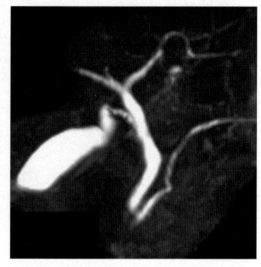

Patient 3:

Patient 4:

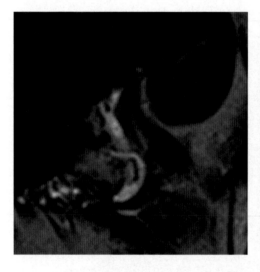

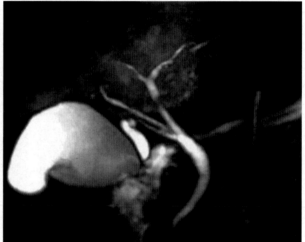

    A. Conventional biliary anatomy
    B. Low and medial insertion of the cystic duct
    C. Posterior right hepatic duct draining into left hepatic duct
    D. Hepatocystic duct
    E. Biliary trifurcation

33 A patient with a history of liver transplant with hepaticojejunostomy was evaluated with MRI. Normal arterial flow was identified at Doppler ultrasound. What is the most likely diagnosis?

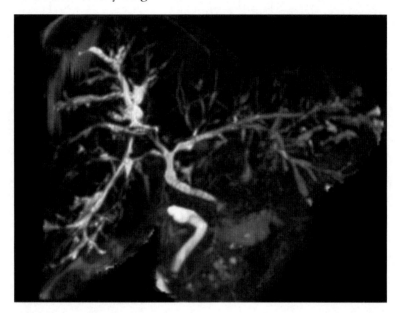

   A. Ischemic cholangiopathy
   B. Choledocholithiasis
   C. Multifocal cholangiocarcinoma
   D. Recurrent primary sclerosing cholangitis

34 Match the biliary findings indicated by the arrows in patients 1 to 4 with the correct description (A to D). Each option may be used once.

Patient 1:

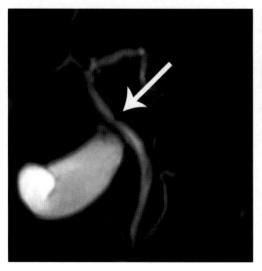 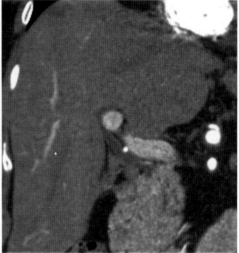

Patient 2:

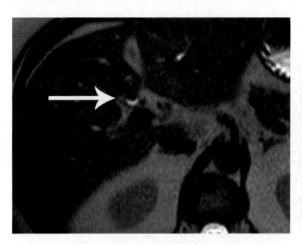

Patient 3:

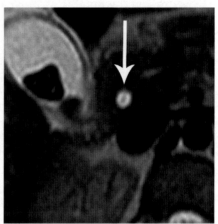

Patient 4:

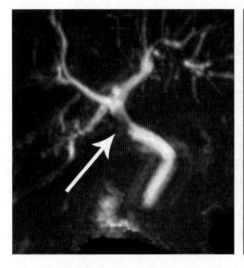
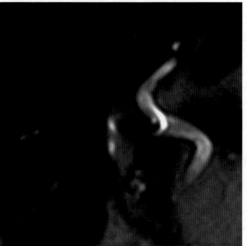

A. Pneumobilia
B. Surgical clip
C. Crossing vessel
D. Bile flow artifact

ANSWERS AND EXPLANATIONS

1 **Answer B.** The ultrasound image shows multiple small echogenic foci in the gallbladder wall associated with **comet tail artifact** (arrows). In the gallbladder, this indicates the presence of cholesterol crystals and is diagnostic for adenomyomatosis. An adenomatous polyp or gallbladder carcinoma typically appears as nonspecific soft tissue thickening or nodularity without shadowing or comet tail artifact. A gallstone is dependent, echogenic, and associated with posterior acoustic shadowing.

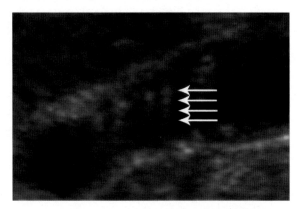

Gallbladder adenomyomatosis is a form of hyperplastic cholecystosis with intramural diverticula (Rokitansky-Aschoff sinuses) in a thickened gallbladder wall. This hyperplasia is a **noninflammatory and nonneoplastic** condition. These sinuses retain bile and develop cholesterol deposits responsible for the comet tail artifact. Adenomyomatosis is thought to be an asymptomatic incidental finding.

Comet tail artifact occurs when echoes reverberate between two parallel and highly reflective surfaces as shown in the following diagram. The successive reverberating echoes return to the transducer later than expected and are mapped erroneously at a greater distance from the anterior gallbladder wall. The later the returning echo, the more attenuated the amplitude, resulting in a comet tail shape of the artifact with the **characteristic short, V-shaped distal tapering. Comet tail artifact is distinct from ring down artifact, which occurs behind gas-containing structures and appears long without tapering.** The mechanism of ring down artifact is different, representing a single continuous echo from resonance of fluid trapped among air bubbles.

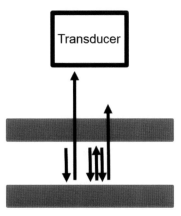

Mechanism of comet tail artifact.

References: Baad M, Lu ZF, Reiser I, et al. Clinical significance of US artifacts. *Radiographics* 2017;37(5):1408–1423.

Boscak AR, Al-Hawary M, Ramsburgh SR. Best cases from the AFIP: adenomyomatosis of the gallbladder. *Radiographics* 2006;26(3):941–946.

2 **Answer C.** Coronal and axial T2W images from an MRCP demonstrate two dark filling focal defects in a mildly prominent common bile duct. The axial image shows **dependent location** of the filling defect. Findings are consistent with **choledocholithiasis**. There is also cholelithiasis, with a stone seen in the gallbladder.

Up to one-third of patients with gallstones develop symptoms, which may include biliary colic, cholecystitis, cholangitis, or pancreatitis. Ultrasound is usually the initial imaging modality performed in patients with right upper quadrant pain and suspected biliary pathology. Choledocholithiasis accounts for the majority of cases of biliary obstruction, most often migrating from the gallbladder. Patients with suspected choledocholithiasis without direct visualization of a ductal stone on ultrasound may proceed to MRCP or ERCP for further evaluation.

MRCP has a high sensitivity of about 90% for choledocholithiasis, compared to 20% to 60% for ultrasound. The stones are visualized as dark filling defects surrounded by bright bile on the heavily T2W images of MRCP. The stones may be round or have a faceted appearance with angular margins. **Stones impacted in the ampulla may be missed or misdiagnosed as ampullary lesions due to the lack of surrounding fluid.** Tiny stones ≤3 mm may still be hard to detect even on thin-slice MRCP.

Pneumobilia would appear as a nondependent hypointensity with air–fluid meniscus on axial images, highlighting the importance of careful correlation with axial images to make the distinction with choledocholithiasis. Cholangiocarcinoma or ampullary carcinoma may present as a soft tissue mass or a stricture. With ascariasis, the parasites can be seen in the bile duct as a linear filling defect.

References: Irie H, Honda H, Kuroiwa T, et al. Pitfalls in MR cholangiopancreatographic interpretation. *Radiographics* 2001;21(1):23–37.

Yeh BM, Liu PS, Soto JA, et al. MR imaging and CT of the biliary tract. *Radiographics* 2009;29(6):1669–1688.

3 **Answer A.** Findings are consistent with **acute (calculous) cholecystitis** as follows:

- The gallbladder is **distended** with shadowing **gallstones** (long black arrow) as well as sludge.
- The gallbladder **wall is thickened** and edematous with a striated appearance and measures >3 mm as delineated by the calipers.
- The gallbladder **wall is vascular** (short white arrows) on the color Doppler image, indicating inflammation.
- **Pericholecystic fluid** is identified (long white arrow).
- Information not provided is that the patient had a **positive sonographic Murphy sign**, with maximum tenderness during compression with the transducer over the gallbladder.

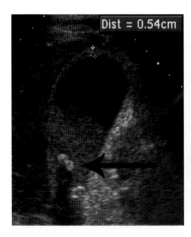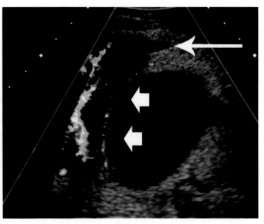

Although the individual imaging features of acute cholecystitis (AC) on ultrasound are nonspecific, identification of multiple features increases diagnostic confidence with overall excellent (>80%) sensitivity and specificity. **While it is considered a sensitive indicator, the sonographic Murphy sign has a relatively low specificity for AC. Furthermore, a negative sonographic Murphy sign does not reliably exclude AC** in diabetic patients with neuropathy or patients who have received pain medication or sedation.

Among the answer choices, acute hepatitis and adenomyomatosis also cause gallbladder wall thickening but are less likely given this constellation of findings. Adenomyomatosis is usually an asymptomatic incidental finding. Other causes of diffuse gallbladder wall thickening are listed in the table below.

Patients with AC may present with right upper quadrant pain, fever, and leukocytosis. A gallstone that is persistently impacted in the cystic duct or gallbladder neck causes gallbladder obstruction and distention. Subsequently, inflammation of the gallbladder wall is induced by the accumulated bile salts or superinfection. **AC can progress to life-threatening complications, which are best evaluated by CT, including gas formation, gangrene, hemorrhage, and perforation.** Definitive treatment for AC is cholecystectomy.

Causes of Diffuse Gallbladder Wall Thickening	
Inflammation	• Acute cholecystitis (calculous and acalculous) • Chronic cholecystitis • Hepatitis
Fluid	• Ascites in the setting of cardiac, hepatic, and renal disease (e.g., congestive heart failure, cirrhosis, nephrotic syndrome) • Fluid overload (e.g., aggressive fluid resuscitation)
Soft tissue	• Adenomyomatosis (a type of hyperplastic cholecystosis) • Neoplasm (gallbladder carcinoma)
Blood	• Injury • Hemorrhagic cholecystitis

References: American College of Radiology. ACR Appropriateness Criteria: right upper quadrant pain. Published 1996. Updated 2018. Available at https://acsearch.acr.org/docs/69474/Narrative. Accessed August 9, 2020.

O'Connor OJ, Maher MM. Imaging of cholecystitis. *AJR Am J Roentgenol* 2011;196(4): W367–W374.

4 **Answers**

Patient 1: C. Gallstone
Patient 2: D. Gallbladder carcinoma
Patient 3: B. Sludge
Patient 4: A. Hematoma

This series reviews the diagnosis of intraluminal gallbladder pathology. Ultrasound is the primary imaging modality for evaluation of the gallbladder. **Color Doppler images should be interpreted with caution.** Problem solving by acquiring additional ultrasound images or by evaluating with a different modality may help make the right diagnosis.

There are foci of mixed color Doppler signal on the gallstone in patient 1 and within the sludge that fills the gallbladder in patient 3. These foci represent **twinkling artifact** that can be seen posterior to a highly reflective material with a rough or granular surface, such as a gallstone, cholesterol deposits, kidney stone, or foreign body. **Cholesterol crystals and stones can produce twinkling as well as the color comet tail artifact**, which is a tapering V-shaped reverberation artifact of alternating colors posteriorly as shown below, analogous to the gray scale version. Depending on its composition, a gallstone may or may not demonstrate these artifacts. This noncalcified gallstone is not visible on the accompanying CT, and a gallstone does not need to be calcified to demonstrate an echogenic surface and twinkling. Usually the diagnosis of a gallstone is made with confidence on gray scale imaging alone, with an echogenic surface and clean posterior acoustic shadowing.

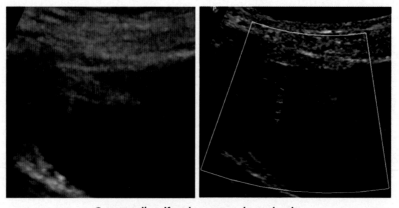

Comet tail artifact in gray scale and color.

These color artifacts can mimic vascular flow leading to misdiagnosis of gallbladder carcinoma. In **patient 3 with cholesterol-laden sludge filling the gallbladder**, correlation with the contrast-enhanced CT reveals no suspicious enhancing mass, with the density of gallbladder contents only mildly greater than simple fluid at 28HU. **A color Doppler cine clip would show nonvascular twinkling, and spectral Doppler interrogation would reveal noise**, as shown on a different patient below. **True vascular flow would demonstrate an arterial or venous waveform.** The visibility of twinkling artifacts may be affected by multiple technical parameters. The artifact may be more prominent with the use of lower frequency transducers and placement of the focus posterior to the echogenic structure.

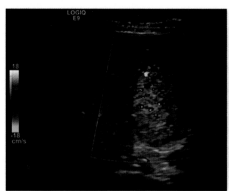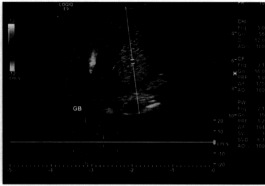

Twinkling artifact in a different patient with gallbladder sludge shows noise with spectral Doppler interrogation.

In **patient 2 with gallbladder carcinoma**, there is no detectable color Doppler flow within the heterogeneous polypoid fundal mass. However, subsequent MR imaging reveals enhancement, confirming neoplasm. **Ultrasound may not reliably identify vascular flow in a gallbladder neoplasm.** In a patient with a nonmobile soft tissue mass, a short interval follow-up or further evaluation with CT or MRI may be warranted to differentiate neoplasm from tumefactive sludge. **The general consensus is that polyps 1 cm or larger should undergo cholecystectomy.** Management for smaller polyps is more variable, but American College of Radiology guidelines suggest yearly follow-up for polyps measuring 7-9 mm, with no follow-up for polyps 6mm or smaller.

Patient 4 has gallbladder hematoma on the ultrasound and CT performed a few days after liver biopsy. There is high-density material on CT. The mass is heterogeneous on ultrasound with no vascular flow demonstrated, and the finding is new from 1 month prior. While sludge can have this appearance, the most likely diagnosis is hemorrhage into the biliary system in the setting of recent liver biopsy.

References: Ghersin E, Soudack M, Gaitini D. Twinkling artifact in gallbladder adenomyomatosis. *J Ultrasound Med* 2003;22(2):229–231.

Kamaya A, Tuthill T, Rubin JM. Twinkling artifact on color Doppler sonography: dependence on machine parameters and underlying cause. *AJR Am J Roentgenol* 2003;180(1):215–222.

Kim HC, Yang DM, Jin W, et al. Color Doppler twinkling artifacts in various conditions during abdominal and pelvic sonography. *J Ultrasound Med* 2010;29(4):621–632.

Mellnick VM, Menias CO, Sandrasegaran K, et al. Polypoid lesions of the gallbladder: disease spectrum with pathologic correlation. *Radiographics* 2015;35(2):387–399.

5 **Answer A.** Biliary strictures are commonly malignant due to pancreaticobiliary carcinoma, but benign causes include hepatobiliary surgery, pancreatitis, and cholangitis. **Up to 90% of cases of benign biliary stricture are iatrogenic related to hepatobiliary surgery, most commonly the sequela of cholecystectomy.** Risk factors for biliary injury during cholecystectomy include variant ductal anatomy, bleeding, inflammation in the surgical bed, and other factors that complicate surgery such as obesity.

References: Katabathina VS, Dasyam AK, Dasyam N, et al. Adult bile duct strictures: role of MR imaging and MR cholangiopancreatography in characterization. *Radiographics* 2014;34(3):565–586.

Raman SP, Fishman EK, Gayer G. Chapter 81: Postsurgical and traumatic lesions of the biliary tract. In: Gore RM, Levine MS (eds). *Textbook of gastrointestinal radiology*, 4th ed. Philadelphia, PA: Elsevier/Saunders, 2015:1348–1391.

6a **Answer A.** The patient's CT and MRCP show a collection of fluid and gas in the cholecystectomy bed. This is not uncommon and may be a postoperative finding that resolves spontaneously. However, **in a patient with signs and**

symptoms of peritonitis, this collection could represent a bile leak or abscess that requires intervention. There is no high density or extravasation of IV contrast to suggest pseudoaneurysm or active hemorrhage. A gallbladder remnant may be left behind if adhesions or variant anatomy prevents complete removal of the gallbladder but should be small rather than filling the length of the gallbladder fossa. A duplicated (accessory) gallbladder is a very rare congenital anomaly that should not be a primary consideration and presumably would have been recognized and removed at cholecystectomy.

If the diagnosis is unclear, an HIDA scan may be useful to confirm a bile leak. MRCP with a hepatobiliary agent such as gadoxetate disodium (Eovist, Bayer HealthCare Pharmaceuticals) has also been used to help diagnose and localize bile leaks, as 50% of this contrast agent is taken up by hepatocytes and excreted into the biliary system during the hepatobiliary phase. Treatment of bile leaks may involve a combination of endoscopic, percutaneous, and surgical intervention.

References: Melamud K, LeBedis CA, Anderson SW, et al. Biliary imaging: multimodality approach to imaging of biliary injuries and their complications. *Radiographics* 2014;34(3):613–623.

Raman SP, Fishman EK, Gayer G. Chapter 81: Postsurgical and traumatic lesions of the biliary tract. In: Gore RM, Levine MS (eds). *Textbook of gastrointestinal radiology*, 4th ed. Philadelphia, PA: Elsevier/Saunders, 2015:1348–1391.

6b **Answer D.** Two months later, the MRCP and the following ERCP reveal the **sequela of biliary injury with a stricture causing high-grade obstruction** (arrow) at the biliary hilum near the cholecystectomy clips. There is no surrounding fluid collection on the MR or extravasation on the ERCP to indicate a recurrent bile leak. (The round area of contrast on the ERCP represents contrast in the duodenum.) The time course and the preceding events are not consistent with either cholangiocarcinoma or sclerosing cholangitis.

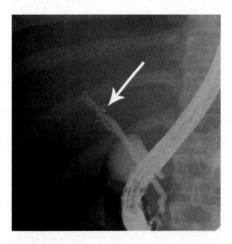

The most common locations for postcholecystectomy strictures are at the junction of the cystic duct with the common duct and at the biliary hilum. **Although these strictures are benign, they can be difficult to manage.** Treatment includes ERCP for stent placement, but recurrence is common. Surgical intervention with hepaticojejunostomy may eventually be required.

References: Katabathina VS, Dasyam AK, Dasyam N, et al. Adult bile duct strictures: role of MR imaging and MR cholangiopancreatography in characterization. *Radiographics* 2014;34(3):565–586.

Raman SP, Fishman EK, Gayer G. Chapter 81: Postsurgical and traumatic lesions of the biliary tract. In: Gore RM, Levine MS (eds). *Textbook of gastrointestinal radiology*, 4th ed. Philadelphia, PA: Elsevier/Saunders, 2015:1348–1391.

7 **Answers.**
Patient 1: B. Emphysematous cholecystitis
Patient 2: A. Cholelithiasis
Patient 3: C. Porcelain gallbladder

There are features on ultrasound that help differentiate gallbladder gas from calcification. However, correlation with CT may be required for diagnosis. **CT is highly sensitive and specific for the detection of gas and calcifications.**

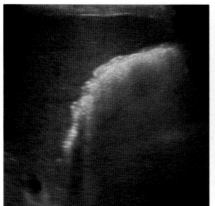 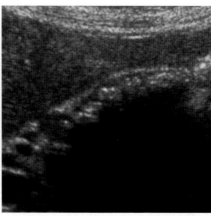 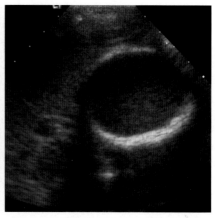

Dirty shadowing (emphysematous cholecystitis), wall–echo–shadow complex (gallstones), and porcelain gallbladder.

Patient 1 has **emphysematous cholecystitis**. Hyperechoic gas is seen in the wall of the gallbladder. The white streaks posterior to the gas on ultrasound represent **"dirty shadowing" with ring down artifacts**, as opposed to the clean, sharp, black shadowing seen posterior to calculi and wall calcification. Ring down artifacts are the result of resonance of fluid trapped among gas bubbles, producing a continuous echo displayed as a long, nontapering streak. **These should not be mistaken for the comet tail artifacts seen with adenomyomatosis, which are short and tapered with a V-shape.** Gas in the gallbladder lumen may be mobile, whereas gas trapped in the gallbladder wall tend to be restricted from moving.

Emphysematous cholecystitis is a serious complication of acute cholecystitis, with gangrene and perforation contributing to a relatively high mortality rate of 15%. **The most common risk factor is diabetes**, which is present in up to 50% of patients. Emphysematous cholecystitis is seen in men two to three times more frequently than in women, whereas gallstones and acute cholecystitis overall occur more frequently in women than in men. It is speculated that cystic artery compromise allows superinfection with a gas-forming organism such as *Clostridium* species and *E. coli*. Treatment is emergent cholecystectomy. If the patient is unable to undergo immediate surgery, percutaneous cholecystostomy is an option until surgery is feasible.

Patient 2 demonstrates the **"wall–echo–shadow complex"** on ultrasound **consistent with a gallbladder filled with stones**. The "wall" of the gallbladder is a thin echogenic white line. Just deep to the wall, the "echo" represents the lobulated contour of the stones, which cause a **clean posterior acoustic "shadow."** Shadowing helps in the diagnosis of stones and is better appreciated with higher-frequency transducers and the **focal zone placed at the level of the stone**. While stones are usually mobile with changes in patient positioning, impacted stones and numerous tightly-packed stones may be restricted from movement.

On CT, stones have variable density and appearance. **CT is less sensitive than ultrasound and MRI for the detection of gallstones.** CT has a sensitivity of 75%, compared to ultrasound sensitivity of 95% for stones >2 mm. Patient 2 has gallstones with rim calcification and internal gas, features that allow visualization on CT. Conventional abdominal radiographs are insensitive, with only 15% to 20% of gallstones detectable.

Patient 3 has a **porcelain gallbladder**, which refers to calcification in the gallbladder wall. It is a **sequela of chronic cholecystitis**, and involvement may be diffuse or segmental. **The association of porcelain gallbladder with gallbladder carcinoma in 1% to 6% of cases is real but significantly lower than previously believed**. A thin layer of echogenic calcium in the wall may not completely attenuate the ultrasound beam, as seen in this case, allowing visualization of the lumen and posterior wall of the gallbladder. If the wall calcification is thicker, there is greater attenuation of the ultrasound beam and more shadowing, which may be more difficult to distinguish from a gallbladder full of stones. Porcelain gallbladder may be visible on radiographs, as shown in the following image from the same patient.

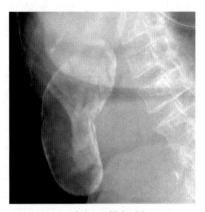

Porcelain gallbladder.

References: Grand D, Horton KM, Fishman EK, et al. CT of the gallbladder: spectrum of disease. *AJR Am J Roentgenol* 2004;183(1):163–170.

Patel NB, Oto A, Thomas S. Multidetector CT of emergent biliary pathologic conditions. *Radiographics* 2013;33(7):1867–1888.

Zulfiqar M, Shetty A, Tsai R, et al. Diagnostic approach to benign and malignant calcifications in the abdomen and pelvis. *Radiographics* 2020;40(3):731–753.

8 **Answer C.** ERCP in this patient with primary sclerosing cholangitis (PSC) reveals diffuse intra- and extrahepatic biliary ductal stricturing. The fibrosis has progressed such that the ducts are very thin and virtually obliterated, resulting in the **"pruned tree" appearance**. More commonly, patients with PSC have alternating intrahepatic biliary stenosis and dilations that result in beading. The extrahepatic ducts and gallbladder may also be involved.

The majority of patients (70% to 90%) with PSC have inflammatory bowel disease, and diagnosis is usually made in young patients at age 30 to 40 years. PSC is more strongly associated with ulcerative colitis (UC) than Crohn disease. PSC is a chronic inflammatory and fibrosing disease of the biliary ducts with a 10% to 15% lifetime risk of cholangiocarcinoma. **Surveillance with MRCP helps identify progression of strictures that require intervention to relieve obstruction or tissue sampling to evaluate**

for cholangiocarcinoma. PSC may progress to cirrhosis and require liver transplantation.

Other diseases can have the appearance of PSC with multiple biliary strictures as follows:

- Ascending (pyogenic) cholangitis is most commonly caused by *E. coli* infection in the setting of biliary obstruction.
- Autoimmune cholangitis (IgG4-related sclerosing cholangitis) can have the same appearance as PSC but diagnosed in older patients.
- AIDS cholangiopathy should be considered in the setting of AIDS.

References: Khoshpouri P, Habibabadi RR, Hazhirkarzar B, et al. Imaging features of primary sclerosing cholangitis: from diagnosis to liver transplant follow-up. *Radiographics* 2019;39(7):1938–1964.

Saich R, Chapman R. Primary sclerosing cholangitis, autoimmune hepatitis and overlap syndromes in inflammatory bowel disease. *World J Gastroenterol* 2008;14(3):331–337.

9a **Answer B.** This is a **choledochal cyst** (also known as a choledochal malformation), with fusiform dilation of the extrahepatic bile duct demonstrated on MRCP. This is consistent with type I cyst according to the Todani classification. Since a choledochal cyst is in continuity with the bile duct, the other choices are incorrect. A bile duct can empty into a periampullary duodenal diverticulum, but this would occur distally. **Patients with choledochal cysts may have an abnormal pancreaticobiliary junction.** In this case, a long common channel of the pancreatic and biliary ducts was noted at ERCP (not shown). Occasionally, other imaging can help confirm communication with the biliary tree, including ERCP, HIDA scan, and hepatocyte phase of an MRI using Eovist contrast agent.

Choledochal cysts are a group of uncommon abnormalities manifesting as biliary ductal dilation. The Todani classification is based on morphology, location, and number of cysts. Alternative classification systems have been proposed that are based on the different causes of cystic dilation, which have different clinical implications. The five types in the Todani classification are listed below. There are other subtypes that are not fully included here.

Todani Classification of Choledochal Cysts (Malformations)	
Type I (most common, 80%–90%)	Single fusiform dilation of part or entire extrahepatic duct
Type II	True diverticulum with a narrow stalk projecting from extrahepatic bile duct
Type III (choledochocele)	Dilation of extrahepatic bile duct within duodenal wall
Type IV (second most common, 10%)	IVa: cysts involving both intra- and extrahepatic ducts
	IVb: multiple dilatations/cysts of extrahepatic ducts only
Type V (Caroli disease)	Multiple dilatations/cysts of intrahepatic ducts only

9b **Answer B.** This choledochal cyst contains a biliary **stone**. The ultrasound, MR, and CT images show a dependent focus internally. On ultrasound, this focus is echogenic with clean posterior acoustic shadowing. This particular stone is hyperdense on noncontrast and postcontrast CT images. There is no increase in density after IV contrast administration to indicate an enhancing lesion such as cholangiocarcinoma. A cholesterol polyp would be a gallbladder finding, not a ductal finding. Cholesterol polyps may be echogenic on ultrasound but without posterior shadowing. Cholesterol polyps may show comet tail artifact since they are nonneoplastic in the spectrum of adenomyomatosis. A hematoma is typically heterogeneous without shadowing.

Biliary stasis and chronic inflammation within choledochal cysts contribute to complications including **malignant transformation, stone formation, cholangitis, pancreatitis, and fibrosis.** The most feared complication of choledochal cyst is malignant transformation. Types I and IV are associated with the highest risk of cholangiocarcinoma, thought to be related to high association with abnormal pancreaticobiliary junction. This abnormal junction results in chronic inflammation from reflux of pancreatic secretions. **Risk of malignancy in the biliary system (most commonly cholangiocarcinoma in adults) is reduced but not eliminated with cyst resection.** The approach to the treatment of type III cysts (choledochoceles) differs from the other types. Symptomatic choledochoceles can often be treated effectively with decompression by endoscopic sphincterotomy alone given their low risk of malignancy.

References: Banks JS, Saigal G, D'Alonzo JM, et al. Choledochal malformations: surgical implications of radiologic findings. *AJR Am J Roentgenol* 2018;210(4):748–760.

Ono A, Arizono S, Isoda H, et al. Imaging of pancreaticobiliary maljunction. *Radiographics* 2020;40(2):378–392.

Santiago I, Loureiro R, Curvo-Semedo L, et al. Congenital cystic lesions of the biliary tree. *AJR Am J Roentgenol* 2012;198(4):825–835.

10 **Answer A.** This patient was clinically diagnosed with **acute hepatitis** (AH). There is marked thickening of the gallbladder wall secondary to the adjacent liver inflammation. **The decompressed lumen is an important clue that this is not acute cholecystitis.** Acute cholecystitis (AC) is a result of obstruction of gallbladder drainage, so the lumen should be distended unless the gallbladder has ruptured. Wall thickening in this case measures up to 2.5 cm. On CT, the wall demonstrates a thin enhancing inner mucosal layer and a prominent low-density edematous submucosal layer. This edematous wall maintains the shape of the gallbladder and is not pericholecystic fluid. On ultrasound, the submucosal edema can result in a lattice-like appearance within the wall that should not be mistaken for sloughed intraluminal membranes of gangrenous cholecystitis. On CT, there is no disruption of the mucosal layer or heterogeneity of the wall thickening on CT to suggest gangrenous cholecystitis or gallbladder carcinoma. No gallstones were identified on US or CT. After the patient recovered from AH, the wall thickening resolved.

Gallbladder wall thickening (defined as >3 mm) is a common finding associated with acute hepatitis. **In some cases, the wall thickening is more prominent along the wall abutting the inflamed liver.** Other causes of wall thickening besides cholecystitis include secondary edema (congestive heart failure, cirrhosis, nephrotic syndrome, and fluid resuscitation), adenomyomatosis, and gallbladder cancer. In AH and secondary edema, the liver may demonstrate periportal edema along the intrahepatic portal tracts. Distinguishing these entities from AC is important to avoid unnecessary surgery. When the diagnosis is unclear on US and CT, nuclear medicine HIDA scan can help determine if there is gallbladder obstruction that would suggest AC over other causes of wall thickening.

References: Brook OR, Kane RA, Tyagi G, et al. Lessons learned from quality assurance: errors in the diagnosis of acute cholecystitis on ultrasound and CT. *AJR Am J Roentgenol* 2011;196(3):597–604.

Runner GJ, Corwin MT, Siewert B, et al. Gallbladder wall thickening. *AJR Am J Roentgenol* 2014;202(1):W1–W12.

11 **Answer A.** This patient with **Caroli disease** has multiple intrahepatic cystic structures in the liver. The **"central dot" sign** (arrows) is identified in the cystic lesions, corresponding to enhancing central portal radicles and characteristic of Caroli disease. The differential diagnosis of multiple small cystic lesions in the liver may include simple hepatic cysts, biliary hamartomas, microabscesses, and biliary papillomatosis, but those entities do not show the central dot sign.

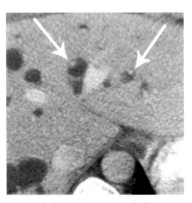

Central dot sign in Caroli disease.

Caroli disease, also known as communicating cavernous biliary ectasia and **Todani type V choledochal cyst, is an autosomal recessive disorder along the spectrum of fibropolycystic liver disease.** Arrest or derangement during embryogenesis of the ductal plate leads to abnormal development with inflammatory dilatation of the intrahepatic bile ducts. Extrahepatic ducts are spared.

- Caroli *disease* is the simple form and presents in young adults with involvement of the larger intrahepatic ducts. This leads to focal or diffuse cystic changes of the intrahepatic bile ducts, which may have a fusiform or saccular appearance, as seen in this case.
- **The complex form of the disease involves both the larger and smaller ducts leading to Caroli *syndrome* and includes features of both Caroli disease and a disease known as congenital hepatic fibrosis (CHF).** Caroli syndrome most often presents in infancy or early childhood. CHF represents involvement of only the smaller peripheral ducts, with nonspecific imaging findings such as splenomegaly and other signs of portal hypertension without cystic lesions apparent.

Complications of Caroli disease include **stone formation, cholangitis, abscess, cirrhosis, and increased risk for cholangiocarcinoma.** If the disease is limited, partial hepatectomy of the involved segment is curative. If diffuse, symptomatic treatment with endoscopic therapy, biliary bypass procedures, or liver transplantation can be considered.

References: Brancatelli G, Federle MP, Vilgrain V, et al. Fibropolycystic liver disease: CT and MR imaging findings. *Radiographics* 2005;25(3):659–670.

Banks JS, Saigal G, D'Alonzo JM, et al. Choledochal malformations: surgical implications of radiologic findings. *AJR Am J Roentgenol* 2018;210(4):748–760.

12 **Answer A.** CT images show acute cholecystitis with diffuse gallbladder wall thickening and rim-calcified stone impacted at the neck/cystic duct junction. Intrahepatic biliary ductal dilation caused by the stone is identified above this level, consistent with Mirizzi syndrome. The distal CBD below this level is decompressed. **Mirizzi syndrome occurs from extrinsic compression of the extrahepatic bile duct related to a calculus impacted at the gallbladder**

neck or cystic duct. The obstruction may be caused by the stone itself or due to associated chronic inflammation, scar, or fistulization. Initial treatment may be ERCP for stone removal and stenting prior to cholecystectomy. Open cholecystectomy is preferred as the degree of inflammation increases the risk of biliary injury with laparoscopic technique.

References: Katabathina VS, Dasyam AK, Dasyam N, et al. Adult bile duct strictures: role of MR imaging and MR cholangiopancreatography in characterization. *Radiographics* 2014;34(3):565–586.

Patel NB, Oto A, Thomas S. Multidetector CT of emergent biliary pathologic conditions. *Radiographics* 2013;33(7):1867–1888.

13a **Answer B. Autoimmune cholangitis.**

13b **Answer D.** This patient was diagnosed with autoimmune cholangitis (AIC), also known as IgG4-related sclerosing cholangitis. **AIC is characterized by a lymphocytic infiltrate rich in IgG4-positive plasma cells and is highly steroid responsive.** Initial CT and MRI demonstrate marked wall thickening diffusely involving the extrahepatic duct, causing obstruction with intrahepatic ductal dilation. **The stricture is long and smooth with visible lumen despite the severity of wall thickening, features that are highly suggestive of AIC.** The possibility of AIC was suggested based on imaging before the patient underwent ERCP and stenting to relieve the initial obstruction. Biopsies were negative for malignancy. After treatment with steroids, follow-up MRI shows significant decrease in wall thickness as well as resolution of obstruction.

Imaging features of AIC overlap with cholangiocarcinoma (CCA) and other types of cholangitis. AIC can present as a focal mass or a shorter segment, indistinguishable from cholangiocarcinoma (CCA). Diagnosis can be difficult and often relies on imaging findings and supportive evidence, such as **elevated serum or tissue IgG4 levels** (found in some but not all patients) and response to steroids. The amount of tissue obtained at biopsies is frequently inadequate for definitive diagnosis. Unfortunately, some patients with AIC undergo surgical resection assuming malignancy, but the surgery is not curative. **Identifying other IgG4-related diseases in the same patient such as autoimmune pancreatitis and retroperitoneal fibrosis increases suspicion for AIC.** Rate of relapse is high and may require additional treatment with steroids or other immunomodulatory drugs. If untreated, AIC in a small percentage of cases can progress to cirrhosis.

Regarding the other answer choices, there is no surgical change that would indicate resection or liver transplant. CCA or PSC are challenging to treat medically and neither would be expected to have this degree of response to therapy in this time period. **PSC presents in younger patients approximately 30 to 40 years old, while AIC presents in older patients approximately 60 to 70 years old as in this case.** The strictures in primary sclerosing cholangitis (PSC) tend to be shorter and multifocal with intervening segments of dilation, resulting in an irregular beaded appearance. Even when PSC demonstrates pruned tree appearance with longer strictures, the thickness of the wall is less prominent when compared to AIC.

References: Madhusudhan KS, Das P, Gunjan D, et al. IgG4-related sclerosing cholangitis: a clinical and imaging review. *AJR Am J Roentgenol* 2019;213(6):1221–1231.

Martínez-de-Alegría A, Baleato-González S, García-Figueiras R, et al. IgG4-related disease from head to toe. *Radiographics* 2015;35(7):2007–2025.

14 **Answer A.** This series of cases reviews benign gallbladder pathology. This patient has **gangrenous cholecystitis**, which is a serious complication of acute cholecystitis. **Complications of acute cholecystitis are best evaluated by CT.** The CT images show a distended gallbladder with a calcified stone (arrow) on the sagittal image impacted in the gallbladder neck. The gallbladder wall is thickened with pericholecystic fluid and inflammatory fat stranding. The wall is irregular and heterogeneously enhancing, with discontinuity of mucosal enhancement (short arrow) and intramural fluid collections.

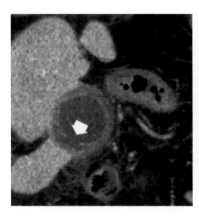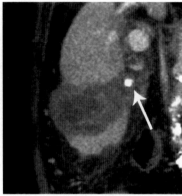

An impacted stone causes gallbladder overdistention, which can lead to gangrene. Findings of gangrenous cholecystitis are as follows:

- **Perfusion defects in the wall**, demonstrated as decreased or discontinuous wall enhancement as seen in this case, have been found to have 80% accuracy in the diagnosis of gangrenous cholecystitis.
- **Heterogeneity of the wall** is due to hemorrhage, necrosis, and abscess formation.
- **Membranes in the lumen** represent sloughed mucosa.
- **Pericholecystic abscesses** can also be seen in cases of perforation.

In some cases, the degree of heterogeneous irregular thickening and enhancement as well as pericholecystic extension may mimic gallbladder carcinoma. Xanthogranulomatous cholecystitis, a rare and severe form of chronic cholecystitis, can be associated with nodular xanthogranuloma formation in the gallbladder wall.

References: Bennett GL. Chapter 77: Cholelithiasis, cholecystitis, choledocholithiasis, and hyperplastic cholecystoses. In: Gore RM, Levine MS (eds). *Textbook of gastrointestinal radiology*, 4th ed. Philadelphia, PA: Elsevier/Saunders, 2015:1348–1391.

Patel NB, Oto A, Thomas S. Multidetector CT of emergent biliary pathologic conditions. *Radiographics* 2013;33(7):1867–1888.

15 **Answer G.** Findings are consistent with a perihepatic **abscess associated with a dropped gallstone**. There is a fluid collection posterior to the right hepatic lobe with an enhancing rim. Within this collection, there is a dependent rim-calcified stone with angular margins that causes posterior acoustic shadowing on the ultrasound. There are surgical clips in the gallbladder fossa consistent with prior cholecystectomy.

Gallstones may be inadvertently dropped during laparoscopic cholecystectomy. Complications from these stones are thought to occur in fewer than 10% of cases. The most common complication of dropped gallstones is abscess formation, typically in the perihepatic region or the abdominal wall at the laparoscopic port sites. Sinus tracts or fistulas to adjacent organs or spaces can develop. **Because a substantial number of gallstones are not visible on CT, findings may be confused with neoplasms** such as sarcoma or ovarian cystic tumor when there is enhancement.

Patients can present months or years after cholecystectomy. Treatment is percutaneous or surgical drainage with complete removal of the gallstone. **Infection recurs if the gallstone nidus is not removed.**

References: Ramamurthy NK, Rudralingam V, Martin DF, et al. Out of sight but kept in mind: complications and imitations of dropped gallstones. *AJR Am J Roentgenol* 2013;200(6):1244–1253.

Raman SP, Fishman EK, Gayer G. Chapter 81: Postsurgical and traumatic lesions of the biliary tract. In: Gore RM, Levine MS (eds). *Textbook of gastrointestinal radiology*, 4th ed. Philadelphia, PA: Elsevier/Saunders, 2015:1442–1459.

16 **Answer I.** The first image is a 3D MIP from MRCP showing a small cystic structure continuous with the cystic duct representing a **remnant gallbladder infundibulum after cholecystectomy.** The second image is a thin-section coronal MRCP image demonstrating choledocholithiasis in the distal CBD, which is causing intra- and extrahepatic biliary ductal dilation. **Choledocholithiasis can occur when stones are inadvertently retained in the remnant or bile ducts after cholecystectomy. Stones can also develop and come to medical attention years after cholecystectomy, with or without a remnant gallbladder.** A remnant gallbladder after laparoscopic cholecystectomy is not uncommon due to technical difficulties identifying anatomic landmarks or severity of gallbladder inflammation precluding complete removal. These findings can be responsible for "postcholecystectomy syndrome" in patients with abdominal pain, dyspepsia, and other gastrointestinal symptoms. In the immediate postoperative setting, the differential diagnosis of a fluid collection in the gallbladder fossa communicating with the cystic duct is a bile leak.

References: Hoeffel C, Azizi L, Lewin M, et al. Normal and pathologic features of the postoperative biliary tract at 3D MR cholangiopancreatography and MR imaging. *Radiographics* 2006;26(6):1603–1620.

Raman SP, Fishman EK, Gayer G. Chapter 81: Postsurgical and traumatic lesions of the biliary tract. In: Gore RM, Levine MS (eds). *Textbook of gastrointestinal radiology*, 4th ed. Philadelphia, PA: Elsevier/Saunders, 2015:1442–1459.

17 **Answer C.** This patient has a **Phrygian cap.** It represents a folding of the gallbladder fundus that is the most common normal variant of gallbladder shape. It is of no clinical significance. The gallbladder wall is thin and unremarkable. The name refers to the resemblance to hats worn by the inhabitants of ancient Phrygia, which is now Turkey.

Reference: Gore RM, Taylor AJ, Ghahremani GG. Chapter 76: Anomalies and anatomic variants of the gallbladder and biliary tract. In: Gore RM, Levine MS (eds). *Textbook of gastrointestinal radiology*, 4th ed. Philadelphia, PA: Elsevier/Saunders, 2015:1340–1347.

18 **Answer H. Bouveret syndrome is the subtype of gallstone ileus associated with duodenal or gastric outlet obstruction.** The thick-walled gallbladder has foci of pneumobilia as a result of fistulization (long arrow on first image below) to the duodenal bulb. A large, faintly hyperdense gallstone (short arrows) fills the duodenal bulb. The stomach is filled with fluid. An inflamed gallbladder can fistulize to adjacent bowel, and gallstones can pass through this fistula. If large (>2.5 cm), the stones can cause bowel obstruction, most commonly at the ileocecal valve. Diagnosis is usually made on CT scan during evaluation of suspected bowel obstruction. **The obstructing stone may be overlooked** if the gallstone is similar in density to debris or bowel fluid.

The diseased gallbladder is easily mistaken for bowel, or it can be so contracted that it is dismissed as resected. In this case, the CT findings were initially misinterpreted as a duodenal ulcer with contained perforation and the gallstone unrecognized. The patient was managed conservatively but weeks later presented with distal migration of the 4.5-cm gallstone and small bowel obstruction (shown below on the second and third images).

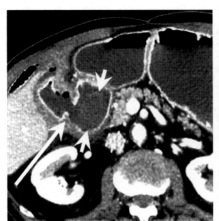
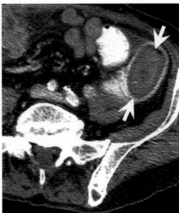
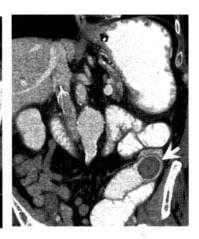

Rigler triad refers to the findings of pneumobilia, bowel distention, and ectopic gallstones seen in gallstone ileus. In patients with pneumobilia without history of sphincterotomy or biliary surgery, the gallbladder fossa and bowel should be carefully examined for subtle findings of fistulizing gallstone disease. **Elderly women** are the typical patient demographic.

References: Brennan GB, Rosenberg RD, Arora S. Bouveret syndrome. *Radiographics* 2004;24(4):1171–1175.

Gan S, Roy-Choudhury S, Agrawal S, et al. More than meets the eye: subtle but important CT findings in Bouveret's syndrome. *AJR Am J Roentgenol* 2008;191(1):182–185.

19 **Answer B.** There are multiple small cysts arranged in a ring pattern at the gallbladder fundus on these T2W MR images consistent with the **"pearl necklace" sign**. This sign has been found to have a specificity >90% for **adenomyomatosis**. Adenomyomatosis is a form of hyperplastic cholecystosis. (The other form is cholesterolosis, which can manifest as cholesterol polyps.) Hyperplastic cholecystoses are noninflammatory and nonneoplastic. Increased pressure from a functional obstruction is thought to be the cause of invagination of hyperplastic epithelium into the gallbladder wall. These invaginations form the Rokitansky-Aschoff sinuses, which have the appearance of cystic spaces and contain trapped bile.

Adenomyomatosis can be **localized (usually at the fundus), diffuse, or segmental.** The segmental form can be seen as **contraction of the wall** that narrows the gallbladder lumen. The wall thickening **can mimic gallbladder carcinoma if the cystic components are not appreciated**. On ultrasound, the identification of comet tail reverberation artifact from the cholesterol crystals in the gallbladder wall is diagnostic for adenomyomatosis. The accuracy for identifying the fluid-filled Rokitansky-Aschoff sinuses confirming adenomyomatosis is highest with T2W MRI/MRCP at >90%, followed by CT and ultrasound. On ultrasound, the fundus may not be well evaluated due to reverberation artifact from the abdominal wall obscuring the near field. The following images show the cystic appearance of Rokitansky-Aschoff sinuses (arrows) on ultrasound and CT in different patients.

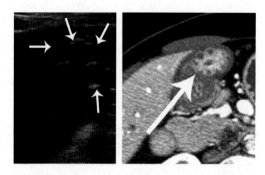

References: Haradome H, Ichikawa T, Sou H, et al. The pearl necklace sign: an imaging sign of adenomyomatosis of the gallbladder at MR cholangiopancreatography. *Radiology* 2003;227(1):80–88.

Levy AD, Murakata LA, Abbott RM, et al. From the archives of the AFIP. Benign tumors and tumor-like lesions of the gallbladder and extrahepatic bile ducts: radiologic-pathologic correlation. Armed Forces Institute of Pathology. *Radiographics* 2002;22(2):387–413.

20 **Answers:**
Patient 1: A. Pneumobilia
Patient 2: C. Periportal edema
Patient 3: B. Portal venous gas
Patient 4: E. Biliary obstruction
Patient 5: A. Pneumobilia

This series of cases reviews the differential diagnosis of branching structures in the liver, typically involving the biliary tree or portal veins. Pneumobilia on CT in patient 1 and radiograph in patient 5 is seen as branching linear hypodensities of air. **Pneumobilia tends to accumulate centrally consistent with the direction of bile flow toward the hilum and within the left lobe in cross-sectional imaging because the left lobe is antidependent in the supine position.**

Causes of pneumobilia are listed in the following table. **In patients with biliary intervention, pneumobilia is an expected persistent normal finding.** If subsequent follow-up imaging shows disappearance of the pneumobilia, recurrent obstruction from stent dysfunction, anastomotic stricture, or recurrent tumor should be suspected.

Causes of Pneumobilia	
Iatrogenic	• ERCP with sphincterotomy, stenting • Surgery with biliary-enteric anastomosis
Traumatic	
Spontaneous biliary-enteric fistula or communication	• Peptic ulcer disease • Gallstone ileus • Recent passage of gallstone
Infection	• Liver abscess communicating with biliary tree • Cholangitis with gas-forming organism (rare)

Patient 2 has periportal edema on CT. When the portal vein is seen in cross section, this is evident as a circumferential halo of edema. When the portal vein is seen longitudinally, **periportal edema is demonstrated as parallel linear hypodensities (arrows) on both sides of the portal vein.** In contradistinction, a dilated duct is seen along one side of portal vein branch. There is hepatic parenchymal edema with heterogeneity on this contrast-enhanced CT. Periportal edema in this patient was due to aggressive fluid resuscitation, but it may be seen in conditions such as congestive heart failure, acute hepatitis, trauma, and liver transplantation.

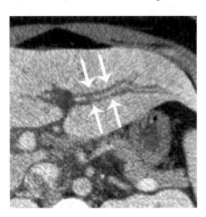

Patient 3 has extensive portal venous gas in the liver. **Because the direction of portal flow is hepatopetal toward the capsule, portal venous gas is most evident peripherally**, in the small branches near the liver capsule. CT is the most sensitive imaging modality for gas, and even very small foci are detectable. Occasionally, gas can be detected in larger portal veins or the mesenteric veins. Portal venous gas is often seen in conjunction with pneumatosis. **The implication of portal venous gas (and pneumatosis) depends on the clinical scenario, and prognosis may not be as dire as previously believed.** The primary concern is ischemic bowel. With early detection now possible, the mortality in patients with mesenteric ischemia accompanied by portal venous gas is decreased to <50%. Other causes of portal venous gas include hepatic abscess, bowel diverticulitis, inflammatory bowel disease, necrotizing pancreatitis, trauma, bowel obstruction, and caustic ingestion. The patient in this case had ingested a caustic substance, which disrupted the gastric mucosa, but there was no life-threatening ischemia.

Patient 4 has **biliary obstruction** as shown by intrahepatic ductal dilation in the left lobe of the liver. This is the **"double-barrel shotgun" sign** of the dilated duct visible parallel to a branch of the portal vein. Attempt should be made to follow the duct as far centrally as possible to identify the site of obstruction.

Portal vein thrombosis (not one of the cases in this series) can cause branching hypodensity along the expected course of the veins. Accompanying altered perfusion in the surrounding parenchyma may be seen.

References: Messmer JM, Levine MS. Chapter 12: Gas and soft tissue abnormalities. In: Gore RM, Levine MS (eds). *Textbook of gastrointestinal radiology*, 4th ed. Philadelphia, PA: Elsevier/Saunders, 2015:178–196.

Shah PA, Cunningham SC, Morgan TA, et al. Hepatic gas: widening spectrum of causes detected at CT and ultrasound in the interventional era. *Radiographics* 2011;31(5): 1403–1413.

Tirumani SH, Shanbhogue AK, Vikram R, et al. Imaging of the porta hepatis: spectrum of disease. *Radiographics* 2014;34(1):73–92.

21 **Answers:**
Patient 1: D. Acute cholecystitis
Patient 2: A. Within normal limits
Patient 3: B. Acute high-grade bile duct obstruction
Patient 4: C. Bile leak
Patient 5: D. Acute cholecystitis

Patient 2 has an HIDA scan within normal limits. There is prompt uptake of radiotracer by the liver, followed by excretion into the common bile duct at about 10 minutes, into the gallbladder at 15 minutes, and into the small bowel at 20 minutes after injection of ^{99m}Tc hepatobiliary iminodiacetic acid. On this image obtained at less than half an hour, all these structures are visualized. The interpretation of HIDA scans requires correlation with the clinical symptoms and scenario.

Patient 1 has findings compatible with **acute cholecystitis with nonvisualization of the gallbladder after 4 hours, implying obstruction of the cystic duct**. Patient 5 underwent a morphine-augmented HIDA scan and also has findings compatible with acute cholecystitis. At 60 minutes, the gallbladder was not visualized. At that point, alternatives to delayed imaging include intravenous administration of 0.04 mg/kg morphine over 1 to 3 minutes or 0.02 μg/kg of cholecystokinin (CCK) in normal saline infused over 15 to 30 minutes. Morphine induces contraction of the sphincter of Oddi to facilitate gallbladder filling in the setting of patent cystic duct. **If the gallbladder is still not seen 30 minutes after morphine injection, findings are compatible with acute cholecystitis**, as the case with patient 5. CCK injection would cause gallbladder contraction and emptying, also facilitating gallbladder filling with radiotracer in the setting of a patent cystic duct.

In patient 5, an additional finding is the rim of increased activity (arrows) at the right inferior margin of the liver at the gallbladder fossa. **This rim sign suggests spread of inflammation to the liver and is highly specific for complicated cholecystitis.** This patient was taken to the operating room and was found to have perforated gangrenous cholecystitis. Also incidentally noted on the postmorphine image is activity below the left lobe of the liver (arrowhead). This represents reflux of bile from the duodenum into the stomach, which can be a normal finding in small quantities of 15% or less.

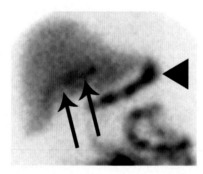

Sensitivity of hepatobiliary scintigraphy for acute cholecystitis is about 90%. False-positive studies are often due to chronic cholecystitis, with fluid or stones preventing adequate radiotracer accumulation in the gallbladder. Nonfilling could also be due to prolonged fasting or hepatocellular dysfunction. False negatives may occur if the inflammation arises in the gallbladder itself, as suspected in some cases of acalculous cholecystitis, rather than inflammation secondary to cystic duct obstruction.

Patient 3 has findings compatible with an **acute high-grade bile duct obstruction**. There is uptake of radiotracer by the liver parenchyma; however, there is **no excretion into the intra- or extrahepatic bile ducts even at 60 minutes.** There has been **clearance of tracer from the blood pool**, with no activity seen in the heart. In this case, the patient had choledocholithiasis, and the severity of the acute obstruction created pressures high enough to prevent radiotracer excretion. The differential diagnosis of nonvisualization of the biliary tree includes hepatocellular dysfunction or intracanalicular cholestasis from a variety of causes such as drug toxicity, sepsis, and cholangitis.

A finding that can distinguish hepatocellular dysfunction from acute high-grade biliary obstruction is poor clearance of tracer from the blood pool.

The following HIDA scan shows findings of hepatocellular dysfunction. The image obtained at 57 to 60 minutes in a patient with a right hepatectomy shows uptake in the remaining left lobe of the liver without biliary excretion. However, in contradistinction to the case of acute high-grade obstruction, there is persistent activity in the cardiac blood pool (arrow). Normally, blood pool activity is cleared by the liver and no longer seen after 10 minutes. The patient returned 24 hours later for a delayed image shown on the right, which revealed activity in the small bowel, confirming hepatocellular dysfunction and a patent biliary system.

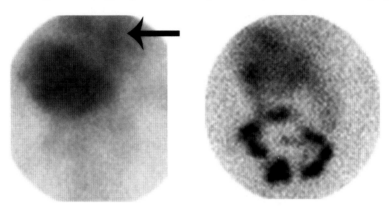

Patient 4 had a recent laparoscopic cholecystectomy and presented on postoperative day 3 with right upper quadrant pain. Fluid was identified in the gallbladder fossa and peritoneal cavity on CT (not shown). Hepatobiliary scintigraphy confirms a bile leak. Radiotracer is seen along the right hepatic margin accumulating in the paracolic gutter when the patient was placed in the right lateral decubitus position. The leak is also seen on the subsequent supine image.

Chronic cholecystitis (no case shown) is thought to be caused by intermittent obstruction of the cyst duct and gallbladder dysmotility, resulting in recurrent episodes of subacute cholecystitis. Chronic cholecystitis is in the differential diagnosis of right upper quadrant pain but is difficult to diagnose. The gallbladder may be small and contracted with a thickened wall, and 95% of cases are associated with cholelithiasis. At hepatobiliary scintigraphy, there may be delayed filling of the gallbladder. **A gallbladder ejection fraction (GBEF) of >50% is normal, but GBEF of <35% at CCK-augmented HIDA scan is suggestive of chronic cholecystitis or biliary dyskinesia.** (GBEF = (baseline activity − activity after CCK infusion)/baseline activity.) Sphincter of Oddi dysfunction, cystic duct syndrome, or medication may also decrease GBEF.

References: Ziessman HA, O'Malley JP, Thrall JH, et al. Chapter 13: Gastrointestinal system. In: Ziessman HA, O'Malley JP, Thrall JH, et al. (eds). *Nuclear medicine*, 4th ed. Philadelphia, PA: Elsevier/Mosby, 2014:288–321.

Ziessman HA, Tulchinsky M, Lavely WC, et al. Sincalide-stimulated cholescintigraphy: a multicenter investigation to determine optimal infusion methodology and gallbladder ejection fraction normal values. *J Nucl Med* 2010;51:277–281.

22 **Answer C.** There is irregular, asymmetric gallbladder wall thickening with heterogeneous enhancement. Foci of gas are also identified internally. This patient has a perforated gallbladder carcinoma. It can be difficult to differentiate complicated cholecystitis from invasive gallbladder carcinoma by imaging, and discovery of carcinoma may be made at the time of cholecystectomy. **Imaging findings such as significantly enlarged porta hepatic lymph nodes and other metastatic disease are more specific for malignancy and help make the diagnosis of adenocarcinoma over**

perforated cholecystitis. Gallbladder carcinoma is more common in women, and peak incidence is in patients 70 to 75 years of age. The majority of cases are associated with gallstones and thought to arise from chronic gallbladder inflammation. Other risk factors include choledochal cysts, abnormal pancreaticobiliary junction, and primary sclerosing cholangitis.

The most common presentation of gallbladder carcinoma seen in 40% to 65% of cases is a large heterogeneously enhancing mass replacing the gallbladder. **The gallbladder can be difficult to recognize, and a neoplasm centered in the gallbladder fossa can mimic a hepatic mass.** Involvement of the liver includes direct invasion as well as hepatic metastases. The second most common imaging presentation of gallbladder carcinoma is a polypoid lesion in the gallbladder, followed by focal or diffuse wall thickening. Other malignancies involving the gallbladder are rare, including metastases (melanoma, breast carcinoma, and hepatocellular carcinoma), lymphoma, carcinoid, and sarcoma.

References: Furlan A, Ferris JV, Hosseinzadeh K, et al. Gallbladder carcinoma update: multimodality imaging evaluation, staging, and treatment options. *AJR Am J Roentgenol* 2008;191(5):1440–1447.

Liang JL, Chen MC, Huang HY, et al. Gallbladder carcinoma manifesting as acute cholecystitis: clinical and computed tomographic features. *Surgery* 2009;146:861–868.

23a **Answer A.** The ultrasound image shows shadowing echogenic structures in the right hepatic lobe, which can be seen with stones and gas. (On occasion, echogenic fat can shadow as well.) Contours are lobulated with clean rather than dirty posterior acoustic shadowing, favoring stones over gas. The noncontrast CT scan confirms that the echogenic structures correspond to high-density foci consistent with **multiple calculi arranged in a branching pattern. Biliary stones may or may not be visible on CT.**

23b **Answer D.** Intrahepatic stones are uncommon, and the extent of disease and number of stones in this case are pathognomonic for **recurrent pyogenic cholangitis** (formerly known as oriental cholangiohepatitis). The T2W MRI shows multiple stones as dark filling defects within the dilated bright intrahepatic biliary ducts. **T1 hyperintensity can be found in pigment stones with high protein content or in stones with certain types of calcification.** Strictures of the peripheral biliary ducts with disproportionate dilation of the central ducts are visualized. Long-standing biliary obstruction can lead to liver abscesses, portal vein thrombosis, strictures, intrahepatic stones, and eventual liver parenchymal atrophy. Intraductal calculi are present in 80% of cases. Patients have an **increased risk of cholangiocarcinoma**, which develops in 5% to 18% of cases.

Recurrent pyogenic cholangitis is a progressive biliary disease characterized by recurrent episodes of bacterial cholangitis. Etiology is unclear, but the initial event is thought to be a parasitic infection that predisposes to biliary stasis and stone formation. There is a **higher prevalence in patients of Asian descent**. In this case, the patient immigrated from the Philippines.

Regarding the other answer choices, the vascular structures such as the visualized IVC are signal voids on the T2W "dark blood" spin echo sequence, not bright like the dilated ducts. Gas would be dark on both T1W and T2W images and rise to the nondependent surface. Ascariasis manifests as long tubular filling defects.

References: Catalano OA, Sahani DV, Forcione DG, et al. Biliary infections: spectrum of imaging findings and management. *Radiographics* 2009;29(7):2059–2080.

Heffernan EJ, Geoghegan T, Munk PL, et al. Recurrent pyogenic cholangitis: from imaging to intervention. *AJR Am J Roentgenol* 2009;192(1):W28–W35.

24a **Answer B.** ERCP images show areas of intrahepatic biliary ductal stricturing and dilation. This imaging appearance can be seen in primary or secondary sclerosing cholangitis. In the setting of AIDS with low CD4 count, these findings are compatible with AIDS cholangiopathy. **AIDS cholangiopathy is usually the result of an opportunistic infection, most commonly *Cryptosporidium* and *Cytomegalovirus* species**, although other pathogens such as *Microsporidia* have also been implicated. No infectious agent can be identified in up to half of patients. The majority of patients affected have **CD4 counts below 100/mm³**, and the incidence has decreased since the advent of effective antiretroviral therapy. Patients usually present with pain, while fever and jaundice are less common because obstruction is usually partial.

The spectrum of disease in AIDS cholangiopathy also includes acalculous cholecystitis (also caused by opportunistic infection), lymphoma, Kaposi sarcoma, and cholelithiasis. The medical treatment of the underlying opportunistic infection does not appear to significantly improve symptoms or cholangiopathic abnormalities. Epstein-Barr virus (HHV-4), the etiology of infectious mononucleosis, has not been directly associated with AIDS cholangiopathy. It has been associated with lymphomas (including posttransplant lymphoproliferative disorder) and nasopharyngeal carcinoma.

References: Bilgin M, Balci NC, Erdogan A, et al. Hepatobiliary and pancreatic MRI and MRCP findings in patients with HIV infection. *AJR Am J Roentgenol* 2008;191(1):228–232.

Katabathina VS, Dasyam AK, Dasyam N, et al. Adult bile duct strictures: role of MR imaging and MR cholangiopancreatography in characterization. *Radiographics* 2014;34(3):565–586.

24b **Answer A.** The majority (60% to 70%) of patients with AIDS cholangiopathy have papillary stenosis related to inflammation caused by the pathogen. This is most often accompanied by findings of sclerosing cholangitis but some have papillary stenosis in isolation. **The combination of papillary stenosis with intrahepatic strictures has been described as being highly suggestive of AIDS cholangitis.** Ultrasound and MRCP are helpful in the initial identification of biliary abnormalities and patient selection for ERCP.

Endoscopy with ERCP is appropriate for further evaluation and treatment of suspected papillary stenosis and cholangitis. Endoscopy allows direct visualization of the papilla, assessment of contrast flow, and biopsy of suspicious lesions. On ERCP, the criteria for papillary stenosis include CBD diameter >8 mm and distal tapering of the terminal 2 to 4 mm of duct, along with abnormal contrast retention. **Technically, there are no established criteria on MRCP for papillary stenosis, although a dilated duct above a short segment of terminal tapering is suggestive in the appropriate clinical setting.** The treatment of AIDS cholangiopathy is usually endoscopic, with sphincterotomy for papillary stenosis and stents for strictures.

References: Bilgin M, Balci NC, Erdogan A, et al. Hepatobiliary and pancreatic MRI and MRCP findings in patients with HIV infection. *AJR Am J Roentgenol* 2008;191(1):228–223.

Katabathina VS, Dasyam AK, Dasyam N, et al. Adult bile duct strictures: role of MR imaging and MR cholangiopancreatography in characterization. *Radiographics* 2014;34(3):565–586.

25 **Answer D.** These are **peribiliary cysts**, which are usually nonobstructing incidental findings in patients with cirrhosis or other underlying severe liver disease. (Note the nodular liver margin consistent with cirrhosis best demonstrated on the coronal CT image.) These cysts **do not communicate with the lumen** but arise in the ductal wall and adjacent connective tissues, thought to represent dilated peribiliary glands. The T2W MR images demonstrate the **classic configuration of small cysts with hairline-thin walls, clustered in the periportal region along the major central bile ducts**. These are of no clinical significance, but **peribiliary cysts can be**

mistaken for obstructed bile ducts, complex cystic masses, or periportal edema. CT (as shown) and US may not be able to demonstrate that these represent individual cysts. Primary sclerosing cholangitis (or other cholangitis) can have beaded morphology due to multifocal strictures with intervening duct dilation but typically have irregular appearance and scattered distribution.

References: Baron RL, Campbell WL, Dodd GD. Peribiliary cysts associated with severe liver disease: imaging-pathologic correlation. *AJR Am J Roentgenol* 1994;162(3):631–636.

Katabathina VS, Flaherty EM, Dasyam AK, et al. "Biliary Diseases with Pancreatic Counterparts": cross-sectional imaging findings. *Radiographics* 2016;36(2):374–392.

26 **Answer: E. Choledocholithiasis** can be diagnosed on CT if the gallstone has characteristic calcification or gas, and is surrounded by a rim of bile. When the density of the gallstone overlaps that of soft tissue, choledocholithiasis can mimic neoplasm. In those cases, ERCP or CT with pre- and postcontrast imaging to detect enhancement can help distinguish between gallstone and neoplasm. **If the gallstone is not initially identified on CT, narrowing the window settings may help detect a faint rim of a nearly isodense stone within the dilated duct.** MRCP would help demonstrate a filling defect in the duct. Ultrasound can detect choledocholithiasis in some cases, but evaluation of the distal duct can be limited. The triradiate configuration of the clefts of gas in a gallstone may produce the classic "Mercedes-Benz" sign (arrow) as seen on the following coronal CT image of the gallbladder in a different patient.

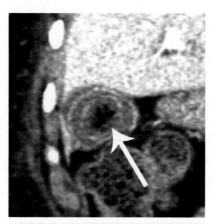

Mercedes-Benz sign in gallstone.

References: Anderson SW, Lucey BC, Varghese JC, et al. Accuracy of MDCT in the diagnosis of choledocholithiasis. *AJR Am J Roentgenol* 2006;187(1):174–180.

Raman SP, Fishman EK. Abnormalities of the distal common bile duct and ampulla: diagnostic approach and differential diagnosis using multiplanar reformations and 3D imaging. *AJR Am J Roentgenol*. 2014;203(1):17–28.

27 **Answer B.** There is an obstructing mass-forming cholangiocarcinoma (CCA) at the biliary hilum (known as a **Klatskin tumor** in this location). CCA is a primary adenocarcinoma of the biliary ducts. The thick-slab coronal MRCP shows signal dropout at the biliary hilum. Thin-slice coronal MRCP image demonstrates the corresponding soft tissue mass. **Because CCA tends to be fibrotic, enhancement may be progressive and more prominent on delayed phase CT and MRI.** The differential diagnosis may include metastatic adenopathy in the porta hepatis from another source.

CCA is classified by anatomic location by the American Joint Committee on Cancer and by morphology by the World Health Organization as shown in the following table. These classifications help determine prognosis and help direct appropriate management.

Classification of Cholangiocarcinoma	

Anatomic	• Intrahepatic
	  o Peripheral to secondary bifurcation of R or L hepatic duct
	  o Hepatectomy for resection
	• Hilar (also known as "Klatskin tumor")
	  o Most common location (50%–65% of CCA)
	  o Hilum including R/L hepatic ducts and common duct down to level of cystic duct bifurcation
	  o Bile duct resection often with hepatectomy
	• Distal extrahepatic
	  o Below the origin of the cystic duct
	  o Pancreaticoduodenectomy for resection

Morphologic	• Mass forming • Periductal infiltrating • Intraductal growing (least common)

CCA is the second most common primary hepatobiliary malignancy after hepatocellular carcinoma. Patients are typically in their 50s to 70s and present with painless jaundice. **Cases are often sporadic, but risk factors for CCA include chronic inflammatory conditions** such as primary sclerosing cholangitis, choledochal cysts, intrahepatic biliary stone disease, parasitic infection, and biliary-enteric anastomosis. Complete resection is curative, but because CCA is difficult to diagnose early, complete resection may not be possible and prognosis is generally poor. CT, MRI, and in some cases PET/CT imaging are useful in determining resectability and in staging. Ancillary treatment includes stenting, radiation, and chemotherapy.

References: Chung YE, Kim MJ, Park YN, et al. Varying appearances of cholangiocarcinoma: radiologic-pathologic correlation. *Radiographics* 2009;29(3):683–700.

Engelbrecht MR, Katz SS, van Gulik TM, et al. Imaging of perihilar cholangiocarcinoma. *AJR Am J Roentgenol* 2015;204(4):782–791.

28 | **Answer B.** The patient has cholangiocarcinoma (CCA) in the intrapancreatic segment of the common bile duct (arrows). Morphology is the **periductal infiltrating type of CCA** with enhancing circumferential wall thickening resulting in an obstructing stricture.

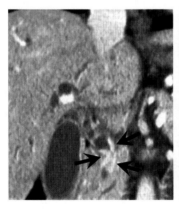 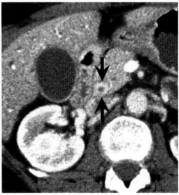

Differential diagnosis of strictures with wall thickening and enhancement includes primary sclerosing cholangitis and the various types of secondary cholangitis (e.g., ascending, IgG4-related (autoimmune), and AIDS cholangitis). **Because even small CCAs can cause biliary ductal dilation, unexplained**

segmental ductal dilation (with or without lobar atrophy) should raise suspicion for CCA even if a tumor is not visible. Correlation with history, clinical factors, and brush biopsy at the time of endoscopic stent placement may be needed. Repeated biopsy may be necessary as sensitivity is limited by the submucosal spread of this tumor. It is best to perform cross-sectional imaging before biliary stent placement, as the stent can induce secondary ductal wall thickening and enhancement confounding evaluation of the extent of disease.

The least common morphologic type of CCA is the intraductal growing type (shown below in a different patient). This type of CCA arises in polypoid precursors such as intraductal papillary neoplasm of the bile duct (IPN-B) or intraductal tubulopapillary neoplasm (ITPN). IPN-B is analogous to intraductal papillary mucinous neoplasm (IPMN) of the pancreas. An enhancing polypoid mass (arrows) fills the lumen and causes upstream duct dilation. **Downstream ducts may also be dilated if the tumor produces mucin.** Intraductal neoplasms grow more slowly and have a **better prognosis than the other types of CCA**. Resection may reveal a combination of benign, dysplastic, or malignant tissue. The main differential diagnosis of a mass-like intraluminal filling defect includes stones (as well as other debris or blood clots), which do not enhance. Metastases are much less common.

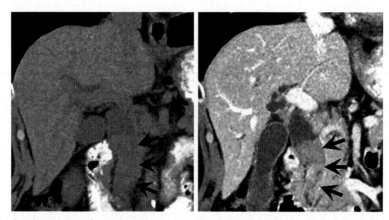

Intraluminal enhancing polypoid mass representing intraductal growing CCA arising in IPN-B.

References: Chatterjee A, Lopes Vendrami C, Nikolaidis P, et al. Uncommon intraluminal tumors of the gallbladder and biliary tract: spectrum of imaging appearances. *Radiographics* 2019;39(2):388–412.29.

Itri JN, de Lange EE. Extrahepatic cholangiocarcinoma: what the surgeon needs to know radiographics fundamentals online presentation. *Radiographics* 2018;38(7):2019–2020.

29 **Answer D.** An ampullary carcinoma is demonstrated. There is biliary ductal dilation down to the ampulla where there is an enhancing polypoid mass (arrows) protruding into the duodenal lumen shown on the following axial and coronal images.

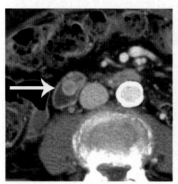 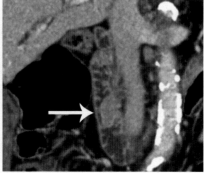

Ampullary and periampullary neoplasms may not be well visualized on imaging since they can be small and/or obscured by normal decompressed duodenum. **Improving duodenal distention with water can improve visualization** of ampullary masses. Patients may require endoscopy and ERCP to evaluate for an occult obstructing lesion.

The differential diagnosis of an enlarged, "bulging" papilla (>10 mm diameter) includes papillitis, intraductal papillary mucinous neoplasm (IPMN), or choledochocele. Papillitis is inflammation that may be caused by an impacted stone or a cholangitis, especially in AIDS cholangitis in which papillary stenosis is a salient feature. The mucin produced by an intraductal papillary neoplasm (usually from the pancreas but sometimes from the bile ducts) can distend the papilla and be seen extruding from the orifice at endoscopy. A choledochocele is a type III choledochal cyst representing cystic dilation of the most distal aspect of the CBD.

Ampullary neoplasms are defined as tumors that occur distal to the confluence of the CBD and pancreatic duct. Tumors that occur within 1 to 2 cm of the ampulla of Vater may be of ampullary, pancreatic, biliary, or duodenal origin. These are referred to as "periampullary" neoplasms if it is not possible to determine the origin at histology. CBD dilation is seen in about 75% of cases, with a smaller percentage showing pancreatic ductal dilation. **The "double-duct" sign referring to dilation of both ducts is most commonly associated with pancreatic ductal adenocarcinoma but can also be seen with ampullary and periampullary neoplasms.** These malignancies if resectable require a Whipple procedure.

References: Kim S, Lee NK, Lee JW, et al. CT evaluation of the bulging papilla with endoscopic correlation. *Radiographics* 2007;27(4):1023–1038.

Nikolaidis P, Hammond NA, Day K, et al. Imaging features of benign and malignant ampullary and periampullary lesions. *Radiographics* 2014;34(3):624–641.

30 **Answer A.** Ultrasound and MRCP show a mildly dilated CBD with a serpiginous, tubular filling defect (arrows) consistent with ascariasis.

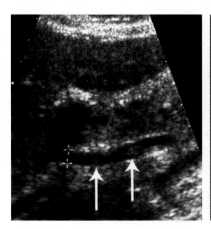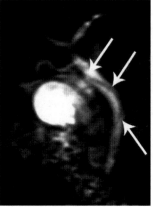

The differential diagnosis of a tubular filling defect includes a stent, debris, or hemobilia. Bile flow artifact is usually faint and exactly central, most evident in the single-shot fast spin echo series, and not apparent when correlating with other series or planes.

Ascaris lumbricoides is the most common parasitic infestation in the world affecting humans. It is most often seen in tropical and subtropical locations but relatively uncommon in the United States and other developed countries. Ascariasis most commonly presents as bowel obstruction from a mass of worms. The worms can migrate from the bowel into the pancreaticobiliary tree through the duodenal papilla, causing **ductal obstruction with cholangitis and pancreatitis. Hepatic abscess** may be seen in severe cases. Treatment is antiparasitic medical therapy and surgical removal of the worms.

References: Lim JH, Kim SY, Park CM. Parasitic diseases of the biliary tract. *AJR Am J Roentgenol* 2007;188(6):1596–1603.

Yeh BM, Chang WC. Chapter 80: Inflammatory disorders of the biliary tract. In: Gore RM, Levine MS (eds). *Textbook of gastrointestinal radiology*, 4th ed. Philadelphia, PA: Elsevier/Saunders, 2015:1427–1441.

31 **Answer C.** The patient has developed layering high density in the gallbladder after recent intravenous administration of iodinated contrast, consistent with vicarious excretion. Most of the contrast is excreted by the kidneys, but a small amount is excreted into the biliary tree. **Vicarious excretion is a common phenomenon.** It is more likely to be visible on a subsequent CT in the setting of decreased renal function, higher contrast dose, and reduced gallbladder emptying (such as in the fasting state). Since it can also be seen in patients with normal serum creatinine levels, it does not necessarily indicate impaired renal function.

Layering high density in the gallbladder can be seen with milk of calcium and hemorrhage. Milk of calcium is a thick substance containing calcium carbonate that can accumulate in the setting of chronic cystic duct obstruction. It would not be expected to develop in 13 hours between the two scans. Hydrops is marked distention of the gallbladder with mucus. This can occur in some cases of chronic cystic duct obstruction. There is no wall thickening or pericholecystic fluid to suggest acute cholecystitis.

References: Boland GWL, Halpert RD. Chapter 8: Gallbladder. In: Boland GWL, Halpert RD (eds). *Gastrointestinal imaging: the requisites*, 4th ed. Philadelphia, PA: Elsevier/Saunders, 2014:315–346.

Krauthamer A, Maldjian PD. Visualization of noncalcified gallstones on CT due to vicarious excretion of intravenous contrast. *J Radiol Case Rep* 2008;2(2):5–8.

32 **Answers:**
Patient 1: C. Posterior right hepatic duct draining into left hepatic duct
Patient 2: A. Conventional biliary anatomy
Patient 2: B. Low and medial insertion of the cystic duct
Patient 4: D. Hepatocystic duct

Biliary ductal variants are associated with increased risk of bile duct injury at the time of surgery (e.g., liver transplant donation, hepatectomy, laparoscopic cholecystectomy). Recognition at MRCP may help surgical planning.

In patient 1, the right posterior hepatic duct drains into the left hepatic duct (arrow in the following image). **This patient also demonstrates a parallel course of the cystic duct (arrowheads), which may be mistaken for a single dilated common duct** on imaging.

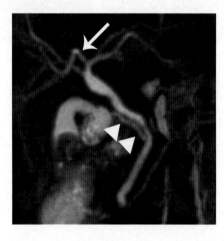

Patient 2 has conventional biliary anatomy, which occurs in about 60% of the population.

Patient 3 has a low and medial insertion of the cystic duct. The cystic duct crosses the common duct from right to left to enter the medial side, at the lower third of the common duct.

Patient 4 has a hepatocystic duct, with a duct from the right lobe traveling through the hepatocystic space draining into the cystic duct (arrows on image below). In contradistinction, small ducts that travel through the gallbladder fossa are considered a subtype of subvesical duct (formerly known as ducts of Luschka) extending from the right lobe and draining into the gallbladder or other ducts. Also incidentally noted in this patient is a nonobstructing impression on the common hepatic duct (arrowhead), which correlated with a normal crossing vessel on other MRCP images (not shown). This is clinically insignificant and should not be mistaken for a stricture. Biliary trifurcation is another ductal variant among the answer choices (not shown).

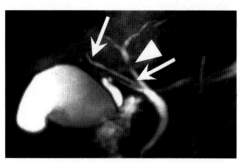

References: Catalano OA, Singh AH, Uppot RN, et al. Vascular and biliary variants in the liver: implications for liver surgery. *Radiographics* 2008;28:359–378.

Yu J, Turner MA, Fulcher AS, et al. Congenital anomalies and normal variants of the pancreaticobiliary tract and the pancreas in adults: part 1, Biliary tract. *AJR Am J Roentgenol* 2006;187(6):1536–1543.

33 **Answer D.** MRCP in this patient who had a liver transplant for primary sclerosing cholangitis (PSC) shows widespread multifocal intrahepatic ductal irregularity and stricturing. Among the choices presented, these findings are most consistent with **recurrent PSC. Ischemic cholangiopathy is also an important cause of nonanastomotic strictures** in liver transplant patients, but this is less likely, although not excluded in the setting of normal arterial flow on Doppler ultrasound. **Secondary cholangitis (not among the answer choices) can have a similar appearance, including ascending (pyogenic) cholangitis and immunologic cholangitis from chronic or acute rejection.** Recurrent PSC develops in 5% to 20% of patients who undergo liver transplant for PSC. Progression of disease may require retransplantation.

The recipient's distal CBD has been ligated and is seen as a blind-ending duct that remains in the pancreatic head. In this patient with PSC, resection of the diseased CBD was required and a hepaticojejunostomy was performed at the time of transplant (common hepatic duct to jejunum with Roux-en-Y reconstruction) rather than a biliary–biliary anastomosis. No choledocholithiasis or other filling defects are seen in the ducts. Cholangiocarcinoma is not the correct answer choice as it is not this diffuse.

Biliary strictures are an important complication of liver transplants. The reported incidence is 5% to 15% in cadaveric transplants and up to 30% in living donor transplants. Strictures may be anastomotic or nonanastomotic. **Anastomotic strictures account for 75% to 90% of cases as a result of fibrosis or ischemia.** In patients who have had liver transplant with biliary–biliary anastomosis, some discrepancy can be normally expected between the caliber of the donor and recipient ducts that can mimic a stricture. Nonanastomotic strictures are often multiple and longer. Nonanastomotic strictures are usually vascular in etiology and can be macroangiopathic due to hepatic artery thrombosis or microangiopathic due to factors such as prolonged ischemia time, donor cardiac death, vasopressors, and immunogenic. Treatment options of biliary strictures include balloon angioplasty, stenting, and resection with reanastomosis.

References: Horrow MM, Huynh ML, Callaghan MM, et al. Complications after liver transplant related to preexisting conditions: diagnosis, treatment, and prevention. *Radiographics* 2020;40(3):895–909.

Khoshpouri P, Habibabadi RR, Hazhirkarzar B, et al. Imaging features of primary sclerosing cholangitis: from diagnosis to liver transplant follow-up. *Radiographics* 2019;39(7):1938–1964.

34 **Answers:**
Patient 1: C. Crossing vessel
Patient 2: A. Pneumobilia
Patient 3: D. Bile flow artifact
Patient 4: B. Surgical clip

This series of cases illustrates common biliary pitfalls on MRCP that may mimic pathology. Recognition and correlation with other series or prior studies can confirm the pitfalls and prevent unnecessary ERCP.

The finding in patient 1 is caused by a **normal crossing vessel**. 3D MRCP image demonstrates **eccentric slight focal narrowing of the common hepatic duct not causing biliary obstruction**. A coronal image from the arterial phase of the prior CT scan shows a bright focus in the porta hepatis representing the hepatic artery (arrow) seen in cross section as it travels between the common duct and the portal vein.

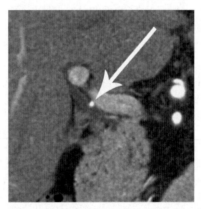

Crossing vessel adjacent to the common duct.

In this case, we happen to have a prior CT that reveals this normal anatomy, but careful correlation with the thin slices on MRCP and familiarity with the normal anatomic relationship are usually adequate. If the MRCP protocol includes a "bright blood" steady-state free precession T2W sequence (e.g., FIESTA or TrueFISP), this vessel may be visible as a bright structure overlapping the duct. Some findings are more easily recognized on CT, such as cholecystectomy clips and biliary stents.

Patient 2 has pneumobilia. **Gas is dark on all MR sequences.** On this axial image, the gas rises to the **nondependent** aspect of bile duct and produces an **air–fluid level with a meniscus**. Stones are also dark but are typically dependent within the duct. Pneumobilia may mimic choledocholithiasis on coronal images because the nondependent position of the gas is not appreciated. It is important to correlate any filling defects on coronal series with thin-slice axial images to avoid this pitfall.

The axial image from an MRCP on patient 3 demonstrates a **bile flow artifact**. This artifact typically appears as a **tiny faint dot in the center of the duct on axial images or occasionally as a thin central linear filling defect on coronal images**. This artifact is common on the **half-Fourier single-shot spin echo** (e.g., HASTE or SSFSE) sequences, which are among the main diagnostic sequences in MRCP. This is an ultrafast sequence acquired with data from a single echo, but it is susceptible to motion such as bile flow that occurs within the time of the slice acquisition, resulting in signal loss. **Correlation with other planes and multishot sequences should show no true filling defects.** The effects of motion on multishot sequences are averaged and cancel out over the multiple echoes that contribute to slice acquisition. Choledocholithiasis is typically in the dependent portion of the duct, not suspended in the center of the duct. In ascariasis, the parasite is a serpiginous linear filling defect within the duct.

Patient 4 has a pseudostricture related to **susceptibility artifact from a cholecystectomy clip**. Surgical clips are dark on all MR series. The artifact associated with the metal is larger than the clip itself. **This "blooming" may affect the adjacent bile duct causing signal dropout.** The thin coronal MRCP image reveals a dark transverse line (arrows) representing the clip. The bright bands bracketing the clip on the left and right sides represent surrounding image distortion.

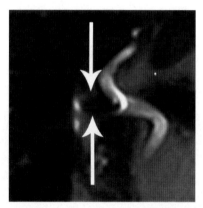

Cholecystectomy clip with susceptibility artifact.

References: Hoang PB, Huang SY, Song AW, et al. Chapter 9: Motion, pulsation, and other artifacts. In: Mangrum WI (ed). *Duke review of MRI physics*, 2nd ed. Philadelphia, PA: Elsevier, Inc., 2019: 91–105.

Irie H, Honda H, Kuroiwa T, et al. Pitfalls in MR cholangiopancreatographic interpretation. *Radiographics* 2001;21(1):23–37.

Katabathina VS, Dasyam AK, Dasyam N, et al. Adult bile duct strictures: role of MR imaging and MR cholangiopancreatography in characterization. *Radiographics* 2014;34(3):565–586.

Yeh BM, Liu PS, Soto JA, et al. MR imaging and CT of the biliary tract. *Radiographics* 2009;29(6):1669–1688.

QUESTIONS

1 On this CT image from a 47-year-old woman with resolving acute pancreatitis, match each labeled retroperitoneal structure (A to F) with the corresponding anatomic description (1 to 6). Each option may be used only once.

1. Anterior renal fascia
2. Posterior renal fascia
3. Lateroconal fascia
4. Anterior pararenal space
5. Perirenal space
6. Posterior pararenal space

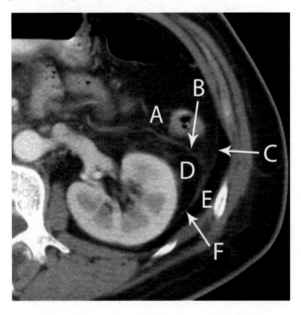

2 The CT images below are from an 82-year-old woman with abdominal distention. No intravenous contrast was given because of renal insufficiency. What is the most likely diagnosis?

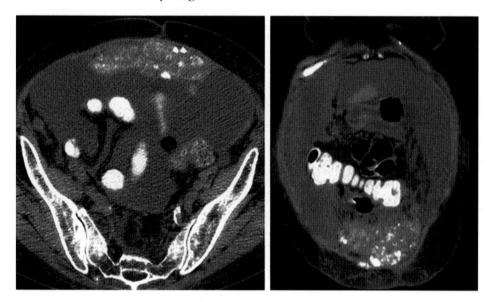

A. Colon carcinoma
B. Lymphoma
C. Mesothelioma
D. Ovarian carcinoma

3 An axial image from a contrast-enhanced abdominopelvic CT performed on a 53-year-old man following blunt injury to the abdomen is shown. Which of the following best explains the findings?

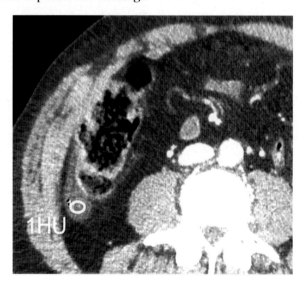

A. Jejunal injury
B. Postbulbar duodenal injury
C. Occult solid organ laceration
D. Abdominal ascites from cirrhosis

4 An 84-year-old woman presents with nausea and vomiting. What is the finding on the following abdominal radiograph and CT scan?

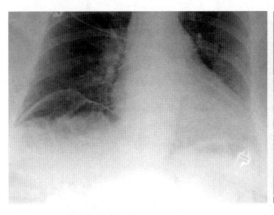 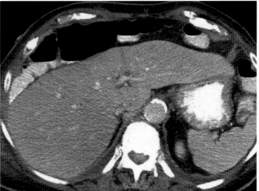

A. Gastric perforation
B. Small bowel obstruction
C. Colonic interposition
D. Morgagni hernia

5 A 55-year-old man with a history of a Whipple procedure for resection of ampullary carcinoma was evaluated with CT scans. The CT on the left was obtained 3 weeks after surgery, and the CT on the right was obtained 18 months later. What is the abnormality in the left anterior abdomen?

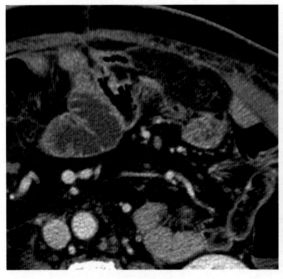 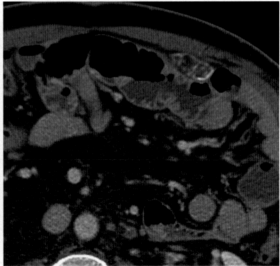

A. Fat necrosis
B. Liposarcoma
C. Abscess
D. Peritoneal carcinomatosis

6 A 60-year-old woman presents with abdominal pain, distention, and constipation. Images from a CT scan are shown below. No malignant cells were identified in the fluid obtained at paracentesis. What is the most likely etiology of the imaging findings?

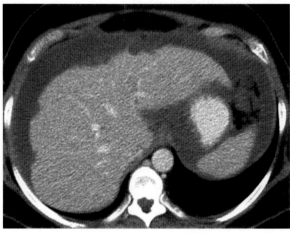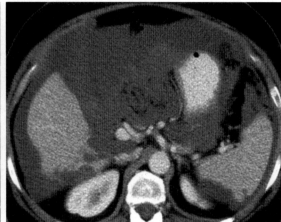

A. Cirrhosis with portal hypertension
B. Appendiceal neoplasm
C. Intraperitoneal bladder rupture
D. Sclerosing encapsulating peritonitis

7 A patient presented with gastrointestinal bleeding. A finding was noted on the CT shown below. After further workup, the patient did not require treatment, and findings were stable at 3 years. This condition may be seen as part of a multisystemic process in association with which of the following diseases?

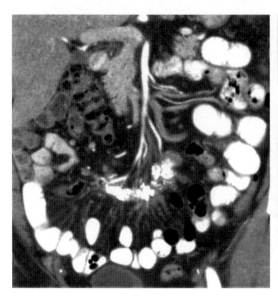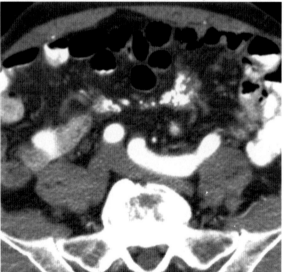

A. Retroperitoneal fibrosis
B. Tuberous sclerosis
C. Whipple disease
D. Graft versus host disease

8 A 74-year-old man presents with abdominal pain and vomiting. What is the diagnosis?

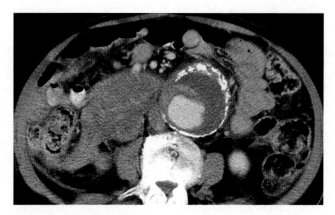

A. Ruptured aortic aneurysm
B. Leiomyosarcoma of the inferior vena cava
C. Lymphoma
D. Type II endoleak

9 What is the finding on the following radiograph?

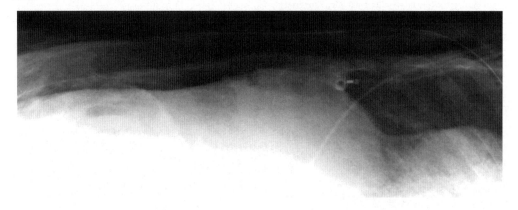

A. Ascites
B. Colonic obstruction
C. Pneumoperitoneum
D. Loculated pleural effusion

10a A 27-year-old patient was stabbed in the upper left flank. He is hemodynamically stable. What of the following imaging studies is the best screening test in this patient for findings requiring laparotomy?

A. FAST (focused assessment with sonography in trauma)
B. Noncontrast abdominopelvic CT
C. Venous phase abdominopelvic CT
D. Abdominopelvic CT with intravenous and rectal contrast

10b Subsequent CT was performed with "triple contrast"—IV, rectal, and oral contrast. What is the deepest structure penetrated by the left flank stab wound?

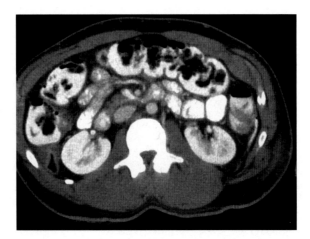

A. Left kidney
B. Descending colon
C. Retroperitoneal fat
D. Subcutaneous tissues

11a A 55-year-old man with a history of total colectomy and J-pouch reconstruction for ulcerative colitis is now 4 days status post surgery for ileostomy takedown. Which statement is most likely TRUE about the appearance of the abdomen on the following radiograph?

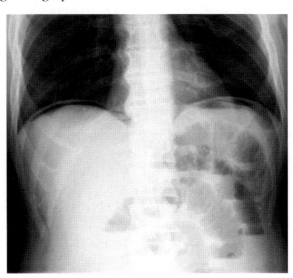

A. The patient requires surgical exploration.
B. The patient requires percutaneous drainage.
C. Findings are within expectations for the postoperative state.
D. Findings are most likely related to mechanical ventilation.

11b What sign is demonstrated in the right upper quadrant on the following supine AP abdominal radiograph?

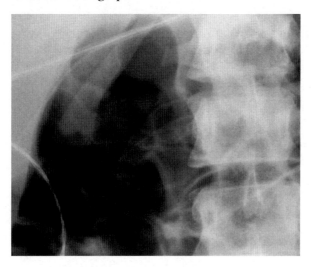

A. Rigler sign
B. Falciform ligament sign
C. Football sign
D. Inverted V sign

12 A 31-year-old woman with a history of inflammatory bowel disease and Caesarean section presents with pelvic and back pain. An MRI was performed. What is the most likely diagnosis?

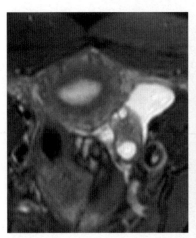 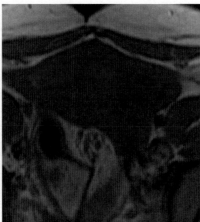 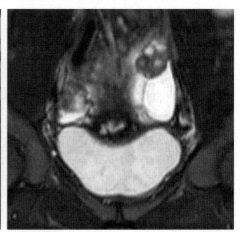

Axial FS T2W, axial T1W, and coronal FS T2W MRI.

A. Colonic duplication cyst
B. Peritoneal inclusion cyst
C. Congenital mesothelial cyst
D. Mature cystic teratoma

13 For the finding associated with the IVC in patients 1 to 3, select the most likely diagnosis (A to E). Each option may be used once or not at all.

Patient 1. Axial and coronal images from contrast-enhanced CT.

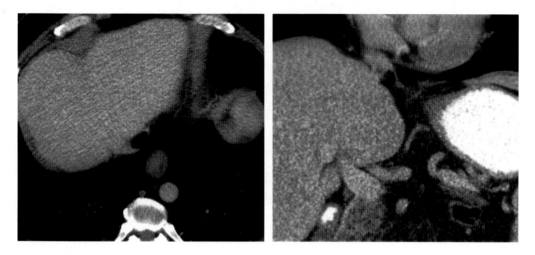

Patient 2. Axial and coronal images from contrast-enhanced CT.

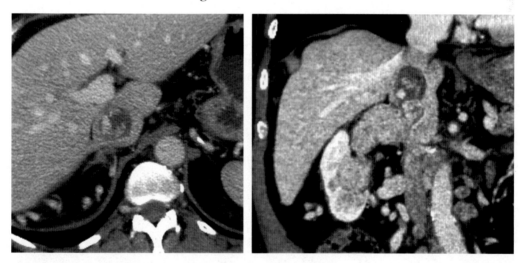

Patient 3. Axial, coronal, and axial images from multiphase contrast-enhanced CT.

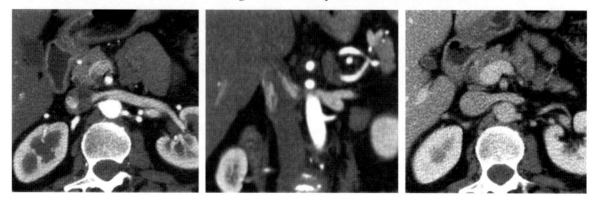

    A. Mixing artifact
    B. Pseudolipoma
    C. Bland thrombus
    D. Tumor thrombus
    E. Primary IVC sarcoma

14 A 57-year-old man undergoes a CT for the evaluation of diarrhea. What is the most likely diagnosis of the finding on the following CT image?

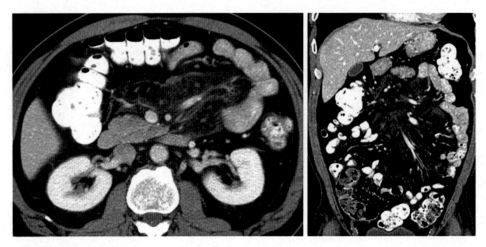

A. Liposarcoma
B. Lymphoma
C. Desmoid tumor
D. Sclerosing mesenteritis

15 Images from a CT scan in a patient with lower abdominal and back pain are shown below. No malignancy was found on subsequent evaluation. This disease process most commonly affects which group of patients?

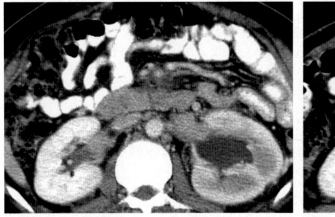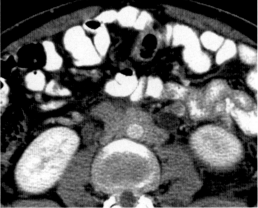

A. Men aged 20 to 30
B. Women aged 20 to 30
C. Men aged 40 to 60
D. Women aged 40 to 60

Match the images for the patients in Questions 16 to 19 with the most likely diagnosis (A to D). Each option may be used only once.

A. Testicular carcinoma metastases
B. Lymphoma
C. Paraganglioma
D. Lymphangioma

16 A 34-year-old man with epigastric pain and early satiety. Axial and coronal CT images are shown.

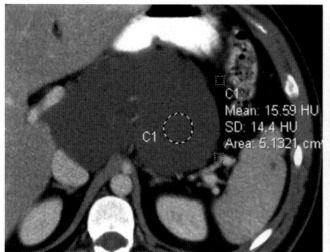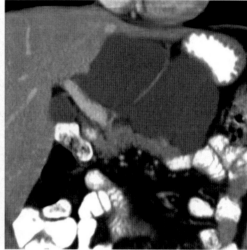

17 A 70-year-old man with back pain.

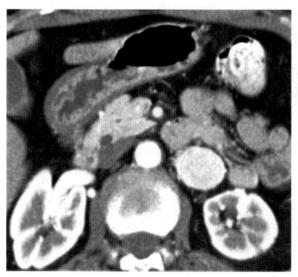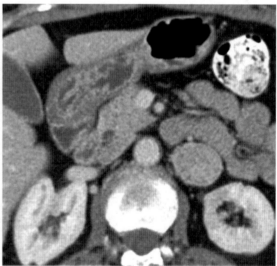

18 A 63-year-old man with fatigue.

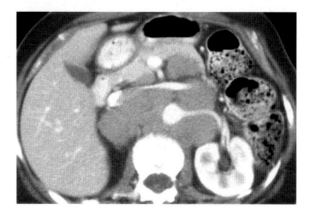

19 A 33-year-old man with back pain.

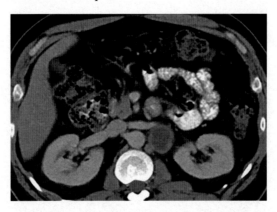

20 A 53-year-old man complains of right lower quadrant pain. What is the most likely diagnosis?

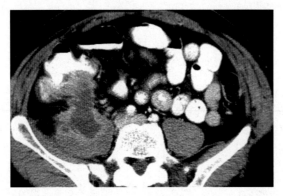

A. Meckel diverticulitis
B. Schwannoma
C. Colon carcinoma
D. Hematoma

21 A 74-year-old man remains hospitalized several days after aortobifemoral bypass graft surgery, which was complicated by a large hemorrhage. The patient has acutely developed renal failure. A CT scan is performed with enteric contrast administered through the gastrostomy tube but no IV contrast. What is the most likely diagnosis?

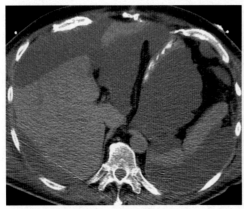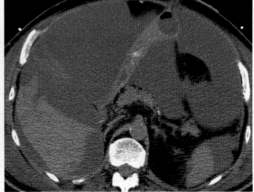

A. Splenic laceration
B. Gastric perforation
C. Pseudomyxoma peritonei
D. Abdominal compartment syndrome

22 A 53-year-old man presents with right flank pain for over 6 months. Ultrasound was performed, which showed a mass. Further evaluation was performed with CT and MRI. What is the most likely diagnosis?

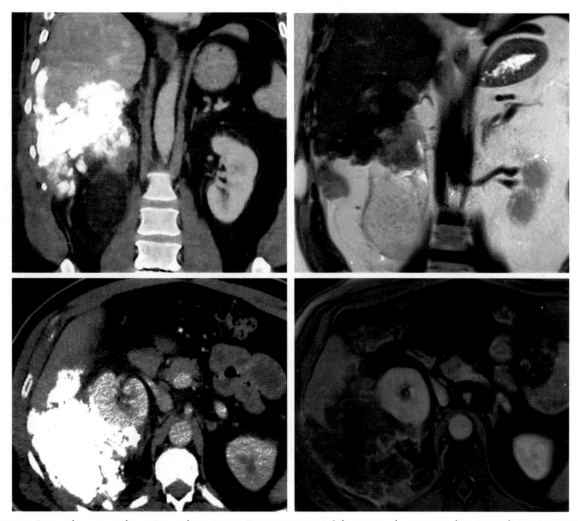

Top row: Coronal venous phase CT and T2W MRI. **Bottom row:** Axial venous phase CT and venous phase FS T1W MRI.

    A. Angiomyolipoma
    B. Renal cell carcinoma
    C. Chondrosarcoma
    D. Liposarcoma

ANSWERS AND EXPLANATIONS

1 **Answers: A4; B1; C3; D5; E6; F2.**

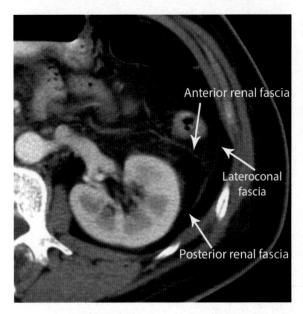

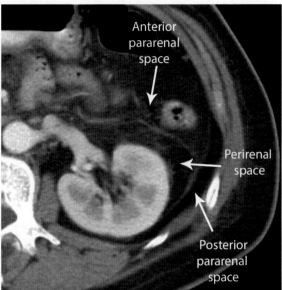

The retroperitoneum can be subdivided into the anterior pararenal space, the perirenal (or perinephric) space, and the posterior pararenal space, which are separated by fascial planes. The fascial trifurcation is the fusion site of the anterior renal fascia (Gerota fascia), posterior renal fascia, and lateroconal fascia and is typically located posterior to the ascending and descending colon. **The multilayered fascia is potentially expansile, is normally 1 to 3 mm in thickness, and may either serve as conduits or barriers for disease spread** in the abdomen and pelvis.

The **anterior pararenal space** is bounded by the posterior parietal peritoneum anteriorly, the anterior renal fascia posteriorly, and the lateroconal fascia laterally. It is contiguous across the midline and contains the ascending colon, the descending colon, the 2nd to 4th portions of the duodenum, and the pancreas.

The **perirenal (or perinephric) spac**e is bounded by the anterior renal fascia anteriorly and the posterior renal fascia posteriorly. It contains the kidneys, renal pelves, proximal ureters, adrenal glands, and fat. The septae of Kunin are fibrous lamellae located in the perirenal space, some of which extend from the renal capsule to the renal fasciae. They may serve as conduits of disease spread.

The **posterior pararenal space** is bounded by the posterior renal fascia anteriorly, the transversalis fascia posteriorly, and the psoas muscle medially. It contains fat and is contiguous with properitoneal fat of the abdomen anteriorly and laterally.

References: Torigian DA, Kitazono MT. Abdomen. In: Torigian DA, Kitazono MT (eds). *Netter's correlative imaging: abdominal and pelvic anatomy*. Philadelphia, PA: Elsevier, 2013:13–108.

Torigian DA, Ramchandani P. CT and MRI of the retroperitoneum. In: Haaga JR, Lanzieri CF, Gilkeson RC (eds). *CT and MRI imaging of the whole body*, 5th ed. Philadelphia, PA: Elsevier, 2009:1953–2040.

2 **Answer D.** There is omental caking with nodular calcifications, most likely peritoneal carcinomatosis from ovarian cancer in this female patient. This appearance may mimic bowel with oral contrast. **Calcifications may be seen in**

both serous and mucinous ovarian neoplasms. Peritoneal carcinomatosis can be "wet" with associated ascites as in this case or "dry" with little to no visible ascites. Mucinous colon cancer is the most common cause of calcified hepatic metastases, but is a less common cause of calcified peritoneal carcinomatosis.

Tumors of ovarian and gastrointestinal origin are the most common causes of carcinomatosis. CT findings of peritoneal carcinomatosis include subtle infiltration of the omental or mesenteric fat; soft tissue nodules; peritoneal nodular thickening and enhancement; ascites; and abdominopelvic organ invasion. Lymphoma with peritoneal involvement and peritoneal mesothelioma can manifest as omental caking, but they are not associated with calcification unless treated. Malignant peritoneal mesothelioma is a rare and often rapidly fatal malignancy, with the main risk factor being prior asbestos exposure.

CT is the study of choice for the evaluation of peritoneal and mesenteric pathology. **Common sites of peritoneal implants are in the dependent aspects of the pelvis (rectouterine pouch of Douglas in women or rectovesical space in men), ileocecal region, paracolic gutters, subhepatic space, subphrenic space, and root of the mesentery.** Patients can develop multifocal small bowel obstruction from tumor implants. Peritoneal carcinomatosis is incurable and predominantly treated with chemotherapy. In patients with ovarian and primary peritoneal carcinomatosis, cytoreductive surgery has been shown to increase survival.

In the United States, **tuberculosis and other causes of granulomatous peritonitis (e.g., fungal infection) should be considered in the setting of peritoneal nodularity** in immunocompromised patients, with or without calcification. Spontaneous bacterial peritonitis (SBP) can be associated with peritoneal thickening and enhancement but is typically smooth (arrows on the following image). SBP usually occurs in patients with cirrhosis and ascites. Likewise, peritoneal calcifications associated with nongranulomatous benign causes of peritoneal disease (such as prior bacterial peritonitis, secondary hyperparathyroidism, and chronic peritoneal dialysis) are typically smooth and sheet-like rather than nodular. Clinical correlation is important as **smooth enhancement does not exclude peritoneal malignancy.**

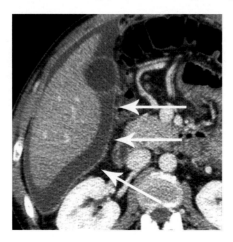

References: Marques DT, Tenório de Brito Siqueira L, Franca Bezerra RO, et al. Resident and fellow education feature: imaging evaluation of peritoneal disease: overview of anatomy and differential diagnosis. *Radiographics* 2014;34(4):962–963.

Zulfiqar M, Shetty A, Tsai R, et al. Diagnostic approach to benign and malignant calcifications in the abdomen and pelvis. *Radiographics* 2020;40(3):731–753.

3 **Answer A.** The findings are compatible with jejunal injury. There is intraperitoneal free fluid, which is low density, as well as two small foci of pneumoperitoneum in the antidependent abdomen (arrows). **In the acute**

blunt trauma setting, the combination of low-density free fluid and free air requires consideration of three things: **(1) intraperitoneal bowel injury** (not postbulbar duodenum, ascending/descending colon, or rectum, which are extraperitoneal), **(2) intraperitoneal bladder rupture (if patient has been catheterized, introducing gas into the urine)**, and **(3) diagnostic peritoneal *lavage*** if the patient's hospital performs this procedure. (Of note, diagnostic peritoneal *aspiration* involves aspiration only and not instillation of fluid, so the free fluid cannot be attributed to that procedure.) Free air should be absent with ascites from cirrhosis and with solid organ laceration, and the latter should result in hemoperitoneum, not low-density free fluid. Assuming a diagnostic peritoneal lavage was not performed, a patient with hematuria should have **CT cystogram to exclude intraperitoneal bladder rupture**, and there should be strong **consideration for laparotomy to identify a traumatic bowel injury**.

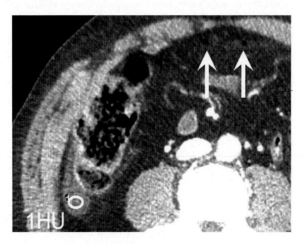

References: Bekker W, Kong VY, Laing GL, et al. The spectrum and outcome of blunt trauma related enteric hollow visceral injury. *Ann R Coll Surg Engl* 2018;100:290–294.

Firetto MC, Sala F, Petrini M, et al. Blunt bowel and mesenteric trauma: role of clinical signs along with CT findings in patients' management. *Emerg Radiol* 2018;25:461–467.

4 **Answer C.** Interposition of the colon is seen between the liver and the diaphragm. **The interposition of bowel in this location has been called the Chilaiditi sign and is usually an asymptomatic incidental finding. It can mimic pneumoperitoneum** on radiographs. Chilaiditi sign is suggested by the presence of colonic haustra, as demonstrated in this case. Patients would not have the peritoneal signs expected with pneumoperitoneum. Chilaiditi *syndrome* refers to symptomatic cases, which are rare. Patients with Chilaiditi syndrome may have vague abdominal symptoms and respond to conservative care.

Regarding the other answer choices, there is no pneumoperitoneum to suggest perforation of the stomach as discussed above. There is no small bowel obstruction because oral contrast is seen in normal-caliber colon. There is no intrathoracic herniation shown to indicate a Morgagni hernia. A Morgagni hernia is a congenital diaphragmatic hernia in the anteromedial abdomen that is right sided in the majority of cases. Most Morgagni hernias contain fat, but a few contain bowel or other abdominal contents and can become symptomatic if strangulated. Bochdalek hernias, which are also congenital diaphragmatic hernias, are more common than Morgagni hernias but usually occur posterolaterally.

References: Venkataraman D, Harrison R, Warriner S. Abnormal gas pattern under diaphragm. *BMJ Case Rep* 2012:bcr0820114650. doi: 10.1136/bcr.08.2011.4650.

Weng WH, Liu DR, Feng CC, et al. Colonic interposition between the liver and left diaphragm—management of Chilaiditi syndrome: a case report and literature review. *Oncol Lett* 2014;7(5):1657–1660.

5 **Answer A.** This patient had an area of **postoperative fat necrosis (secondary omental infarction)** with subsequent evolution. The first CT shows an elongated circumscribed area of fat stranding (long arrows). The abdominal wall surgical scar (short arrow) is seen nearby. The adjacent small bowel is unaffected by this omental process with no wall thickening. Subsequent CT image shows significant decrease in size (long arrow) and development of rim and internal calcifications. These findings are consistent with evolution and healing of fat necrosis in the omentum.

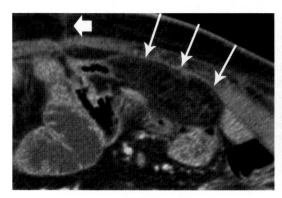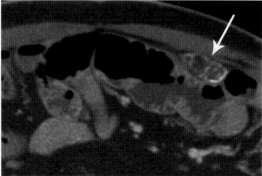

Other etiologies of fat necrosis besides surgery are epiploic appendagitis, primary omental infarction, and adjacent inflammatory processes such as pancreatitis. The following CT in a different patient shows the classic appearance of primary omental infarction in a 31-year-old man, with a large area of fat stranding (arrows), typically > 5 cm. This condition usually occurs in the right lower quadrant because the blood supply to the right lateral free edge of the omentum is less robust. Primary omental infarction is most often seen in young patients 20 to 40 years of age with men more often affected than women, and there may be a history of marathon running. **Treatment of fat necrosis is usually nonsurgical with analgesics for pain control. The exception is omental infarct from omental torsion**, which would be suspected on CT if there is a swirling of the omentum and vessels. Omental torsion is a mechanical phenomenon that requires surgery.

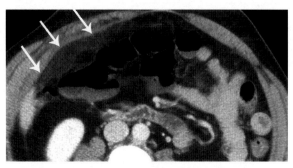

Primary omental infarction in a young man.

Fat necrosis can mimic other answer choices. Malignancies such as peritoneal carcinomatosis and liposarcoma would not spontaneously shrink and calcify in this manner. Patients with acute fat necrosis may present with symptoms resembling acute appendicitis or diverticulitis. The encapsulated appearance can mimic abscess especially in the postoperative setting, but the center of the lesion is fat density, not fluid.

References: Kamaya A, Federle MP, Desser TS. Imaging manifestations of abdominal fat necrosis and its mimics. *Radiographics* 2011;31(7):2021–2034.

Lubner MG, Simard ML, Peterson CM, et al. Emergent and nonemergent nonbowel torsion: spectrum of imaging and clinical findings. *Radiographics* 2013;33(1):155–173.

6 **Answer B.** This patient has pseudomyxoma peritonei, which is an uncommon condition most often caused by a ruptured appendiceal mucinous neoplasm. There is a large volume of low-density fluid. **The multifocal scalloping of the hepatic and splenic margins is a key observation that indicates complex fluid rather than simple ascites.** In classic pseudomyxoma peritonei, cells disseminated from the **rupture of a benign or low-grade neoplasm** produces a large volume of mucin that accumulates in the peritoneal cavity. Rare epithelial cells may be identified in the mucin without overt malignancy. In this case, a benign villous adenoma was found at surgery in the ruptured appendix. A cystic ovarian mass in the setting of pseudomyxoma peritonei may represent a primary ovarian neoplasm responsible for the disease versus peritoneal spread. **Although classic pseudomyxoma peritonei tends to have an indolent clinical course due to its low-grade characteristics, there is high morbidity from the effects of the mucinous fluid on the organs.** Management is predominantly surgical, and patients may require multiple surgeries for small bowel obstruction and other complications.

In contradistinction to classic pseudomyxoma peritonei, peritoneal mucinous carcinomatosis is a high-grade neoplasm with an abundance of cells that are clearly malignant at pathology. The imaging appearance may be similar to classic pseudomyxoma peritonei because the malignancy also produces low-density mucinous ascites. However, peritoneal mucinous carcinomatosis is more aggressive and has a worse prognosis.

In the answer choices, cirrhosis with portal hypertension and intraperitoneal bladder rupture would result in simple-appearing fluid without organ scalloping. Sclerosing encapsulating peritonitis (also known as abdominal cocoon) is a rare chronic inflammatory condition most often seen in patients with a longstanding history of peritoneal dialysis. In this condition, progressive collagen formation and an inflammatory infiltrate tether and encapsulate multiple small bowel loops resulting in bowel obstruction. Surgery is required to free the bowel from the capsule.

The scalloping of the liver margin in the setting of pseudomyxoma peritonei or peritoneal carcinomatosis is distinct from the hepatic nodularity seen with cirrhosis. A subcapsular hepatic or splenic hematoma may scallop the liver contour, but there would be a history of trauma and hemoperitoneum rather than low-density fluid. The diaphragmatic slips (arrows on the following CT image), which are normal muscle bundles that can be seen at the liver margin, should not be confused with the liver scalloping caused by complex ascites or macronodularity in cirrhosis.

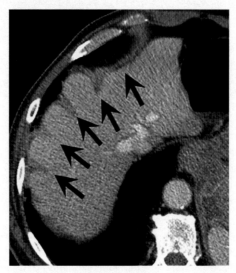

Normal diaphragmatic slips mimicking liver scalloping/nodularity.

References: Leonards LM, Pahwa A, Patel MK, et al. Neoplasms of the appendix: pictorial review with clinical and pathologic correlation. *Radiographics* 2017;37(4):1059–1083.

Levy AD, Shaw JC, Sobin LH. Secondary tumors and tumorlike lesions of the peritoneal cavity: imaging features with pathologic correlation. *Radiographics* 2009;29(2):347–373.

7 **Answer A.** Retractile (fibrosing) mesenteritis is in the spectrum of sclerosing mesenteritis, a condition characterized by chronic mesenteric inflammation. **Some of the fibrosing diseases have recently been recognized as belonging to the spectrum of multisystemic IgG4-related inflammatory diseases,** which are characterized by a lymphoplasmacytic infiltrate rich in IgG4-positive cells. This includes a significant proportion of (but not all) cases of sclerosing mesenteritis and retroperitoneal fibrosis, the correct answer choice.

There is a lobulated mass (arrows) with dense calcifications and spiculated margins tethering the ileal mesentery. The two primary differential diagnoses are carcinoid tumor metastasis and retractile mesenteritis. Both can occur with or without calcifications. The two entities are frequently indistinguishable, with other malignancies also in the differential diagnosis, so further evaluation and/or biopsy is usually required. **A clue to the diagnosis of carcinoid instead of retractile mesenteritis would be visualization of one or more hypervascular primary neuroendocrine neoplasms within the adjacent small bowel, often a subtle finding.** In this case, further evaluation was negative for neuroendocrine tumor or other malignancy, and subsequent stability for years without treatment was consistent with retractile mesenteritis. Patients are commonly asymptomatic, or occasionally present with abdominal pain, weight loss, intestinal obstruction/ischemia, mass, or diarrhea.

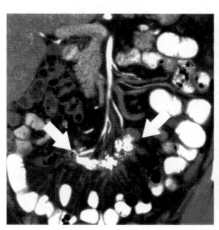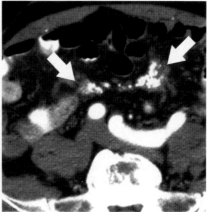

The spectrum of sclerosing mesenteritis at pathology includes:

- Mesenteric panniculitis (inflammation)
- Mesenteric lipodystrophy (fat necrosis)
- Retractile (fibrosing) mesenteritis, considered late stage with more invasive behavior

The differential diagnosis for nodular mesenteric calcification also includes benign and malignant entities. Calcifications can be seen in implants from ovarian cancer and mucinous tumors as well as treated lymphoma. Granulomatous infection or inflammation, such as tuberculosis or sarcoidosis, may be seen as calcified mesenteric lymph nodes.

Regarding the other answer choices, tuberous sclerosis, Whipple disease, and graft versus host disease have not been associated with sclerosing mesenteritis. Tuberous sclerosis is a genetic neurocutaneous disorder with thoracoabdominal findings of lymphangioleiomyomatosis (LAM, with lung cysts), renal angiomyolipomas, renal cysts, and renal cell carcinomas. Whipple disease is an infection with the Whipple bacillus *Tropheryma whipplei* classically presenting with arthralgias and abdominal symptoms. Patients with Whipple disease may have nodular bowel wall thickening and low-density adenopathy. Graft versus host disease is an immune response in the recipient of an allogeneic hematopoietic cell transplant to donor cells. It can involve the gastrointestinal tract with diffuse bowel wall thickening.

References: George V, Tammisetti VS, Surabhi VR, et al. Chronic fibrosing conditions in abdominal imaging. *Radiographics* 2013;33(4):1053–1080.

Martínez-de-Alegría A, Baleato-González S, García-Figueiras R, et al. IgG4-related disease from head to toe. *Radiographics* 2015;35(7):2007–2025.

8 **Answer A.** The most common finding in **ruptured abdominal aortic aneurysm** (AAA) is retroperitoneal hemorrhage (white arrows). This is a surgical emergency. Signs of AAA instability seen in this case include the crescent sign (black arrow) within the mural thrombus and loss of intimal calcification along a section of the wall.

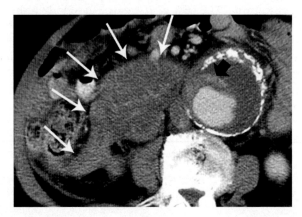

The risk of rupture increases with aneurysm size. The size threshold for AAA repair is in the range of 5.0 to 5.5 cm. **Serial CT scans should be carefully compared to assess for the following signs of instability and impending rupture. The presence of these signs may prompt endovascular and surgical repair.**

Signs of AAA Instability and Impending Rupture	
Finding	Comments
Rapid enlargement	~6 mm in 6 months ~1 cm in 1 year
Crescent sign	Crescent of high density in the mural thrombus • Noncontrast CT: denser than intraluminal blood • Contrast CT: denser than psoas muscle
Wall irregularity	New loss of intimal calcification compared to prior studies Pseudoaneurysm formation
Decreasing thrombus volume	Plaque erosion Luminal outpouching
Perianeurysmal fat stranding	
"Draped aorta" sign	Indicates chronic contained rupture Loss of fat planes between AAA and spine or psoas muscle Outpouching Scalloping of vertebral body indicating chronic bony remodeling

Other causes of retroperitoneal hemorrhage besides AAA rupture include anticoagulation, bleeding diathesis, surgery, trauma, arterial catheterization, or organ pathology with rupture (e.g., ruptured renal angiomyolipoma). CT is often utilized as the initial diagnostic tool in patients with suspected retroperitoneal hemorrhage. **On noncontrast CT, high-attenuation (30 to 70 HU) fluid is typically seen with acute hemorrhage, whereas chronic hemorrhage or acute hemorrhage in patients with anemia may have lower attenuation.** Active arterial hemorrhage or pseudoaneurysms may be seen on contrast-enhanced CT as extravascular foci of high attenuation with density similar to that of aorta. Over time, hematomas decrease in size and density.

The constellation of findings and the shape of the hyperattenuating hematoma accumulating along the retroperitoneal fascial planes are most consistent with AAA rupture rather than a neoplasm like lymphoma or IVC leiomyosarcoma. A type II endoleak is seen after endovascular graft repair of AAA as contrast within the aneurysm sac, but there is no endograft device in this patient.

References: Torigian DA, Ramchandani P. CT and MRI of the retroperitoneum. In: Haaga JR, Lanzieri CF, Gilkeson RC (eds). *CT and MRI imaging of the whole body*, 5th ed. Philadelphia, PA: Elsevier, 2009:1953–2040.

Wadgaonkar AD, Black JH, Weihe EK, et al. Abdominal aortic aneurysms revisited: MDCT with multiplanar reconstructions for identifying indicators of instability in the pre- and postoperative patient. *Radiographics* 2015;35(1):254–268.

9 **Answer C.** There is a layer of lucency (arrows) between the abdominal wall and the right lateral margin of the liver on this left lateral decubitus radiograph. This is consistent with pneumoperitoneum.

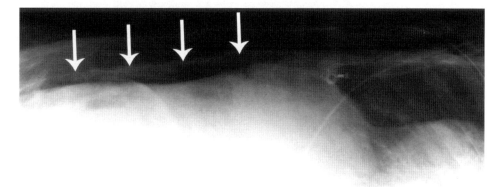

A left lateral decubitus position helps to detect pneumoperitoneum when the patient cannot be imaged in the upright position. A left lateral is preferred over a right lateral decubitus or a cross table supine decubitus because the gas is more readily identified adjacent to the margin of the liver. To optimize sensitivity for pneumoperitoneum, the patient should be lying in the decubitus position for 15 minutes before the image is obtained to allow the gas to rise to the nondependent aspect of the abdomen. These radiographic techniques are performed less frequently now because patients often proceed to CT. **CT is the most sensitive modality for the detection of gas and can also reveal the cause of pneumoperitoneum.**

Ascites is not radiolucent. The gas is not seen within any bowel to indicate the presence of colonic obstruction. Although decubitus radiographs may be used to determine if a pleural effusion is loculated, there is no evidence of a pleural effusion in the visualized portion of the chest.

References: Boland GWL, Halpert RD. Chapter 10: Peritoneum, retroperitoneum, and mesentery. In: Boland GWL, Halpert RD (eds). *Gastrointestinal imaging: the requisites*, 4th ed. Philadelphia, PA: Elsevier/Saunders, 2014:382–406.

Messmer JM, Levine MS. Chapter 12: Gas and soft tissue abnormalities. In: Gore RM, Levine MS (eds). *Textbook of gastrointestinal radiology*, 4th ed. Philadelphia, PA: Elsevier/Saunders, 2015:178–196.

10a **Answer D. Abdominopelvic CT with intravenous (venous phase) and rectal contrast.** In low-velocity penetrating trauma to the upper left flank, the primary concern would be for injuries to the spleen, colon, diaphragm, and pleural space. While a FAST might be positive if there is significant hemorrhage, a negative FAST does not exclude the need for laparotomy, and CT is preferred in a hemodynamically stable patient. A CT with intravenous contrast is preferred to a noncontrast examination, and the addition of rectal contrast allows for detection of full-thickness colonic injuries. The use of oral contrast is more controversial, particularly because of the delay needed to assess more than the most proximal segments of small bowel.

10b **Answer B. Descending colon.** This axial CT image with triple contrast shows hematoma and edema within the subcutaneous tissues of the left flank at the entry site of the flank stab wound. There is hematoma and a small focus of gas in the underlying abdominal wall musculature. The left kidney appears normal, but there is contrast tracking from the lateral wall of the descending colon (arrows), confirming full-thickness colonic wall penetration. Retroperitoneal gas in this case would confirm penetration into the retroperitoneum but would not necessarily mean hollow viscus injury as it would with blunt trauma. **Extravasation of rectal contrast is specific but not sensitive for colonic injury from penetrating trauma.**

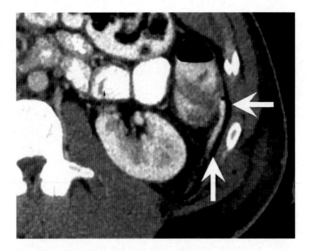

References: Bondia JM, Anderson SW, Rhea JT, et al. Imaging colorectal trauma using 64-MDCT technology. *Emerg Radiol* 2009;16:433–440.

Dreizin D, Boscak AR, Anstadt MJ, et al. Penetrating colorectal injuries: diagnostic performance of multidetector CT with trajectography. *Radiology* 2016;281:749–762.

11a **Answer C.** Pneumoperitoneum seen beneath the diaphragms on this upright radiograph is an expected finding in patient's status post recent abdominal surgery and procedures. This patient whose colon was surgically absent also had dilated small bowel with air–fluid levels, representing postoperative ileus that eventually resolved along with the pneumoperitoneum. **Postoperative gas seen within 10 days on radiographs or within 2 weeks on CT is likely acceptable after abdominal surgery, as long as it is not increasing, and does not require surgical or percutaneous intervention.** Pneumoperitoneum persisting beyond this time period or increasing in volume raises concern for a bowel complication such as anastomotic leak. As little as 1 mL may be detectable beneath the right hemidiaphragm with the proper technique on an upright chest or abdominal radiograph, which includes positioning the patient such that the x-ray beam strikes the diaphragm tangentially.

Barotrauma in the setting of mechanical ventilation is an uncommon cause of pneumoperitoneum. It can be mistaken for a sign of bowel perforation and lead to unnecessary surgical exploration. It should be suspected in an intubated patient when there are other signs of barotrauma such as pneumothoraces, pneumomediastinum, and subcutaneous emphysema, which are not seen in this case.

References: Earls JP, Dachman AH, Colon E, et al. Prevalence and duration of postoperative pneumoperitoneum: sensitivity of CT vs left lateral decubitus radiography. *AJR Am J Roentgenol* 1993;161(4):781–785.

Hindman NM, Kang S, Parikh MS. Common postoperative findings unique to laparoscopic surgery. *Radiographics* 2014;34(1):119–138.

11b **Answer A. Rigler sign (the double wall sign)** is demonstrated on the image, with gas seen on both sides of the bowel wall (arrows) making the wall visible as a thin white line. This is a sign of **pneumoperitoneum**. This appearance is occasionally produced by overlapping segments of gas-filled bowel in the absence of pneumoperitoneum, limiting the accuracy of this sign. The Rigler sign should not be confused with Rigler triad, which indicates gallstone ileus with pneumobilia, small bowel obstruction, and gallstone.

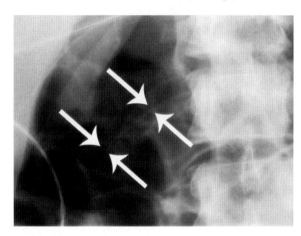

The detection of pneumoperitoneum on a supine AP abdominal radiograph is challenging. Upright and left decubitus radiographs are more sensitive, with CT the most sensitive imaging modality. If detectable on a supine abdominal radiograph, pneumoperitoneum is most often visible in the right upper quadrant adjacent to the liver. The other answer choices are all signs that can be seen with pneumoperitoneum but are less commonly identified than Rigler sign. The falciform ligament sign (white arrows on radiograph and CT images below) is the ligament outlined by gas. The inverted V sign (black arrows) is seen in the pelvis when gas outlines the lateral umbilical folds, which carry the inferior epigastric vessels. The football sign is more often seen in children and refers to a large volume of gas in the abdominopelvic cavity collectively resembling the shape of a football.

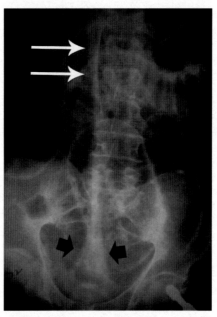

Falciform ligament sign and inverted V sign of pneumoperitoneum.

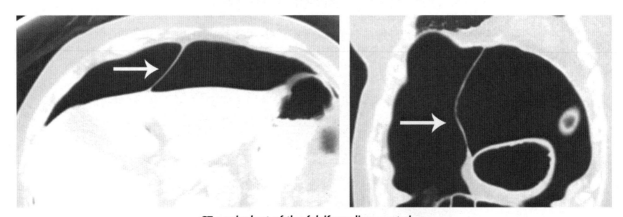

CT equivalent of the falciform ligament sign.

References: Levine MS, Scheiner JD, Rubesin SE, et al. Diagnosis of pneumoperitoneum on supine abdominal radiographs. *AJR Am J Roentgenol* 1991;156(4):731–735.

Messmer JM, Levine MS. Chapter 12: Gas and soft tissue abnormalities. In: Gore RM, Levine MS (eds). *Textbook of gastrointestinal radiology*, 4th ed. Philadelphia, PA: Elsevier/Saunders, 2015:178–196.

12 **Answer B.** Imaging findings and clinical history are consistent with a peritoneal inclusion cyst (PIC), which is also known as a benign cystic mesothelioma. There is a multiseptated cystic structure (white arrows) in the left adnexa, which surrounds the normal left ovary (black arrow). The normal ovary can be identified by its small follicles. This is the **classic "spider web" pattern of peritoneal inclusion cyst with an "entrapped ovary."** The cyst may have thin septations as seen best on the coronal image in this case, and its margins typically conform to the peritoneal cavity as shown.

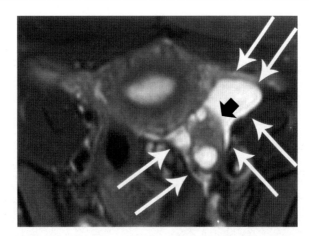

A PIC is an acquired cyst that occurs almost exclusively in **premenopausal women with a history of pelvic inflammation, trauma, or surgery**. Patients may have a history of endometriosis, pelvic inflammatory disease, or inflammatory bowel disease. **The precipitating event causes adhesions that trap fluid around the ovary when follicles rupture as part of normal ovulation.** Treatment in symptomatic cases of PIC is usually initially conservative with oral contraceptives and analgesics. In some cases, transvaginal drainage or laparoscopic surgery may be attempted, but cyst recurrence is common.

Regarding the other answer choices, a duplication cyst of the bowel would be a submucosal mass associated with a segment of bowel, not demonstrated here. A congenital mesothelial cyst is typically a thin-walled unilocular cyst in the mesentery containing simple fluid. It is thought to represent fluid trapped between mesothelial layers of the peritoneum that are incompletely fused. A mature cystic teratoma (dermoid cyst) is diagnosed by the presence of fat. In this case, there is no hyperintensity within the lesion on the non-fat–saturated T1W image to indicate fat.

The differential diagnosis also includes other pelvic and mesenteric cystic lesions. Hydrosalpinx and tuboovarian abscess (TOA) classically have a coiled tube appearance. TOA also shows wall thickening and surrounding inflammation indicating an acute infection. An endometrioma would be hyperintense on T1W images with hypointensity and shading on T2W images, not seen here. **A PIC may be misdiagnosed as an ovarian cystic neoplasm if the entrapped ovary is mistaken for a tumor nodule.** An ovarian cystic neoplasm would not conform to the margins of the peritoneal cavity. A lymphangioma may have a multilocated thin-walled cystic appearance but does not entrap the ovary.

References: Jain KA. Imaging of peritoneal inclusion cysts. *AJR Am J Roentgenol* 2000;174(6):1559–1563.

Moyle PL, Kataoka MY, Nakai A, et al. Nonovarian cystic lesions of the pelvis. *Radiographics* 2010;30(4):921–938.

13 **Answers:**
Patient 1: B. Pseudolipoma
Patient 2: D. Tumor thrombus
Patient 3: A. Mixing artifact

The **IVC pseudolipoma** in patient 1 represents fat that artifactually appears intraluminal in the upper IVC. This appearance may be mistaken for an IVC thrombus. The normal angulated course and tapering of the IVC just below the confluence with the right atrium makes this area susceptible to partial volume averaging artifact with the surrounding fat. **In general, partial volume** averaging artifacts are typically resolved by correlating with a different plane or acquiring images with thinner slices.

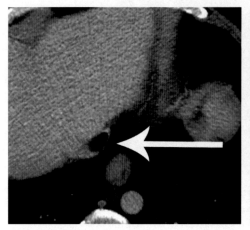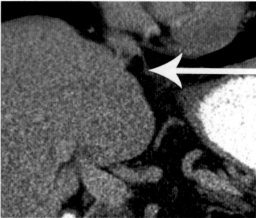

IVC pseudolipoma.

Patient 2 has **tumor thrombus in the IVC**. The thrombus enhances heterogeneously and is outlined by the contrast in the IVC. On the coronal image below, the arrows indicate the renal cell carcinoma (RCC) as well as the associated tumor thrombus expanding the right renal vein and IVC. Perirenal collateral veins have developed due to the venous obstruction. RCC is the most common malignancy with extension into the IVC. **Thrombus does not preclude resection, but the extent of thrombus affects surgical management.** Supradiaphragmatic thrombus requires a combined cardiothoracic and abdominal approach. Bland thrombus would be a nonenhancing filling defect that usually causes little expansion of the vessel. On an abdominal CT, the visualized pulmonary arteries at the lung bases should be inspected for pulmonary emboli if IVC, renal vein, or gonadal vein thrombus is detected.

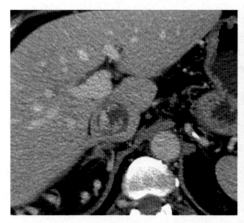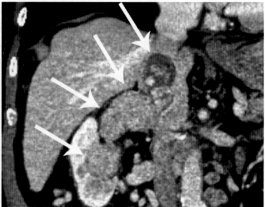

RCC with enhancing tumor thrombus in the renal vein and IVC.

The IVC in patient 3 shows contrast mixing artifact, a finding that occurs near the confluence of vessels. In the arterial phase axial and coronal images, the contrast in the renal veins encounters the unopacified blood in the IVC, resulting in central hypodensity that can mimic IVC thrombus (arrows). The venous phase image confirms a normal IVC with homogeneous luminal enhancement. A 70- to 90-second delay improves uniformity of opacification of the IVC. **This illustrates the importance of phase of enhancement and presence of adjacent vessels when evaluating the vasculature.**

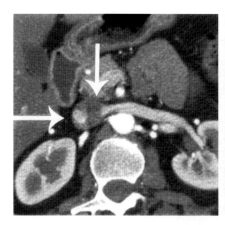 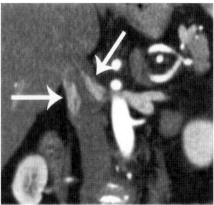 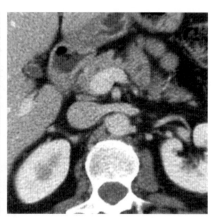

IVC mixing artifact.

Even though liposarcoma is the most common type of retroperitoneal sarcoma, the most common primary malignancy of the IVC is leiomyosarcoma. IVC leiomyosarcoma is a rare malignancy originating from the vessel wall. The following case of a primary IVC leiomyosarcoma shows a mass (long arrows) that is projecting from the IVC (short arrow). Some of these tumors show mainly exophytic growth as demonstrated in this example, while others mainly intraluminal growth. Heterogeneous enhancement and cystic necrosis may be identified. It is difficult to distinguish primary IVC leiomyosarcoma from other retroperitoneal tumors that secondarily encase or invade the IVC such as retroperitoneal sarcoma, metastatic adenopathy, and paraganglioma. The tumor requires aggressive surgery with IVC reconstruction if resectable. Prognosis is poor with about 15% survival at 10 years.

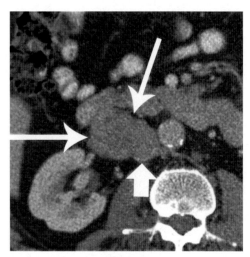

Primary IVC leiomyosarcoma.

References: Smillie RP, Shetty M, Boyer AC, et al. Imaging evaluation of the inferior vena cava. *Radiographics* 2015;35(2):578–592.

Webb EM, Wang ZJ, Westphalen AC, et al. Can CT features differentiate between inferior vena cava leiomyosarcomas and primary retroperitoneal masses? *AJR Am J Roentgenol* 2013;200(1):205–209.

14 **Answer D.** CT images reveal "misty" hazy infiltration of the mesenteric fat of the jejunal mesentery. The area is circumscribed by a curvilinear pseudocapsule, with minimal mass effect upon adjacent small bowel loops. There is sparing of the fat around the undisturbed mesenteric vessels ("fat halo" or "fat ring" sign), and there are multiple subcentimeter mesenteric lymph nodes in the fat. These are all typical features of **mesenteric panniculitis, a subtype of sclerosing mesenteritis.** Sclerosing mesenteritis is usually incidental and asymptomatic, unrelated to this patient's diarrhea. A primary liposarcoma of this size and location would disturb mesenteric vessels. Desmoid tumor does not contain fat.

Although sclerosing mesenteritis is benign, a coexisting malignancy elsewhere may be discovered in some patients. Some cases show histopathologic findings compatible with IgG-4–related disease. If symptomatic, treatment for sclerosing mesenteritis may include surgical resection or immunosuppressive drugs such as steroids. **The lymph nodes within mesenteric panniculitis are typically small. Larger nodes would raise suspicion for malignancy** such as in the following CT image of lymphoma associated with "misty mesentery."

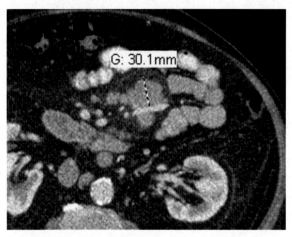

Lymphoma with misty mesentery and enlarged lymph nodes.

Other causes of "misty mesentery" besides mesenteric panniculitis and lymphoma include inflammation (e.g., pancreatitis), edema (e.g., from cardiac, hepatic, or renal disease), and malignancy (e.g., peritoneal carcinomatosis).

References: George V, Tammisetti VS, Surabhi VR, et al. Chronic fibrosing conditions in abdominal imaging. *Radiographics* 2013;33(4):1053–1080.

McLaughlin PD, Filippone A, Maher MM. The "misty mesentery" mesenteric panniculitis and its mimics. *AJR Am J Roentgenol* 2013;200(2):W116–W123.

15 Answer C. This patient has retroperitoneal fibrosis (RPF). There is confluent soft tissue anterior and lateral to the abdominal aorta, with sparing posterior to the aorta (long arrows). This tissue obstructs the left ureter (short arrow) causing hydronephrosis. RPF is most commonly seen in patients 40 to 60 years old with male to female ratio of 3:1.

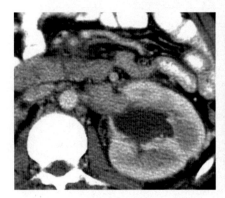
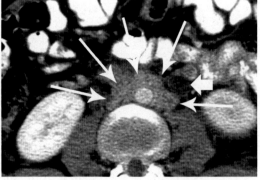

RPF is most commonly identified around the abdominal aorta and common iliac arteries. In the acute stage of RPF, enhancement may be seen along with

MRI T2 hyperintensity reflecting edema. In the chronic/inactive stage, the soft tissue mass is hypovascular with low T2 signal intensity. Posterior sparing is not specific for RPF, since adenopathy from benign and malignant causes can also show posterior sparing. However, **if posterior soft tissue is identified, the process is unlikely to be RPF** and is most likely lymphadenopathy.

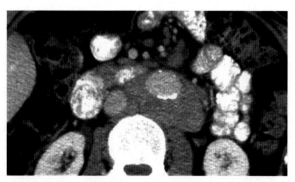

Lymphadenopathy posterior to aorta in lymphoma.

RPF is an uncommon condition initially recognized as a fibrotic process that results in obstructive uropathy. **Some cases that were previously idiopathic are now believed to be part of the spectrum of IgG4-related inflammatory diseases** listed in the table below. About a third of cases of RPF have **known etiologies including autoimmune disease, radiation, medications** such as ergot alkaloids for migraines, **malignancy** such as lymphoma or metastases, **asbestos** exposure, and retroperitoneal **hemorrhage**. Treatment is with steroids and immunosuppressants. Symptomatic relief with stenting can be performed in patients with obstructive uropathy. In refractory cases, surgeries including ureterolysis and transposition are considered.

Spectrum of IgG4-Related Diseases	
Abdomen	• Chronic periaortitis (which includes retroperitoneal fibrosis and aortitis)
	• Autoimmune pancreatitis
	• Autoimmune hepatitis
	• Sclerosing cholangitis
	• Sclerosing mesenteritis
	• Tubulointerstitial nephritis and glomerulonephritis
Chest	• Sclerosing mediastinitis
	• Pulmonary inflammatory pseudotumor
	• Interstitial pneumonitis, pleuritis, and pericarditis
Head and Neck	• Orbital pseudotumor
	• Riedel thyroiditis
	• Sclerosing dacryoadenitis and sialadenitis
	• Hypophysitis and pachymeningitis
Others	• Sclerosing mastitis, prostatitis, orchitis

References: Caiafa RO, Vinuesa AS, Izquierdo RS, et al. Retroperitoneal fibrosis: role of imaging in diagnosis and follow-up. *Radiographics* 2013;33(2):535–552.

George V, Tammisetti VS, Surabhi VR, et al. Chronic fibrosing conditions in abdominal imaging. *Radiographics* 2013;33(4):1053–1080.

16 **Answer D.** There is a cystic mass located between the stomach and the pancreas with features consistent with **lymphangioma**, a benign cystic neoplasm. Walls are imperceptible walls and fluid is simple (density measuring 20 HU or less). The **"vessel penetration" sign** is present (arrows), with vessels passing through relatively undisturbed.

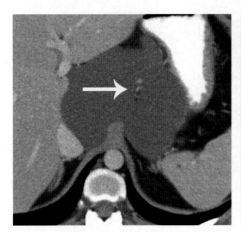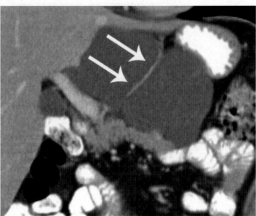

Lymphangiomas may be unilocular or multilocular with a round, lobulated, or elongated appearance. The walls or septations may calcify. **Occasionally, density measurements reveal negative Hounsfield units because of the lipid in chyle.** With growth, hemorrhage, or infection, lymphangiomas can become symptomatic and appear complex on imaging, mimicking abscess, or cystic neoplasm. Treatment if symptomatic is surgical resection.

References: Levy AD, Cantisani V, Miettinen M. Abdominal lymphangiomas: imaging features with pathologic correlation. *AJR Am J Roentgenol* 2004;182(6):1485–1491.

Yang DM, Jung DH, Kim H, et al. Retroperitoneal cystic masses: CT, clinical, and pathologic findings and literature review. *Radiographics* 2004;24(5):1353–1365.

17 **Answer C.** This patient has a **paraganglioma (also known as an extra-adrenal pheochromocytoma)** along the expected course of the organ of Zuckerkandl. There is an ovoid left para-aortic mass with **classic hypervascular enhancement** on the arterial phase image on the left. The differential diagnosis includes a hypervascular metastasis, sarcoma, and Castleman disease. However, paragangliomas can have a **range of atypical features with cystic, hemorrhagic, or calcified components.** On MRI, appearance T1 and T2 signal intensity are variable, and the classic "light bulb" marked T2 hyperintensity only occurs in a minority of cases.

Paragangliomas can occur anywhere along the sympathetic chain from base of the skull to the bladder. In the retroperitoneum, they are frequently found along the organ of Zuckerkandl, which runs from above the superior mesenteric artery to the aortic bifurcation. **[68]Ga-DOTATATE PET/CT is emerging as the radionuclide functional imaging study of choice** over ^{123}I-metaiodobenzylguanidine (MIBG) for diagnosis and staging of abdominal somatostatin receptor (SSTR)–positive neuroendocrine tumors, including paragangliomas and pheochromocytomas. Positive tumors would be amenable to treatment with peptide receptor radionuclide therapy targeted to SSTRs including as lutetium 177 (^{177}Lu)–labeled or yttrium 90 (^{90}Y)–labeled DOTATATE SSTR analogues.

Patients may present with the classic triad of headache, diaphoresis, and tachycardia with positive 24-hour urine catecholamines and metanephrines. The suggestion of a paraganglioma is important as **alpha- and beta-adrenergic blockade is recommended prior to biopsy to prevent hypertensive**

crises and arrhythmias. Extra-adrenal pheochromocytomas are more likely to be malignant and metastasize than adrenal lesions. Up to 40% of pheochromocytomas and paragangliomas may be familial, higher than previously believed, and those patients may benefit from periodic whole-body screening.

References: Elsayes KM, Narra VR, Leyendecker JR, et al. MRI of adrenal and extraadrenal pheochromocytoma. *AJR Am J Roentgenol* 2005;184(3):860–867.

Withey SJ, Perrio S, Christodoulou D, et al. Imaging features of succinate dehydrogenase-deficient pheochromocytoma-paraganglioma syndromes. *Radiographics* 2019;39(5):1393–1410.

18 **Answer B.** There is bulky lymphadenopathy in the retroperitoneum and mesentery in this patient with lymphoma. The appearance of lymphadenopathy is often nonspecific, but occasionally, there are clues to the diagnosis. **The vessels show little narrowing and excellent contrast opacification despite the bulk of surrounding adenopathy, reflecting the pliable nature of lymphoma and consistent with the "vessel penetration" sign.** The layering of the vessels among the lymphadenopathy on this axial image is also an example of the "sandwich" or "hamburger" sign of lymphoma.

Untreated lymphoma is typically of homogeneous soft tissue density as seen in this case; however, bulky lymphoma may occasionally appear inhomogeneous. Aside from the imaging appearance, the patient's age removes testicular carcinoma metastases from primary consideration.

References: Lin E. Chapter 16: Retroperitoneum, vessels, and nodes. In: Lin E, Coy DL, Kanne JP (eds). *Body CT: the essentials*. New York, NY: McGraw-Hill, 2015:231–240.

Nishino M, Hayakawa K, Minami M, et al. Primary retroperitoneal neoplasms: CT and MR imaging findings with anatomic and pathologic diagnostic clues. *Radiographics* 2003;23(1):45–57.

19 **Answer A.** There is an enlarged retroperitoneal lymph node with central low attenuation. Low-density retroperitoneal lymphadenopathy most likely represents testicular carcinoma metastases in this young man. Depending on the clinical setting, the major **differential diagnoses for low-density adenopathy includes metastases (necrotic, cystic, or mucinous) as well as granulomatous infections (fungi, atypical mycobacteria, and tuberculosis).** Patients with Whipple disease and celiac disease may also demonstrate low-density lymphadenopathy, the latter showing fat–fluid levels in a rare condition called cavitary mesenteric lymph node syndrome. Untreated lymphoma usually has a more homogeneous appearance without central low density.

Reference: Paño B, Sebastià C, Buñesch L, et al. Pathways of lymphatic spread in male urogenital pelvic malignancies. *Radiographics* 2011;31(1):135–160.

20 **Answer C.** This patient has a colon cancer in the cecum, which has perforated resulting in a sinus tract extending to the psoas muscle with abscess formation. The iliopsoas muscles are primary hip flexors and are extraperitoneal in location. Patients may have pain exacerbated by hip extension, which stretches the psoas muscle. **Perforated colon cancers can fistulize** to adjacent anatomy including skin, bladder, and vagina. Regarding the other answer choices, Meckel diverticulitis should be associated with the distal ileum not colon. A schwannoma and hematoma would not be expected to behave in this way.

It can be difficult to distinguish among abscess, hematoma, and neoplasm by imaging alone, and clinical history is important. Abscess and neoplasm are most often secondary to direct extension from an adjacent process such as appendicitis, diverticulitis, Crohn disease, tuberculosis, or perforated colon cancer. Hematogenous spread of infection or metastases are less common than direct extension. Spontaneous psoas abscesses are uncommon but occur more often in the pediatric population and should be considered when a child presents with fever, abdominal pain, and limp. Primary mesenchymal tumors such as schwannomas and sarcomas can be found in the psoas muscle.

References: Kim SW, Shin HC, Kim IY, et al. CT findings of colonic complications associated with colon cancer. *Korean J Radiol* 2010;11(2):211–221.

Torres GM, Cernigliaro JG, Abbitt PL, et al. Iliopsoas compartment: normal anatomy and pathologic processes. *Radiographics* 1995;15(6):1285–1297.

21 **Answer D.** This patient has **abdominal compartment syndrome** (ACS), which is a life-threatening condition requiring urgent intervention. There is a large quantity of complex peritoneal fluid. The rapid accumulation of fluid and blood in the peritoneal cavity in this patient after surgery has produced tension with significant mass effect on the visualized organs. There is distortion (black arrows) of the liver, spleen, and stomach, which have angular flattened margins. The IVC (white arrow) is also flattened. The tension compresses vessels throughout the abdomen and pelvis and compromises vascular flow, for example, to the kidneys contributing to acute renal failure. In this case, the liver parenchyma is heterogeneous, which could indicate organ compromise. Diaphragmatic excursion decreases, reducing respiratory function. **Percutaneous or surgical decompression is urgently indicated and can reverse organ failure.**

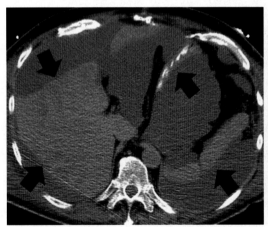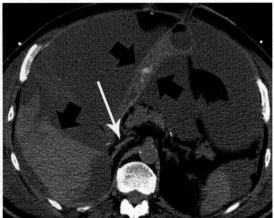

ACS is defined as intra-abdominal pressure of at least 20 mm Hg with dysfunction of at least one thoracoabdominal organ. There is a high mortality rate of 60% to 70%. It is probably underrecognized as it frequently occurs in patients who are critically ill with other reasons for multiorgan dysfunction. **ACS should be considered when there is a rapid increase in fluid or hemorrhage in the peritoneum or retroperitoneum over hours or days, accompanied by signs of mass effect on the internal organs and vessels.** There is usually a history of significant trauma or surgery.

When fluid accumulation occurs more slowly as with cirrhosis or peritoneal carcinomatosis, the abdomen accommodates and ACS does not occur. Regarding the other answer choices, pseudomyxoma peritonei can produce mucinous ascites that causes mass effect, but the effect is usually hepatosplenic scalloping and an indolent course rather than rapid decompensation. There is no splenic laceration demonstrated. There is no oral contrast extravasation or pneumoperitoneum to suggest gastric perforation.

References: Patel A, Lall CG, Jennings SG, et al. Abdominal compartment syndrome. *AJR Am J Roentgenol* 2007;189(5):1037–1043.

Pickhardt PJ, Shimony JS, Heiken JP, et al. The abdominal compartment syndrome: CT findings. *AJR Am J Roentgenol* 1999;173(3):575–579.

22 **Answer D.** This heterogeneous retroperitoneal tumor demonstrates an inferior component of macroscopic fat and a superior component of calcification and enhancing soft tissue. The mass invades the liver and displaces the right kidney. An aggressive fat-containing tumor arising in the retroperitoneum is most likely a **liposarcoma**, which is the **most common retroperitoneal sarcoma.** In this case, the calcifications represent osteosarcomatous **dedifferentiation**.

Regarding the other answer choices, an exophytic renal angiomyolipoma (AML) is a common retroperitoneal mass containing fat, but AMLs typically do not calcify or demonstrate aggressive margins. In addition, there is no renal parenchymal defect demonstrated in the kidney to indicate that this mass is arising from the kidney. As shown below in a different patient with an exophytic AML, the parenchymal defect (long arrow) can be very small even if the AML is large (short arrows).

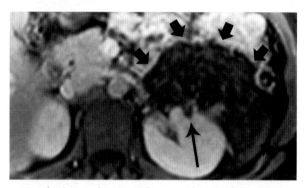

Exophytic renal AML with parenchymal defect sign.

While intracellular *microscopic* fat can be detected in clear cell renal cell carcinoma (RCC), *macroscopic* fat is not typical of RCC. Rare cases of small foci of macroscopic fat in RCC have been described associated with renal sinus invasion, osseous metaplasia, and lipid-producing necrosis. However, these are not major components of the RCC. Rarely chondrosarcoma can be extraskeletal, but there is no fat. The calcifications expected in chondrosarcoma are the classic "arcs and whorls" associated with cartilage.

Liposarcomas can be classified as atypical lipomatous tumor/well-differentiated liposarcoma (WDLS), dedifferentiated liposarcoma (DDLS), myxoid liposarcoma, or pleomorphic liposarcoma. DDLS demonstrates morphological variability including leiomyosarcomatous, rhabdomyosarcomatous, and osteosarcomatous components, among others. Nonfatty solid components can be found in both WDLS and DDLS, and **some liposarcomas show no visible fat. Features suspicious for DDLS include necrosis, calcification, fluid within solid component, and more avid enhancement**. Surgery is the mainstay of treatment, and the only curative approach. The efficacy or chemotherapy and radiation is controversial. DDLS has stronger propensity of lung metastasis and recurrence compared to WDLS.

References: Bhosale P, Wang J, Varma D, et al. Can abdominal computed tomography imaging help accurately identify a dedifferentiated component in a well-differentiated liposarcoma? *J Comput Assist Tomogr* 2016;40:872–879.

Levy AD, Manning MA, Al-Refaie WB, et al. Soft-tissue sarcomas of the abdomen and pelvis: radiologic-pathologic features, Part 1-common sarcomas: from the radiologic pathology archives. *Radiographics* 2017;37:462–483.

QUESTIONS

1 A 64-year-old man was noted to have a palpable abdominal mass while undergoing preoperative evaluation for prostatectomy. What is the diagnosis?

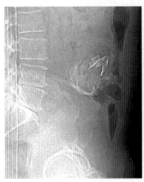 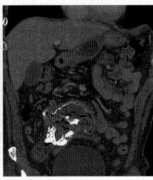 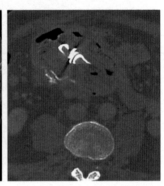

A. Gastrointestinal stromal tumor
B. Gossypiboma
C. Colonic diverticulitis with abscess
D. Liposarcoma

2 A 40-year-old man with a history of renal cell carcinoma undergoes an abdominal CT scan. What is the most likely diagnosis?

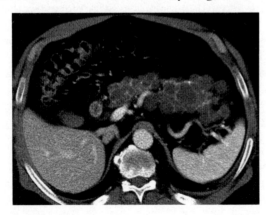

A. Birt-Hogg-Dubé syndrome
B. Tuberous sclerosis
C. von Hippel-Lindau disease
D. Cystic fibrosis

3 A 45-year-old man was evaluated with contrast-enhanced CT. What is the most likely diagnosis?

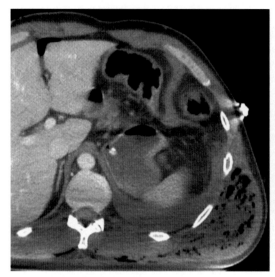 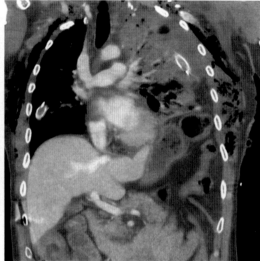

A. Diaphragmatic rupture
B. Hypoplastic left lung
C. Morgagni hernia
D. Tension pneumothorax

4 What is the cause of the following artifact?

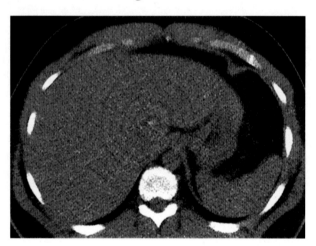

A. Beam hardening
B. Slip ring malfunction
C. Detector element defect
D. X-ray tube arcing

5 Axial image and sagittal image from a contrast-enhanced CT in a 20-year-old woman are shown. Her injuries are classic for which mechanism of trauma?

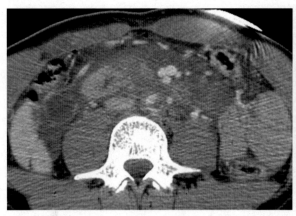
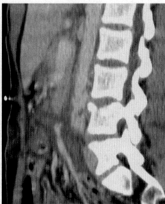

A. Nonaccidental abuse
B. Lap-belt compression
C. Fall from extreme height
D. Hyperextension injury

6 The findings on the following contrast-enhanced CT indicate that the patient presented with which condition?

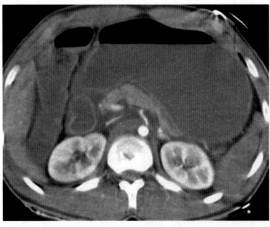
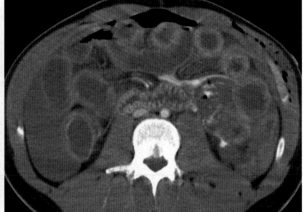

A. Diabetic ketoacidosis
B. Small bowel obstruction
C. Sepsis
D. Trauma

7 A patient presents with the following CT images. Serum angiotensin-converting enzyme (ACE) levels may be markedly elevated in this disease. Which of the following statement is TRUE about this disease?

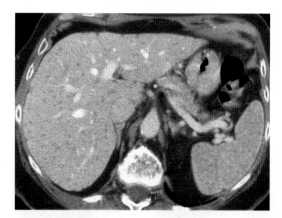

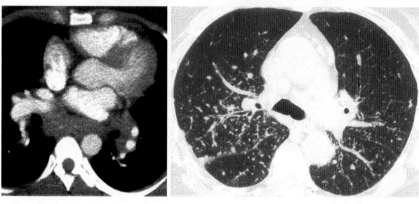

A. The most common radiologic finding is lung involvement.
B. Involvement of the liver and spleen is symptomatic in most cases.
C. The disease is characterized histologically by noncaseating granulomas.
D. The most common cause of death from this disease is central nervous system involvement.

8 This patient with a small bowel polypoid mass found to be a gastrointestinal stromal tumor (GST) was discussed in Chapter 3. A second similar mass is present in a posterior jejunal loop. At surgery, multiple additional GSTs were found. Images through the chest and lower back are shown. What diagnosis do these findings suggest?

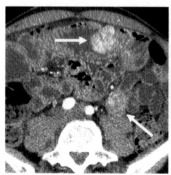
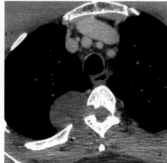
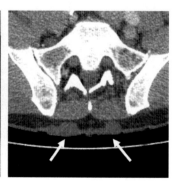

A. Scleroderma
B. Peutz-Jeghers syndrome
C. Gardner syndrome
D. Neurofibromatosis type 1

9 Match the images for patients 1 to 4 with the correct clinical history (A to D) based on the findings shown. Each option may be used only once.

Patient 1:

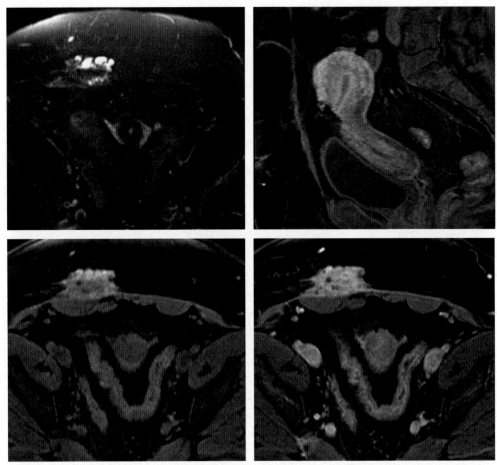

Top row: Axial FS T2W and sagittal FS T1W postcontrast MRI. **Bottom row:** Axial FS T1W pre- and postcontrast MRI.

Patient 2:

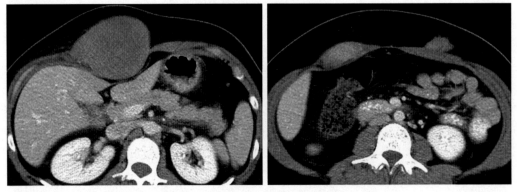

Axial images from contrast-enhanced CT.

Patient 3:

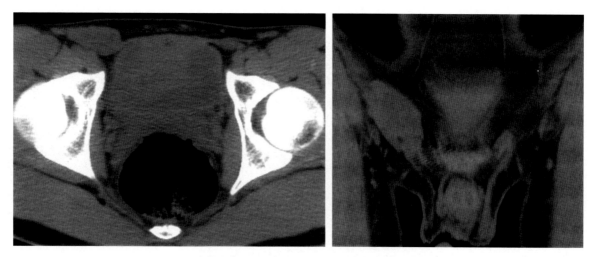

Axial and coronal noncontrast CT images.

Patient 4:

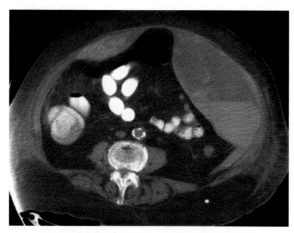

Axial CT without IV contrast.

A. A 93-year-old patient hospitalized for pneumonia and acute renal failure requiring dialysis, now with abdominal pain

B. A 47-year-old patient with cyclical pain along surgical incision

C. A 15-year-old patient with abnormal genital examination

D. A 39-year-old patient status post colectomy

10a A 35-year-old woman presents with abdominal fullness. What is the most likely diagnosis?

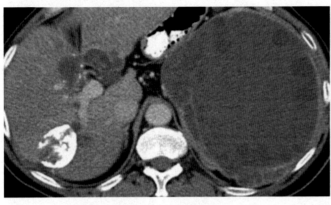 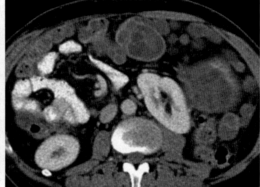

    A. Amebic abscesses
    B. Peritoneal carcinomatosis
    C. Desmoid tumors
    D. Echinococcal cysts

10b What imaging feature is demonstrated on the images in the previous question?
    A. Water lily sign
    B. Hydatid sand
    C. Daughter cysts
    D. Central dot sign

11 Which of the following techniques would decrease the conspicuity of the type of artifacts shown on the following CT images from two different patients?

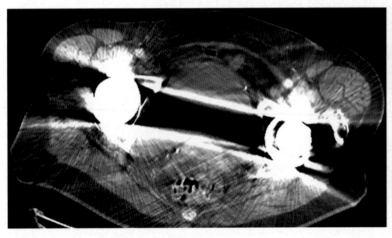 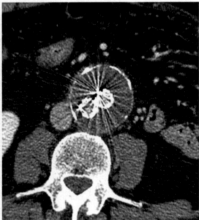

    A. Decreasing the reconstruction slice thickness
    B. Decreasing mAs
    C. Increasing kVp
    D. Decreasing the maximum window of the CT scale

12 What is TRUE about the phenomenon accounting for the signal intensity (arrows) at the margins of the kidneys on this abdominal MR image?

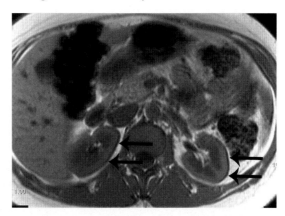

A. It occurs in the frequency-encoding but not the phase-encoding direction.
B. It is caused by out-of-phase protons within the pixels.
C. It can be reduced by shimming.
D. It is more prominent when imaging at 1.5 Tesla compared to 3 Tesla.

13 Two images from an MRI examination and one image from a CT scan on the same patient are presented below. What accounts for the large area of signal loss on the MR images?

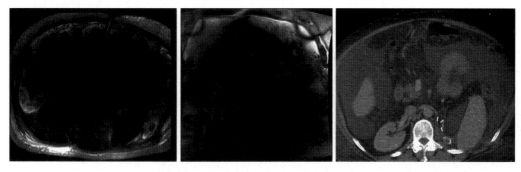

A. Metallic foreign bodies
B. Respiratory motion
C. Pneumoperitoneum
D. Dielectric effect

14 A 51-year-old woman is evaluated with an MRI for a pancreatic lesion. What is the finding incidentally noted in the left kidney?

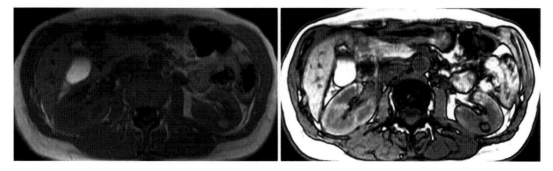

A. Renal cyst
B. Renal angiomyolipoma
C. Clear cell renal cell carcinoma
D. Renal stone

For each patient in questions 15 to 19, identify the MRI artifact. Each option may be used once or not at all:

    A. Metallic susceptibility artifact
    B. Radiofrequency spike artifact
    C. Respiratory motion artifact
    D. Wraparound (aliasing) artifact
    E. Misplaced presaturation pulse
    F. Fluid motion artifact

15 Patient 1:   **16** Patient 2:   **17** Patient 3:

18 Patient 4:   **19** Patient 5:

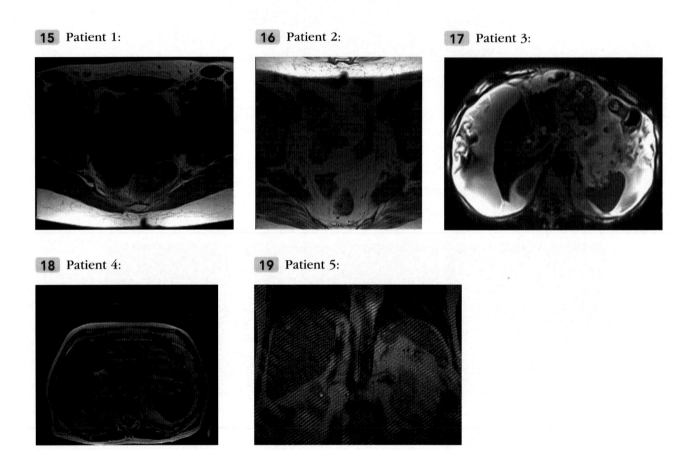

ANSWERS AND EXPLANATIONS

1 **Answer B.** A **gossypiboma** is a retained mass of fabric. This patient had a surgical laparotomy pad inadvertently left behind at appendectomy 18 years ago. The patient was asymptomatic at the time of discovery. Gossypibomas classically have spongiform appearance with **internal foci of gas** and **whorled architecture** of the wavy layers of fabric. A radiopaque marker strip if present makes the diagnosis, and **may be more easily recognized as a foreign body on the scout image (arrow below) rather than individual CT slices.** Chronic gossypibomas may calcify or develop an enhancing fibrous capsule. This enhancement can lead to misdiagnosis as abscess or as a neoplasm such as gastrointestinal stromal tumor or sarcoma. Retained surgical material can act as a nidus for infection.

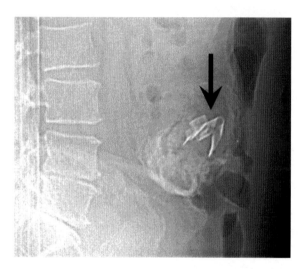

References: Bahrami S, Chow D, Kadell B. Thoracic and abdominal devices radiologists should recognize: pictorial review. *AJR Am J Roentgenol* 2009;193(6 Suppl):S106–S118.

Gayer G, Petrovitch I, Jeffrey RB. Foreign objects encountered in the abdominal cavity at CT. *Radiographics* 2011;31(2):409–428.

2 **Answer C.** There is diffuse cystic replacement of the pancreas in von Hippel-Lindau (VHL) disease, a rare autosomal dominant hereditary disorder that is one of the neurocutaneous syndromes. VHL disease is associated with benign and malignant tumors due to inactivation of the VHL tumor suppressor gene. **The most common cause of mortality is renal cell carcinoma, a neoplasm that occurs in almost half of patients with VHL.** Central nervous system hemangioblastomas (arrow on the following image) are benign vascular tumors, but complications from hemangioblastomas also contribute significantly to morbidity and mortality.

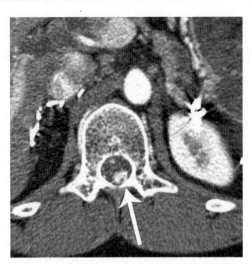

Spinal hemangioblastoma on abdominal CT in patient with VHL. There are surgical clips from resection of bilateral adrenal pheochromocytomas.

Birt-Hogg-Dubé is a neurocutaneous syndrome that is associated with renal cell carcinoma and lung cysts but not pancreatic cysts. Tuberous sclerosis and cystic fibrosis rarely do show pancreatic cysts, but cystic replacement is not a feature, and they have no association with renal cell carcinoma. (Tuberous sclerosis is associated with renal angiomyolipomas.)

There is variable expression of VHL, but asymptomatic family members can be identified by genetic testing. **Multimodality imaging plays a key role in screening for malignancy and other clinically significant manifestations.** About 40 manifestations involving over a dozen organs have been associated with VHL, some of them listed below, including other pancreatic lesions. Pancreatic cysts are the most prevalent manifestation, occurring in 40% to 90% of patients. These cysts are usually asymptomatic but help identify patients with VHL.

Two entities that are rare and essentially pathognomonic for VHL when bilateral are endolymphatic sac tumors and epididymal papillary cystadenomas. Endolymphatic sac tumors are hypervascular and can locally invade and destroy the petrous temporal bone, causing hearing loss. Papillary cystadenomas in the epididymis are mixed solid and cystic tumors, which have no malignant potential and do not require intervention.

Selected Manifestations of von Hippel-Lindau Disease

Pancreatic
- Cysts (most common finding in VHL, typically asymptomatic)
- Neuroendocrine tumors
- Serous microcystic cystadenomas
- (Pancreatic adenocarcinoma)

Neurologic
- Hemangioblastomas (cerebellum is most common location and contribute significantly to morbidity and mortality; also found in the retina, spine, and medulla)
- Endolymphatic sac tumor (tend to be bilateral and can cause hearing loss)

Renal
- Cysts
- Renal cell carcinoma (most common cause of mortality)

Adrenal
- Pheochromocytoma

Other genitourinary
- Papillary cystadenomas of the epididymis (tend to be bilateral, no malignant potential)

References: Ganeshan D, Menias CO, Pickhardt PJ, et al. Tumors in von Hippel-Lindau syndrome: from head to toe-comprehensive state-of-the-art review. *Radiographics* 2018;38(3):849–866.8.

Gosein M, Harris A, Pang E, et al. Abdominal imaging findings in neurocutaneous syndromes: looking below the diaphragm. *AJR Am J Roentgenol* 2017;209(6):1197–1208.

3 **Answer A.** Axial and coronal CT images show discontinuity (arrows) of the left hemidiaphragm consistent with **diaphragmatic rupture**, complicated by herniation of the stomach, transverse colon, spleen, and a small portion of the left hepatic lobe into the left thorax. The left lung is compressed by the herniation and is opacified due to contusion and hemorrhage. The mediastinum is shifted to the right, and no pneumothorax is identified. There is traumatic subcutaneous emphysema in the left chest wall, so congenital pathology such as Morgagni hernia (anterior and medial at cardiophrenic angle) and hypoplastic left lung are not the best choices.

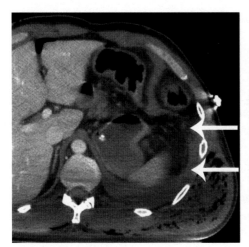 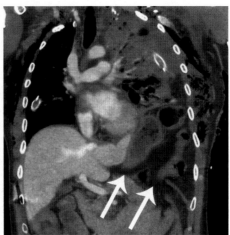

Diaphragmatic injuries are almost always associated with other injuries. **The left diaphragm is ruptured more often** than the right. Evaluation of the integrity of the diaphragm may be challenging, and **correlation of the axial images with CT multiplanar reconstructions in the coronal and sagittal planes** may be helpful. Direct and indirect signs of diaphragmatic rupture have variable sensitivity but excellent specificity >90%. A few of these signs are listed in the table below. Complications of diaphragmatic rupture include bowel incarceration, obstruction, and strangulation; respiratory insufficiency; pneumonia; pleural effusion/empyema; and tension physiology from mediastinal shift. Diaphragmatic rupture **requires surgical repair.**

Signs of Diaphragmatic Rupture	
Direct Signs	**Comments**
Segmental diaphragmatic defect	• Discontinuity with direct visualization of injury
Dangling diaphragm	• Free edge of torn diaphragm deviating toward the center of the body
Absent diaphragm	• Complete absence, nonrecognition, or indistinctness of hemidiaphragm

(Continued)

Signs of Diaphragmatic Rupture (*Continued*)	
Indirect Signs (Related to Consequences of Rupture)	
Herniation through a defect	• Passage of abdominal contents into the pleural or pericardial space • Mimics: Congenital hernias and acquired hernias through hiatus
Collar sign	• Waist-like constriction of herniated structure at the site of rupture
Hump and band sign	• Constriction of the liver through a right-sided rupture
Dependent viscera sign	• Direct contact between the herniated abdominal organs and posterior chest wall

References: Desir A, Ghaye B. CT of blunt diaphragmatic rupture. *Radiographics* 2012;32(2):477–498.

Nason LK, Walker CM, McNeeley MF, et al. Imaging of the diaphragm: anatomy and function. *Radiographics* 2012;32(2):E51–E70.

4 **Answer C.** This is a ring artifact indicating a defective detector element. **It is corrected by recalibration, cleaning, or replacement of the detector.** If the artifact is more subtle, one of the central rings may be mistaken for a mass. The other answer choices do not produce concentric ring artifacts.

Beam hardening causes central low-density areas (cupping) or streaking. The slip ring allows the gantry to rotate smoothly and facilitates transmission of power and data. When there is loss of normal contact between the slip ring and the various stationary CT components, artifactual lines of incomplete data cross the image. X-ray tube arcing can occur with contamination of the tube or the oil surrounding the tube by gas or impurities, resulting in intermittent loss of x-ray output. This may manifest as increased noise and lines across the image.

References: Boas FE, Fleischmann D. CT artifacts: causes and reduction techniques. *Imaging Med* 2012;4(2):229–240.

Triche BL, Nelson JT, McGill NS, et al. Recognizing and minimizing artifacts at CT, MRI, US, and molecular imaging. *Radiographics* 2019;39(4):1017–1018.

5 **Answer B.** This constellation of findings is consistent with lap-belt compression injury. There is abnormal thickening and hypoenhancement of the transverse duodenal segment (short white arrows), which was confirmed at surgery to be completely transected. The CT images show linear intraluminal filling defects within the abdominal aorta (long white arrows). Sagittal images show that the aortic injury is at the same level as a vertebral body fracture (long black arrow). Small bowel injuries and abdominal aortic injuries are each relatively uncommon following blunt trauma. However, **seatbelts, and in particular lap belts, have been implicated in this pattern of blunt abdominal trauma involving flexion–distraction spine injuries, bowel injuries, and abdominal aortic injuries**. There have also been reports of rupture of the spleen, pancreas, kidney, liver, and gravid uterus. Delayed diagnosis can lead to significant morbidity and mortality.

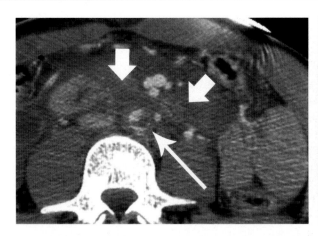
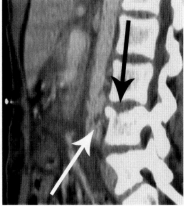

References: Dreizin D, Munera F. Blunt polytrauma: evaluation with 64-section whole-body CT angiography. *Radiographics* 2012;32(3):609–631.

Fadl SA, Sandstrom CK. Pattern recognition: a mechanism-based approach to injury detection after motor vehicle collisions. *Radiographics* 2019;39(3):857–876.

6 **Answer D.** This patient presented with penetrating **trauma** from a gunshot. There is hemoperitoneum as well as pneumoperitoneum with subcutaneous emphysema. In the setting of penetrating trauma, pneumoperitoneum does not always indicate bowel injury. However, in this case, there is **bowel injury** with decreased enhancement of the wall of the jejunum in the left upper quadrant as well as **mesenteric vascular injury with active contrast extravasation** (white arrows).

This patient exhibits the **CT hypotension/hypoperfusion complex ("shock bowel")**. The bowel wall is thickened due to edema and shows prominent mucosal enhancement. The stomach and small bowel are dilated and fluid filled not because of bowel obstruction but because of hypofunction and poor resorption of fluid.

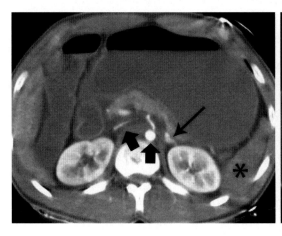
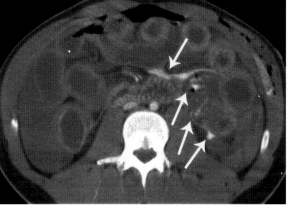

Additional features of the CT hypotension complex other than the bowel findings are less consistently identified. The additional features seen here are:

- Abnormal great vessels (short black arrows) with flattened IVC of <9 mm AP dimension and a diminutive aorta
- Halo sign with rim of low-density fluid surrounding the flattened IVC
- Hyperenhancing adrenal gland (long black arrow)
- Hypoenhancing spleen (asterisk)

Other features of CT hypotension not shown here include:

- Delayed nephrograms
- Hepatic hypoenhancement
- Heterogeneous pancreatic enhancement with surrounding fluid

Although the CT hypotension complex was originally described in trauma, other causes of severe hypotension can produce the same findings, including diabetic ketoacidosis, sepsis, and cardiac arrest. It is more frequently seen in children, including cases of nonaccidental trauma, than in adults. Supportive care is indicated (separate from the traumatic findings in this case, which require surgical attention). **Findings of CT hypotension complex are reversible** and should not be mistaken for ischemic bowel requiring resection.

References: Alexander LF, Hanna TN, LeGout JD, et al. Multidetector CT findings in the abdomen and pelvis after damage control surgery for acute traumatic injuries. *Radiographics* 2019;39(4):1183–1202.

Ames JT, Federle MP. CT hypotension complex (shock bowel) is not always due to traumatic hypovolemic shock. *AJR Am J Roentgenol* 2009;192(5):W230–W235.

7 **Answer C.** These imaging findings associated with elevation of serum angiotensin-converting enzyme (ACE) level are consistent with **sarcoidosis**. There are mediastinal and hilar adenopathy, symmetric perilymphatic/peribronchovascular nodular interstitial lung disease, and numerous small hypoattenuating hepatic and splenic nodules. Sarcoidosis is a systemic inflammatory disease characterized by the development of **noncaseating (nonnecrotizing) granulomas**. The disease has protean manifestations and appears in the differential diagnosis across multiple organ systems. **The constellation of imaging findings may be seen in other granulomatous disease including disseminated infection by mycobacterial and fungal organisms.** Findings also overlap with lymphoma and metastatic disease, but malignancies are unlikely to be bilaterally symmetric or upper lobe predominant. An elevated ACE level is neither highly sensitive nor specific for sarcoidosis, but significant elevation along with these findings supports the diagnosis.

The multisystemic manifestations of sarcoidosis are summarized in the table below. **The most common radiologic finding is intrathoracic adenopathy, found in the majority of patients.** Lymphadenopathy may contain calcifications. **Mortality from sarcoidosis occurs in up to 5% of cases, usually from severe pulmonary or cardiac involvement.**

Abdominal abnormalities may be seen with or without intrathoracic manifestations. **The liver and spleen are the most commonly affected** abdominal viscera at autopsy, although involvement may not be appreciated on imaging and the great majority are asymptomatic. The nodules are hypoenhancing to surrounding parenchyma and hypointense on T1W and T2W MR images. Asymptomatic involvement of the liver and spleen does not require treatment.

Sarcoidosis is of uncertain etiology but may be the result of an exaggerated cellular response to an antigenic trigger. In the United States, the disease is most prevalent in African Americans. There is variability in disease manifestation and natural history, ranging from spontaneous remission to chronic progressive disease. The mainstay of treatment is **corticosteroids**, although in severe cases, immunosuppressive agents such as methotrexate and cyclophosphamide are used.

Manifestations of Sarcoidosis

Anatomic Location	Comments

Chest	• Lymphadenopathy (85%): bilateral hila and mediastinum
	• Lungs (20%): perihilar and upper lobe predominant
	  ○ Peribronchovascular nodular interstitial pattern
	  ○ Confluent opacities
	  ○ End-stage fibrosis
	• Heart: areas of myocardial delayed enhancement on MRI

Abdomen	• Liver and spleen
	  ○ Hepatosplenomegaly
	  ○ Nodules
	  ○ Biliary strictures and cholestasis
	  ○ Cirrhosis
	• Lymphadenopathy (30%)
	• Kidneys (20%)
	  ○ Nephrocalcinosis from hypercalcemia
	  ○ Interstitial and glomerular nephritis
	  ○ Nodules
	• (Pancreas in <5% of cases: pancreatitis, nodules)
	• (Bowel in <5% of cases, mostly stomach: fold thickening, ulcers, nodules)

Pelvis	• (Scrotum: epididymal and testicular nodules in <5% of cases)
Head and neck	• Cervical lymphadenopathy • Lacrimal and parotid glands (panda sign on 67-gallium scintigraphy) • Eyes: uveitis • Central nervous system (10%): basilar predilection involving cranial nerves, leptomeninges, pituitary and hypothalamus, deep white matter, spinal cord
Skin	• Erythema nodosum (red tender nodules) • Lupus pernio (indurated facial plaques)

References: Ganeshan D, Menias CO, Lubner MG, et al. Sarcoidosis from head to toe: what the radiologist needs to know. *Radiographics* 2018;38(4):1180–1200.

Prabhakar HB, Rabinowitz CB, Gibbons FK, et al. Imaging features of sarcoidosis on MDCT, FDG PET, and PET/CT. *AJR Am J Roentgenol* 2008;190(3 Suppl):S1–S6.

8 **Answer D.** All of the listed entities are associated with small bowel findings as well as cutaneous or other soft tissue abnormalities. In this patient, the combination of multiple small bowel GSTs, a circumscribed posterior chest paraspinous mass extending partially into and expanding the neural foramen typical for a schwannoma or neurofibroma, and nodular skin masses suggests **neurofibromatosis type 1**.

Scleroderma findings include small bowel dilatation and closely spaced thin folds ("hidebound" appearance) and skin changes due to excess collagen deposition. Peutz-Jeghers syndrome includes small bowel hamartomatous polyps and adenocarcinomas, and skin changes of mucocutaneous melanin deposits. Gardner syndrome is associated with adenomatous polyps and adenocarcinomas of small bowel (especially the duodenum) as well as soft tissue desmoid tumors.

Neurofibromatosis type 1 (NF-1), also known as von Recklinghausen disease, is a common autosomal dominant neurocutaneous syndrome affecting 1 in 3,000 people. Half of cases are inherited, and the other half are sporadic, with wide variation in penetrance and manifestations. **Gastrointestinal abnormalities are relatively common in NF-1. These include mesenchymal neoplasms, of which neurofibromas are the most common, and gastrointestinal stromal tumors, leiomyomas, and leiomyosarcomas.** Other tumor types include neuroendocrine tumors (especially in the duodenum) and rarely adenocarcinomas.

Selected Features of Neurofibromatosis Type 1	
Central nervous system	• Gliomas, including optic glioma • Meningiomas • Lisch nodules (pigmented hamartomas of the iris)—specific for NF-1 when multiple
Cutaneous	• Café au lait spots • Dermal neurofibromas • Freckling in the axillary and inguinal regions
Abdominal	• Neurofibromas in paraspinal region, mesentery, and bowel • Malignant peripheral nerve sheath tumor (the most common malignancy, seen in 5%–10% of patients) • Gastrointestinal stromal tumors • Paragangliomas (pheochromocytomas and extra-adrenal pheochromocytomas) • Carcinoids in the periampullary region
Musculoskeletal	• Dysplasia of the sphenoid wing or long bones

References: Gosein M, Harris A, Pang E, et al. Abdominal imaging findings in neurocutaneous syndromes: looking below the diaphragm. *AJR Am J Roentgenol* 2017;209(6):1197–1208.

Levy AD, Patel N, Abbott RM, et al. Gastrointestinal stromal tumors in patients with neurofibromatosis: imaging features with clinicopathologic correlation. *AJR Am J Roentgenol* 2004;183(6):1629–1636.

9 | **Answers:**

Patient 1: B. Scar endometriosis in a 47-year-old patient with cyclical pain along surgical incision

Patient 2: D. Desmoid tumors in a 39-year-old patient status post colectomy

Patient 3: C. Undescended testis in a 15-year-old patient with abnormal physical examination

Patient 4: A. Rectus sheath hematomas in a 93-year-old hospitalized patient with new abdominal pain

Diagnoses to consider in patients with abdominal wall masses are listed below.

Differential Diagnosis of Abdominal Wall Masses	
Normal tissue in abnormal location	• Hernia • Undescended testis
"Water"	• Seroma • Sites of subcutaneous injection of medication, which can develop into injection granulomas composed of fat necrosis, scar, and calcification • Sebaceous cysts

Differential Diagnosis of Abdominal Wall Masses (*Continued*)	
"Blood"	• Hematoma
"Pus"	• Abscess
"Cells"	• Benign or low-grade neoplasm ○ Lipoma ○ Scar endometriosis ○ Desmoid tumor (a benign or low-grade nonmetastasizing neoplasm) • Malignant neoplasm ○ Metastases, including a "Sister Mary Joseph nodule" from peritoneal or hematogenous spread to umbilicus ○ Lymphoma ○ Sarcoma

Patient 1 has **scar endometriosis** with abdominal wall pain and lump along her caesarean section incision. **Classically, the pain is cyclical associated with menses,** but some patients may be asymptomatic. Axial MR images show a heterogeneous infiltrative enhancing mass involving the right rectus muscle and subcutaneous fat. The sagittal image demonstrates the dark susceptibility artifact from caesarean section in the low anterior uterus. Scar endometriosis is the result of incorporation of endometriomas into the abdominal wall at the time of gynecologic surgery. **These implants can enhance and show color Doppler vascular flow.** Appearance is variable on T1W and T2W images. The colon has not been resected in this case so choice D is incorrect.

Patient 2 is a **young patient status post total colectomy for familial adenomatous polyposis (FAP) and Gardner syndrome.** The CT shows multiple soft tissue masses in the bilateral abdominal wall consistent with desmoid fibromatosis. Desmoid tumors may also be intra-abdominal involving the mesentery. **They may arise sporadically in the abdominal wall in patients without Gardner syndrome, typically in women of childbearing age, but desmoid tumors are found in about 20% of patients with Gardner syndrome.** There is a **strong association with prior surgery, most commonly a total colectomy.** Desmoid tumors have a spectrum of appearances depending on their underlying composition. Degree of enhancement is variable. Those with a greater amount of collagen have the appearance of soft tissue, while those with greater amount of myxoid components appear more cystic. These tumors are in the spectrum of "deep fibromatosis" and grouped by site of origin into intra-abdominal (including mesenteric), abdominal (wall), and extra-abdominal fibromatosis. Although it is considered a benign or low-grade neoplasm that does not metastasize, desmoid fibromatosis is locally aggressive and may cause complications such as bowel obstruction and fistulas. **The disease is often difficult to locally control, and patients frequently recur despite resection and chemoradiotherapy.** Metastatic disease and lymphoma are in the differential diagnosis of abdominal and mesenteric masses but are less likely given the clinical history.

Patient 3 has an **undescended testis (cryptorchidism).** Only one testis was palpable in the scrotum on physical examination. An ovoid structure is present in the right anterior pelvic wall (arrows on the following images), with the suggestion of a triangular epididymal head at the superior pole on the coronal view. On the normal left side, the spermatic cord (short arrows on the following coronal image) is seen in the inguinal canal extending into the scrotum but not on the cryptorchid right side. **An undescended testis may be atrophic and not recognized as testicular tissue.** In this case, low-dose CT was performed, but an **ultrasound would identify the location of an undescended testis**

without radiation exposure. Even if orchiopexy is performed to relocate the testis, patients with cryptorchidism continue to have increased risk of subfertility and testicular cancer, requiring continued surveillance.

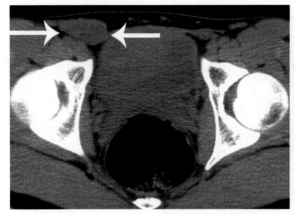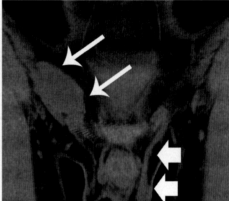

Undescended testis.

Patient 4 with acute pain has bilateral **rectus sheath hematomas**. There are spindle-shaped heterogeneous masses expanding the rectus sheath bilaterally on this CT without IV contrast. There is layering high density in the collection on the left representing a **serum-hematocrit level.** Hematomas of the anterior abdominal wall frequently involve the rectus sheath. Risk factors include trauma, surgery, anticoagulation, and coughing. This patient was being heparinized for dialysis and coughing because of pneumonia. Occasionally, active hemorrhage is identified on a contrast-enhanced examination.

References: Ballard DH, Mazaheri P, Oppenheimer DC, et al. Imaging of abdominal wall masses, masslike lesions, and diffuse processes. *Radiographics* 2020;40(3):684–706.

George V, Tammisetti VS, Surabhi VR, et al. Chronic fibrosing conditions in abdominal imaging. *Radiographics* 2013;33(4):1053–1080.

Gore RM, Ghahremani GG, Donaldson CK, et al. Chapter 112: Hernias and abdominal wall pathology. In: Gore RM, Levine MS (eds). *Textbook of gastrointestinal radiology*, 4th ed. Philadelphia, PA: Elsevier/Saunders, 2015:2053–2076.

10a **Answer D. Echinococcal cysts.**

10b **Answer C.** This patient has disseminated echinococcal infection. There are multiple complex cystic masses with appearance **pathognomonic for echinococcal (hydatid) cysts.** The dominant mass replacing the spleen represents an **encapsulated "mother cyst" with multiple peripheral "daughter cysts"** (short white arrows) arranged in a spoke wheel, or rosette, pattern. The daughter cysts typically demonstrate lower density on CT than the mother cyst. Other complex cysts are seen scattered in the liver and peritoneal cavity (long white arrows). There should be a **history of travel** to underdeveloped parts of the world where this disease is endemic.

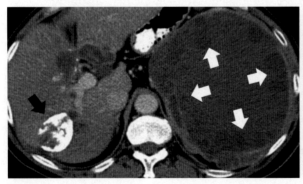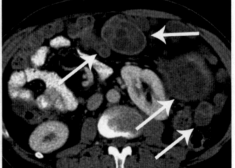

Echinococcal cysts have variable appearance, ranging from simple cysts to complex solid and cystic masses. Lesions with extensive calcification, such as the one in the right lobe of the liver (short black arrow), are more likely to represent involuted inactive cysts. The **"water lily" sign** is also highly specific for echinococcal cysts, referring to sloughing and collapse of the internal membrane within a cyst. **"Hydatid sand"** represents mobile debris that can be seen in the cysts on ultrasound. When imaging features are less specific, the differential diagnosis may include cystic lesions such as abscess or biliary cystadenoma/cystadenocarcinoma (not answer choices). Cystic or necrotic metastases may be considered if there are enhancing soft tissue components. Amebic abscesses are usually unilocular and thick walled, with appearance similar to pyogenic (bacterial) abscesses. The "central dot" sign is an enhancing focus associated with the cystic lesions of Caroli disease.

Hydatid disease is a parasitic infection caused by tapeworms endemic in underdeveloped parts of the world, particularly where sheep are raised. Humans are infected by ingesting water contaminated with dog feces harboring *Echinococcus* eggs. **The liver is the most common site of involvement, seen in 75% to 80% of cases, followed by the lung and spleen**, but widespread dissemination is possible. The World Health Organization's ultrasound classification has five categories and is the most widely used. The system attempts to stage individual cysts as active, transitional, or inactive based on ultrasound appearance in order to direct treatment. **Echinococcal cysts may be complicated by peritoneal rupture, portal obstruction, biliary obstruction, and superinfection.** Treatment options include surgery, percutaneous aspiration, and antiparasitic agents such as albendazole. The antiparasitic agents also prevent anaphylaxis during the procedure.

References: Pakala T, Molina M, Wu GY. Hepatic echinococcal cysts: a review. *J Clin Transl Hepatol* 2016;4(1):39–46.

Zalaquett E, Menias C, Garrido F, et al. Imaging of hydatid disease with a focus on extrahepatic involvement. *Radiographics* 2017;37(3):901–923.

11 **Answer C.** Increasing kVp. Multiple mechanisms account for metal artifacts, such as beam hardening, scatter, photon starvation, edge gradient effects, and narrow window of the CT scale. With photon starvation, not enough photons are reaching the detectors. **Photon starvation** increases with greater density of the material. The resulting dark and bright bands are preferentially oriented in the direction of greatest attenuation—along the path of the hip replacements. **Beam hardening** occurs because lower-energy photons are absorbed more rapidly than higher-energy photons when encountering a high-density material, such that the polychromatic beam that has passed through a material consists of a larger proportion of higher-energy protons. As a result, **the attenuation data along the subsequent path of the beam do not reflect true tissue density, and bands or streaks are seen.** Beam hardening can result in cupping, with the center of an object appearing artifactually lower density than the periphery.

Of note, there is **windmill configuration of the metal artifact in the second image in the setting of helical acquisition**. Dark and bright streaks radiate from the metal at regular intervals and appear to spin from one image to the next. This configuration reflects undersampling in the Z-axis and is a type of aliasing. The number of pairs in the windmill correlates with the number of detectors intersecting the reconstructed imaging plane. This windmill artifact produced by bone is particularly problematic in the head, so CT protocols may use axial rather than helical acquisition to improve intracranial visualization as demonstrated on the images below. Windmill artifact can also be reduced by reducing the pitch.

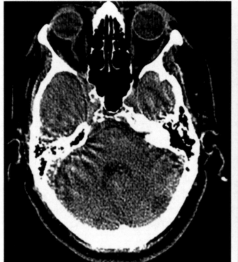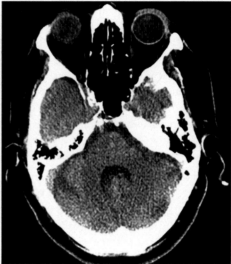

Windmill artifact with helical acquisition, corrected with axial acquisition.

CT scanners are equipped with algorithms that reduce some of the effects of beam hardening and photon starvation. Metal artifact reduction (MAR) reconstruction algorithm as shown below improves visualization of tissues surrounding a hip replacement.

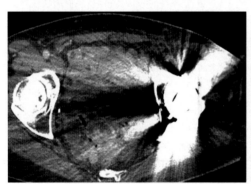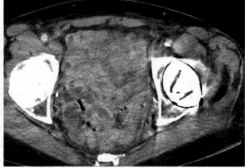

Application of MAR reconstruction algorithm.

Some techniques that reduce the conspicuity of metal artifacts are listed below.

Techniques for Reducing Metal Artifacts on CT	
Technique	**Comments**
Apply metal artifact reduction (MAR) algorithms	• A threshold Hounsfield unit is used to identify metal, then interpolates missing data in projection space from neighboring uncorrupted projections • Primarily suppress artifacts that are due to photon starvation • Iterative reconstruction that can be applied retrospectively

Techniques for Reducing Metal Artifacts on CT (*Continued*)

Technique	Comments
Angle the CT gantry	• To avoid the metal or decrease the distance, the beam travels through the metal
Increase peak voltage (kVp)	• Improves beam penetration through metal • Dual-energy CT scanners acquire images at both low and high kVP • Decreases iodinated contrast enhancement and decreases subject contrast
Decrease (narrow) the collimation	• Smaller focal area = thinner slice acquisition for better spatial resolution
Increase tube current (mAs)	• Decreases noise
Reconstruct with thicker sections	• Decreases noise
Select a smoother reconstruction algorithm (kernel)	• Soft tissue algorithms are smoother than bone algorithms but have less spatial resolution
Extend the CT scale to accommodate the very high density of metal	• Standard maximum window of CT numbers is 4,000 HU, but most metallic implants have density beyond this range that is unable to be reconstructed, causing blurring and distortion • Option to extend scale up to 40,000 HU available on some scanners

References: Katsura M, Sato J, Akahane M, et al. Current and novel techniques for metal artifact reduction at CT: practical guide for radiologists. *Radiographics* 2018;38(2):450–461.12.

Triche BL, Nelson JT, McGill NS, et al. Recognizing and minimizing artifacts at CT, MRI, US, and molecular imaging. *Radiographics* 2019;39(4):1017–1018.

12 **Answer A.** Chemical shift artifacts type I and II are seen where fat and water protons meet inside the body. The dark line seen on the left-sided margin of both kidneys is a **type I chemical shift artifact, a phenomenon seen in the frequency-encoding but not phase-encoding direction.** The frequency-encoding direction in abdominal imaging is usually assigned to the transverse dimension (so that phase encoding can be assigned to the shorter anteroposterior dimension and minimize scan time); therefore, this artifact is usually seen in the transverse dimension. The corresponding bright line at the opposite (right-sided) margin of both kidneys is less conspicuous because of the brightness of the perirenal fat. Whether the black and white lines are seen on the left or right side depends on whether the frequency-encoding gradient is increasing or decreasing from left to right.

Type I chemical shift artifact is due to spatial misregistration. Spatial localization in the frequency direction is inferred by the frequency of precession of the proton. However, **protons in the water process at a slightly different frequency than that of fat. The MRI scanner misrepresents this as a difference in spatial location**, as depicted on the following diagram.

The misregistration is worse (the line is thicker) at 3 Tesla than at 1.5 Tesla because the difference in precession frequency between water and fat protons is larger at greater field strengths. **The artifact may be reduced by increasing the receiver bandwidth or using a fat suppression technique.** Swapping the phase and frequency directions may move the artifact to a different location. Type II chemical shift involves out-of-phase protons within the same pixel. Shimming improves magnetic field homogeneity, which does not improve type I chemical shift artifact.

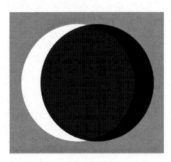

Spatial misregistration in type I chemical shift.

References: Huang SY, Seethamraju RT, Patel P, et al. Body MR imaging: artifacts, k-space, and solutions. *Radiographics* 2015;35(5):1439–1460.

Triche BL, Nelson JT, McGill NS, et al. Recognizing and minimizing artifacts at CT, MRI, US, and molecular imaging. *Radiographics* 2019;39(4):1017–1018.

13 **Answer D.** There is a large area of signal loss in the central abdomen rendering the MR images nondiagnostic. This appearance is consistent with the **dielectric effect (or "standing waves")**. An electric field always coexists with a magnetic field. **Intra-abdominal fluid, such as ascites in this case or amniotic fluid, can promote the formation of a circulating electric field due to its conductive properties** under the influence of the external RF field. This current produces its own magnetic field that interferes with the main magnetic field.

Dielectric artifacts are worse at 3 Tesla than at 1.5 Tesla, because the RF of the transmission field is at a higher frequency. This shortens the wavelengths to a distance that more closely approximates the size of many adult torsos (26 cm at 3 Tesla, compared to 52 cm at 1.5 Tesla). When this occurs, the interactions of the soft tissues with the electric component of an electromagnetic field come into play. Standing waves can develop, causing areas of increased or decreased signal intensity. **The dielectric effect may be seen on one or multiple series**, depending on the field of view and other parameters affecting soft tissue interactions. To reduce the dielectric artifact:

- **Apply dielectric pads** to the patient's body to simulate body mass.
- **Use multichannel transmit arrays**, which tailor the RF waveforms to compensate for the spatial variations.
- **Image at 1.5 Tesla** instead of 3 Tesla.

Metallic foreign bodies cause susceptibility artifact with blooming and signal dropout, but the surgical clips in the left renal fossa on the CT image would not account for the size of the signal loss. Respiratory motion causes repetitive ghosting. Pneumoperitoneum is poorly demonstrated on MRI, and MRI should not be used for detection. Gas is dark on MRI, but there is no pneumoperitoneum on the CT image.

References: Hoang PB, Huang SY, Song AW, et al. Chapter 9: Motion, pulsation, and other artifacts. In: Mangrum WI (ed). *Duke review of MRI physics*, 2nd ed. Philadelphia, PA: Elsevier, Inc., 2019:91–105.

Huang SY, Seethamraju RT, Patel P, et al. Body MR imaging: artifacts, k-space, and solutions. *Radiographics* 2015;35(5):1439–1460.

14 **Answer B.** These are T1W gradient echo in- and out-of-phase images without IV contrast. The appearance of the out-of-phase image is characterized by **type II chemical shift, which manifests as the black boundary artifact (also known as the India ink or etching artifact) around structures with a fat–water interface**. If a mass contains *macroscopic* (not microscopic) fat such as this **renal angiomyolipoma** (AML), its border with the fluid-containing organ will demonstrate the black boundary artifact (arrow) on the out-of-phase image. The macroscopic fat in the AML is bright on both of the non–fat-saturated T1 images. The following image on the right is a fat-saturated T1W image showing that this lesion loses signal intensity, behaving as expected for macroscopic fat.

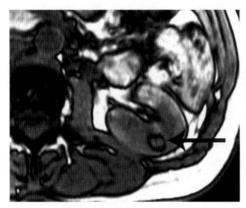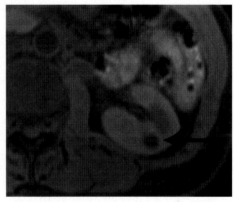

Renal AML with black boundary on out-of-phase T1W and fat saturation on FS T1W image.

A clear cell renal cell carcinoma and other lesions that contain *microscopic* fat should demonstrate an area of signal dropout on the out-of-phase image rather than a thin boundary. A renal stone of this size is usually dark on all MRI sequences. A renal cyst may be T1 hyperintense if it is proteinaceous or hemorrhagic, but the black boundary artifact with renal parenchyma is not associated with such cysts.

Type II chemical shift artifact **occurs in any direction with a fat–water interface, not just the frequency-encoding direction that is seen with type I chemical shift**. The TE is selected such that the fat and water spins located in the same pixel are out of phase, at about 2.3 msec in a 1.5-Tesla magnet. (Timing is different in 3-Tesla magnets.) The signals cancel each other out within a pixel, creating the black boundary artifact. This artifact is not seen when a TE is chosen that achieves an in-phase image (around 4.6 msec, double that of the out-of-phase image) or if fat saturation is applied.

References: Huang SY, Seethamraju RT, Patel P, et al. Body MR imaging: artifacts, k-space, and solutions. *Radiographics* 2015;35(5):1439–1460.

Triche BL, Nelson JT, McGill NS, et al. Recognizing and minimizing artifacts at CT, MRI, US, and molecular imaging. *Radiographics* 2019;39(4):1017–1018.

15 **Answer E.** MRI for patient 1 demonstrates a **misplaced presaturation pulse** ("sat band") across the midpelvis. **Spatial selective presaturation pulses are applied to suppress signal arising outside the area of interest but inside the field of view, so that the signal does not compromise image interpretation.** A sat band placed across the anterior abdominal wall (arrows) can prevent respiratory motion artifact or wraparound artifact. In a sagittal spine series, a sat band may be placed over bowel to reduce motion artifact from bowel peristalsis. A presaturation pulse can also be used to saturate the protons in flowing blood before they enter the volume being evaluated. In time-of-flight MRI, vascular flow in one direction can be eliminated so that flow in other direction is preferentially displayed. **Application of presaturation pulses increases scan time.**

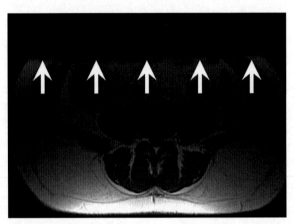

Correctly placed saturation band.

References: Hoang PB, Song AW, Merkle EM. Chapter 5: Frequency and spatial saturation pulses. In: Mangrum WI (ed). *Duke review of MRI physics*, 2nd ed. Philadelphia, PA: Elsevier, Inc., 2019:49–54.

Sheikh-Sarraf M, Nougaret S, Forstner R, et al. Patient preparation and image quality in female pelvic MRI: recommendations revisited. *Eur Radiol* 2020;30:5374–5383.

16 **Answer D.** MRI for patient 2 demonstrates wraparound (aliasing) artifact. A section of the patient's posterior soft tissues and coccyx are superimposed anteriorly. **Wraparound artifact occurs in the phase-encoding direction** when using small fields of view. The signal is not sampled with enough phase-encoding steps to correctly localize the data, and the MRI system erroneously maps these signals to the opposite end of the axis. Because the shorter axis is usually designated the phase-encoding direction to save time during image acquisition, wraparound artifact is usually seen in the anteroposterior direction on 2D axial images of the torso.

Wraparound artifact can also occur in the craniocaudal direction on a 3D sequence. Frequency encoding is performed on one axis and phase encoding on the other two axes (including the slice selection axis in the craniocaudal Z-direction). On the image below, the bowel and lumbar spine from the patient's lower abdomen are superimposed on the heart and lungs from aliasing along the Z-axis. Aliasing in the frequency-encoding direction is no longer encountered in clinical practice. Modern MRI systems prevent this by automatic frequency oversampling, which does not incur a time penalty.

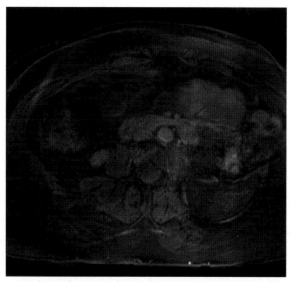

3D wraparound artifact in the Z-axis.

Techniques to Decrease Wraparound Artifact

Technique	Comments
Oversample in the phase-encoding direction	<ul><li>2D wrap: increase field of view (FOV)</li><li>3D wrap: perform slice oversampling in the Z-axis</li><li>Effects:<ul><li>Increases scan time</li><li>Decreases spatial resolution</li><li>Increases signal-to-noise ratio</li></ul></li></ul>
Switch phase- and frequency-encoding directions on 2D sequence	<ul><li>Moves the artifact into a different axis so it does not overlap the area of interest</li><li>Effect:<ul><li>Increases scan time when phase-encoding axis moved from shorter to longer axis</li></ul></li></ul>
Apply presaturation pulses to anatomy outside area of interest	<ul><li>Crushes the signal from outside the area of interest so it does not wrap into image</li><li>Effect:<ul><li>Increases scan time for applying the extra pulses</li></ul></li></ul>

References: Hoang PB, Huang SY, Song AW, et al. Chapter 9: Motion, pulsation, and other artifacts. In: Mangrum WI (ed). *Duke review of MRI physics*, 2nd ed. Philadelphia, PA: Elsevier, Inc., 2019:91–105.

Huang SY, Seethamraju RT, Patel P, et al. Body MR imaging: artifacts, k-space, and solutions. *Radiographics* 2015;35(5):1439–1460.

17 **Answer F.** MRI for patient 3 demonstrates fluid motion artifact. **This artifact is particularly prominent on half-Fourier single-shot spin echo** sequences (e.g., HASTE for Siemens MRI or SSFSE for GE MRI). This ultrafast sequence acquires an image in less than half a second, reducing some motion artifacts such as from respiration. However, **signal is degraded by motion that occurs within the time of slice acquisition.** There can be loss of signal from motion of ascites in this case (arrows on image below) and bile in MRCP. Any fluid-filled structure can demonstrate this artifact, including cysts, gallbladder, bowel, and bladder. **This artifact can simulate pathology such as stones, gas, or soft tissue nodularity.**

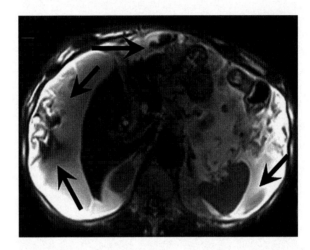

Correlation with multishot sequences helps exclude pathology since they are less prone to this type of motion artifact. **With multishot technique, k-space is filled over multiple TRs such that the random effects of fluid motion are averaged and fluid appears homogeneous**.

References: Hoang PB, Huang SY, Song AW, et al. Chapter 9: Motion, pulsation, and other artifacts. In: Mangrum WI (ed). *Duke review of MRI physics*, 2nd ed. Philadelphia, PA: Elsevier, Inc., 2019:91–105.

Huang SY, Seethamraju RT, Patel P, et al. Body MR imaging: artifacts, k-space, and solutions. *Radiographics* 2015;35(5):1439–1460.

18 **Answer C.** MRI in patient 4 demonstrates respiratory motion artifact. There is repetitive shading and ghosting matching the contour of the anterior abdominal wall. Patient motion, which may be voluntary or involuntary, can cause ghosting, blurring, signal loss, and misregistration. **Motion artifacts are most prominent in the phase-encoding direction**, which is typically anteroposterior in abdominal imaging. Techniques to reduce motion artifacts are listed in the table below.

Techniques to Reduce Motion Artifacts

Technique	Comments
Swap the phase- and frequency-encoding directions	• Maps the artifact in a different direction to avoid the area of interest
Apply presaturation band to moving tissue	• Eliminates signal from the moving tissue that could map into the area of interest
Synchronize acquisition with respiration	• Breath hold • Navigator pulse • Use of bellows with respiratory triggering
Use faster sequences	• Single-shot sequences (faster, partial k-space sampling) • Shorten echo train length on fast spin echo sequences • Parallel imaging
Place patient in prone position	• Reduces excursion of the abdominal wall
Use alternative k-space sampling techniques	• Radial or other k-space acquisition techniques that average the motion throughout the image
Increase number of signal averages	
Use flow compensation techniques	• Gradient moment nulling for vascular flow

References: Hoang PB, Huang SY, Song AW, et al. Chapter 9: Motion, pulsation, and other artifacts. In: Mangrum WI (ed). *Duke review of MRI physics*, 2nd ed. Philadelphia, PA: Elsevier, Inc., 2019:91–105.

Huang SY, Seethamraju RT, Patel P, et al. Body MR imaging: artifacts, k-space, and solutions. *Radiographics* 2015;35(5):1439–1460.

19 **Answer B.** The MRI in patient 5 demonstrates **spike artifact, which is a type of radiofrequency (RF) interference artifact**. Multiple bands are seen across the image with suggestion of a crosshatched "herringbone" pattern. RF interference can occur from sources internal or external to the MRI system.

Spike artifact occurs with corruption of individual data points in k-space from a transient electromagnetic spike, such as a spike generated by gradients applied at high duty cycles, static, or defective light bulbs. **The corrupted data points in k-space are converted into a series of bands on the reconstructed image by Fourier transformation.** A single corrupted data point usually results in a simple straight "corduroy" band pattern, while multiple corrupted points result in a complex crosshatched "herringbone" pattern.

Zipper artifact is different type of RF interference artifact. The MRI suite provides strong RF shielding, but if there is a problem with the enclosure and a periodic RF signal intrudes (rather than a single spike), it will propagate with alternating bright and dark lines resembling a zipper. Zipper artifacts can occur in the phase-encoding, or less commonly, the frequency-encoding direction depending on the cause. Two examples from different patients are shown below. The door of the MRI suite should be checked for adequate seal and monitoring equipment inspected. Additional **troubleshooting of the system and surrounding environment** is required if RF interference artifacts are persistent.

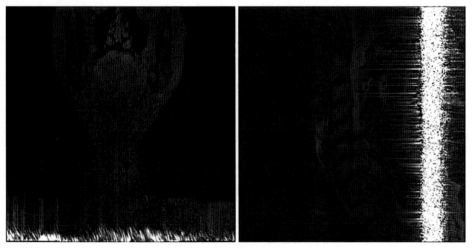

Zipper artifacts.

References: Graves MJ, Mitchell DG. Body MRI artifacts in clinical practice: a physicist's and radiologist's perspective. *J Magn Reson Imaging* 2013;38(2):269–287.

Zhuo J, Gullapalli RP. AAPM/RSNA physics tutorial for residents: MR artifacts, safety, and quality control. *Radiographics* 2006;26(1):275–297.

Note: Page number followed by "*f*" and "*t*" indicates figure and table respectively.